Y0-BXW-908

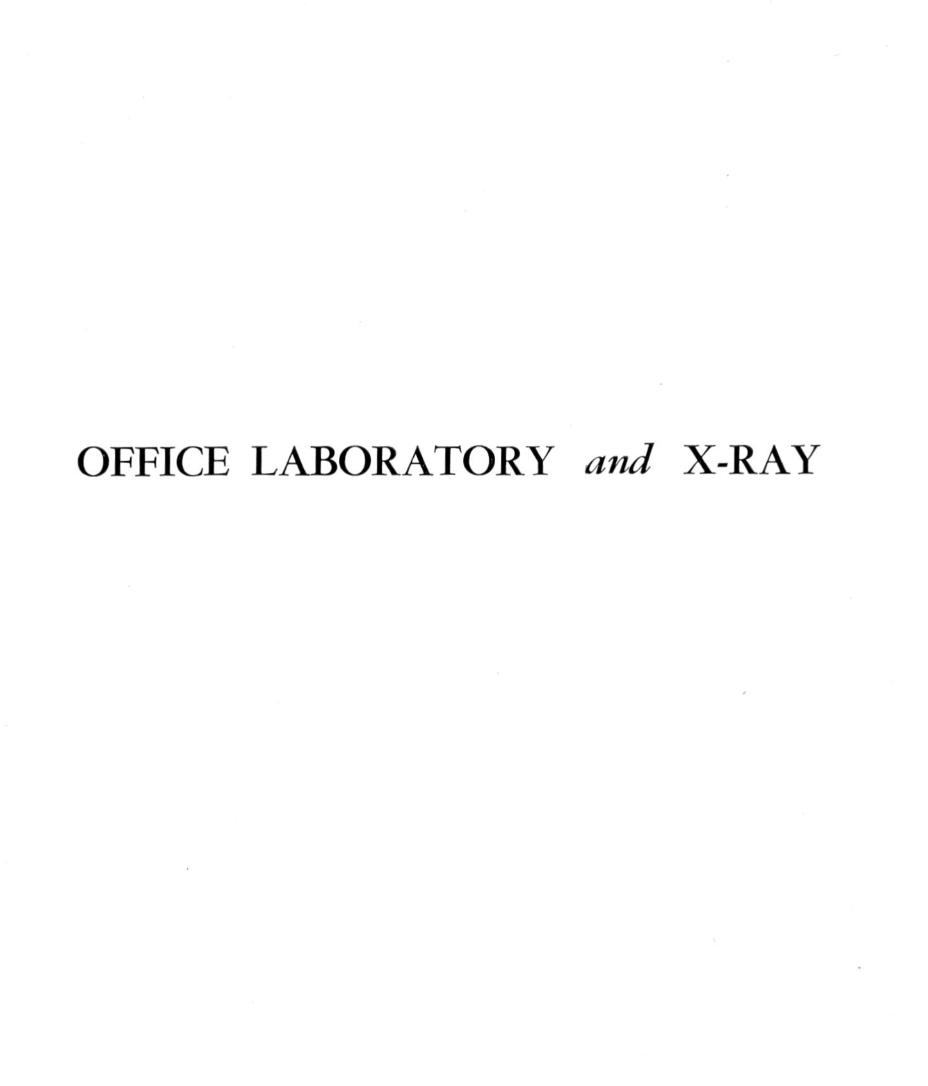

OFFICE LABORATORY *and* X-RAY

Practical use of the

OFFICE LABORATORY *and* X-RAY

Including the Electrocardiograph

by

PAUL WILLIAMSON, M.D.

ST. LOUIS
THE C. V. MOSBY COMPANY
1 9 5 7

LIBRARY OF CONGRESS CATALOG CARD NUMBER 57-12648

PRINTED IN THE UNITED STATES OF AMERICA

DEDICATED WITH LOVE TO FOUR LITTLE STINKERS
WHO ARE LOTS OF FUN:

PAULA, aged 10

LEE, aged 8

NATHAN, aged 6

DAVID, aged 4

Preface

The useful information to be gained from the small office laboratory and x-ray is far more extensive than many physicians achieve with such equipment. Utilization to maximum benefit will greatly increase the scope of office practice and add to diagnostic accuracy.

This book is not a compendium of advanced techniques. No procedure is listed or discussed that cannot be done by a home-trained technician in any office with a minimum of basic equipment. In writing I have assumed that the reader has a reasonable knowledge of the basic techniques and presently owns books devoted to the exact methodology of the tests. My emphasis has been placed on what the results mean and the common sources of error.

As any individual project must be, this work is biased. It is the outcome of an extended critical analysis of the functions and functioning of some several hundred office practices, including my own. The deductions and techniques herein have been useful to me. Perhaps you, too, will find them of service.

There is another aspect to be considered. We doctors seem to have a predilection for gadgetry. Often this is particularly apparent in our use of the laboratory and x-ray. Some of these procedures, while both useful and accurate, are shrouded with custom and followed with almost mystic faith. One purpose of this book is to separate, insofar as possible, the useful from the useless and the factual from the assumed.

The sections dealing with inherent errors in the tests are complete but not extensive. Any test or mechanical procedure is largely worthless if one accepts the result as complete truth without exploring the possible sources of error and taking each into account.

Proper interpretation of the tests and films is the key to successful use of the office laboratory and x-ray. Many times there is a gross difference between what the results seem to mean and what they really do mean. It is for this reason that interpretation is emphasized.

Certain basic equipment is needed to carry out the procedures discussed in this book. In addition to an electrocardiograph and a fluoroscope, an x-ray machine capable of an output of 100 kvp at 100 ma is necessary. Larger machines are of little use in the office but a smaller one will limit your ability to obtain clear films of moving parts.

The office laboratory should have a good microscope and its accessory equipment. A photoelectric colorimeter is an inexpensive and accurate means of doing chemical tests. These two basic instruments, along with a centrifuge, chemical apparatus, sedimentation rack, and a few other similar items, make up an adequate small laboratory.

This book was made possible by the assistance of my wife, Ann, who did the art work, and our associate of many years, Mrs. Kate Broach, who did the library research and manuscript preparation.

I hope this book serves you well.

Paul Williamson, M.D.

Contents

SECTION ONE

Chapter Ten

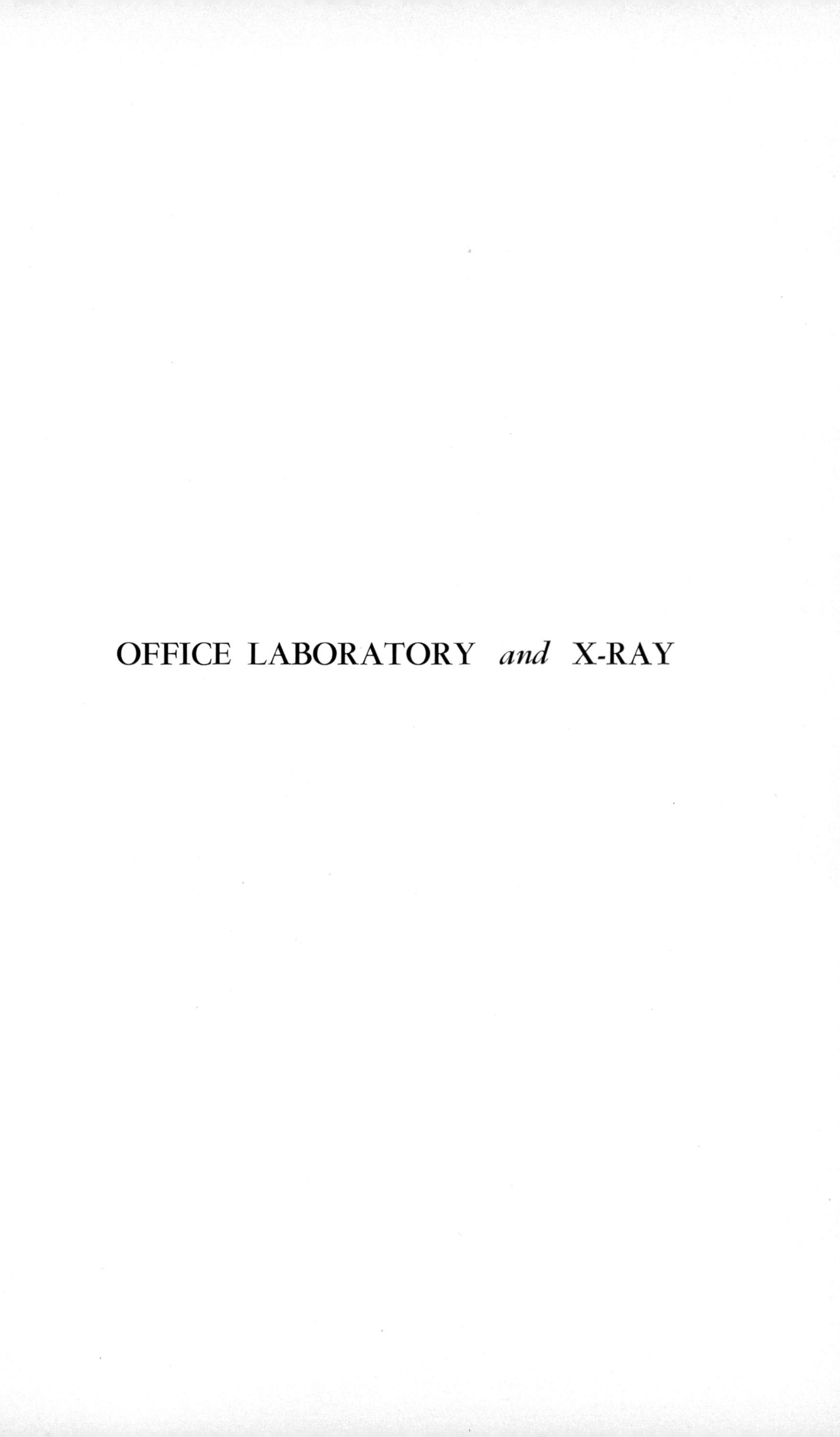

OFFICE LABORATORY *and* X-RAY

Section One

CHAPTER ONE

The Use of Counting Chambers

RED BLOOD CELL COUNT

Technique

Blood is usually obtained from a small stab wound made in the anterolateral aspect of a finger pad, in the lobe of the ear, or in the heel. A common sharp-pointed scalpel blade is used to make the stab incision after cleansing the area with alcohol and waiting a few seconds for the alcohol to dry. The common error in making the wound is to underestimate the thickness of the skin to be perforated and thereby fail to procure adequate blood flow.

A pernicious error on the part of the technician is to squeeze the area to be incised between the fingers in order to prevent pain. This does indeed reduce the minor discomfort but it also has the effect of adding undesirable circulatory and tissue fluid changes. Hold loosely the area to be pricked and make the incision with a quick, stabbing motion. Allow bleeding to occur spontaneously without squeezing the part to cause flow of blood. Applied pressure has the effect of diluting the blood with tissue fluids which are expressed at the same time.

Allow two or three drops of blood to escape and wipe them away with a sterile, dry sponge. Now hold the incision in such a position that a drop of blood will accumulate over it without running down the side of the finger, ear, or heel.

Place the beak of the pipette in this drop of blood and allow capillary action to carry the blood upward to the 0.5 mark. Only rarely need suction be applied to fill the red cell pipette.

Quite often an overfilling occurs, the blood column extending past the 0.5 mark. While laboratory experts shudder at the technique, the easiest means of withdrawing a small amount of blood from the overfilled pipette is to rub the tip of the pipette gently in the palm of one's hand. Needless to say, with some bloods it is wise to use the patient's palm or a damp sponge.

When the column of blood impinges exactly upon the 0.5 mark, wipe the outside of the pipette free of blood and draw the diluent into the pipette until the column of blood and fluid reaches the 101 mark just above the bulb. Then close the pipette at both ends and shake until the blood and diluting fluid are thoroughly mixed.

Normal saline makes an adequate diluent if it is changed frequently. At least every third day the container (a one-ounce bottle) must be emptied, washed, and dried and the saline replaced. A better diluent is Hayem's fluid. This is the formula:

Mercuric chloride	0.5
Sodium sulfate	5.0
Sodium chloride	1.0
Distilled water	200.0

The counting chamber is not filled until several drops have been expelled from the pipette and discarded. The mixture of blood and fluid is then allowed to flow into the space between the counting chamber bed and cover glass until this space is completely filled. There must be no extension of the fluid laterally past the edges of the chamber bed. If this happens, clean the chamber and refill.

When the chamber has been properly charged, put it aside for a few minutes to allow settling. Before counting, examine the slide under low power. If the corpuscles are not evenly distributed, there is an error, and the entire technique should be repeated. If the distribution is even, one then changes to the high dry lens and counts the cells in five squares of the heavily-ruled area like this:

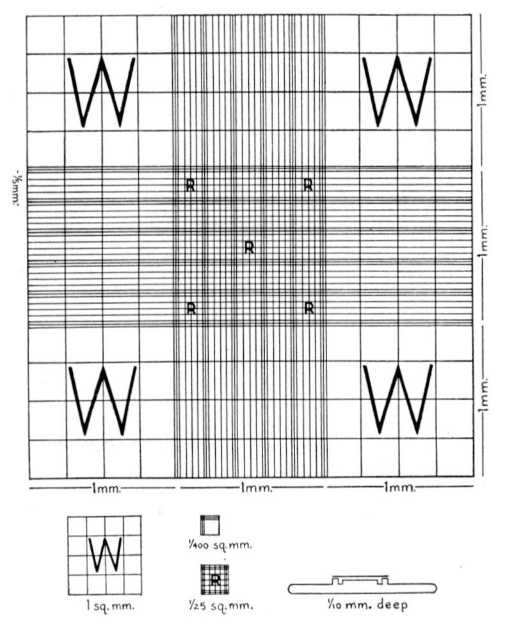

(Gradwohl: Clinical Laboratory Methods and Diagnosis, 1956, The C. V. Mosby Co.)

To the total number of all cells counted in the five squares one adds four ciphers and the count is expressed in millions. Thus: Total 450 cells, 4,500,000. An even more useful expression is to add a decimal point between the first and second numbers. Thus: Total cells 450, 4.5 million.

Of greatest importance in the whole test is the use of scrupulously clean and dry equipment. Most of us now use counting chambers with bright-line ruling of the Neubauer pattern. Such chambers require gentle handling to avoid scratches on the ruled surface. It is entirely feasible to wash them with water and dry with lens paper.

Pipettes should be cleaned by flushing them with water, followed by alcohol and then by ether. A simple venturi suction device can be attached to the laboratory sink and used for this purpose. After rinsing the pipette with ether, air should be sucked through it for at least 10 seconds to make sure that it is completely dry.

Errors

Enumeration of red blood cells is not an accurate test. Assuming perfect technique (which is most unlikely in the office laboratory), the count has a possible, unavoidable mechanical error of about 15 per cent. When a count is reported as 4.5 million, the actual count is between 3.83 and 5.17 million *if the technique has been perfect.* Add to this the technical errors that so frequently creep in and one has a test of little reliability.

Errors in obtaining the blood have been mentioned in the preceding paragraphs. Mistakes in handling the equipment are equally frequent. The common ones are as follows:

1. Slow handling after the blood, but not the diluting fluid, has been allowed to enter the pipette. The result is clotting, with parts of the clot remaining in the capillary portion of the pipette. This must be avoided by rapid handling.

2. Inaccurate dilution. It is not easy to make an exact dilution of red blood cells.

The difficulty of controlling capillary attraction, trouble in exerting proper suction and its elimination at an exact time, difficulty in preventing a slight running back from the pipette into the fluid reservoir, all combine to offer countless chances for error. The only remedy is exacting technique.

3. Improper application of the cover glass to the counting chamber or movement of the glass after the chamber is charged. Again, exacting technique is the only answer.

In summary, one must remember that total errors of as much as 25 per cent are not uncommon in the process of erythrocyte enumeration. The average error in the office laboratory is probably about 15 per cent.

Interpretation

It is essential that the physician realize exactly what information is provided by the red blood count. It gives a rough indication of the number of blood cells *per unit of blood.* In the normal individual this number is inconstant. It varies with a number of compensatory reactions of the body. There are physiologic variations. These basic facts must be understood if proper interpretation of the count is to be made.

The red blood count does not give a positive diagnosis of anemia. The count may be greatly altered by physiologic and pathologic processes which have nothing to do with the various anemias. As an example, dehydration with its consequent hemoconcentration indicates the removal of some of the fluid elements from the blood, not an increase in the number of red blood cells.

In the normal person 1.0 ml. of blood will contain about 0.45 ml. of cellular elements and about 0.55 ml. of fluid. In dehydration the ratio changes due to loss of fluid elements, and the person may show 0.55 ml. of cellular elements and 0.45 ml. of fluid for each 1.0 ml. of blood. If such blood were put in a counting chamber, a spuriously high red count would result.

To take an example in the opposite direction: During the latter trimester of pregnancy there is a physiologic dilution of the blood due to an increase in the fluid elements. When such blood is subjected to a red count, the resulting figure will be low. This indicates an increase in fluid elements, not a decrease in red blood cells. All kinds of complicated treatment are applied in such pregnancy cases in an attempt to treat a disease that is not present. The error is due to an assumption on the part of the physician that the blood count is an absolute indicator of the number of red cells in the body. He may ignore the fact that the red count is just as sensitive to changes in the relative amount of fluid elements in the blood-vascular system as it is to changes in the number of red cells.

There are three states or conditions that seem primarily able to change the red blood count:

1. Changes in oxygen demand by the tissues
2. Changes in fluid balance
3. Disease (including hemorrhage)

The first of these, changes in oxygen demand, is by far the most important in accounting for many changes in blood count. The process is not teleologic, as my statement would imply, but represents some unknown chemical adjustment of the bone marrow and spleen to oxygen partial pressures or saturations. Some of the variations and their causes are interesting.

The best known change is that induced by high altitude. People who live in or who are transient in higher altitudes invariably have an increase in both relative and total number of erythrocytes. While not so well known, the converse is entirely true. People who live under increased air pressure, such as those who spend time in deep mines or caissons, usually have lower red blood counts.

There is even a minor diurnal change which amounts to from 4 to 6 per cent. The sleeping organism creates less demand for oxygen and the count reaches its lowest point about the time of waking. Then, as activity increases throughout the day, there is a slow but steady and appreciable increase in the number of red cells per unit of blood.

Extreme muscular exercise and even the anxiety of psychoneurosis with its attendant increased muscular tension will cause an increase in the number of red blood cells. Obviously, since chemical reactions are speeded by increasing temperature, those people who live in tropical areas are likely to have higher blood counts than those who live in temperate or arctic areas.

In cases where there is slowing of the circulation, with consequent inefficient distribution of oxygen by the blood, there tends to be a compensatory increase in red cells. The best example is cardiac decompensation. If prolonged, even though moderate, decompensation will usually cause a greatly increased count. It is particularly important that the doctor differentiate in his own mind the increased red blood count due to circulatory slowing from the disease known as polycythemia vera. The disease is a medical rarity.

Various diseases of the lung which prevent adequate aeration may cause an increase of compensatory nature. Often in this group of diseases there is an accompanying toxic effect that inhibits blood formation. This makes less likely a marked increase in red blood cell count unless a loss of fluid elements supervenes with consequent hemoconcentration.

A second condition that may cause changes in the red blood count is fluid balance. This is much more readily apparent than the changes in oxygen tension which we have been discussing. The most frequently seen entity is the increased count of minor dehydration. The reasons for it are perfectly apparent and need no elaboration. One aspect of this has more than ordinary interest. In children such a "dehydration count" may effectively cover up an anemia which was the original factor in making the child susceptible to the illness leading to dehydration.

The lowered blood count in the latter trimester of pregnancy is a matter of fluid balance and does not indicate pathology. The same may be true of the patient who mobilizes large quantities of body fluids, such as the cardiac patient in the process of digitalization.

The third factor which must be mentioned is the existence of actual blood pathology. The older definition of the anemias was a lowered red blood count. Today the definition might be changed to read: A lowered amount of hemoglobin per milliliter of blood in the presence of normal fluid balance and the absence of physiologically induced alterations. Admittedly, this is a bit involved but it essentially states the case.

At the opposite end of the scale is polycythemia vera. It is such a rare disease in the average practice that one should be most wary of crediting the diagnosis until extensive confirmation is available. Most polycythemias are attempts at physiologic compensation rather than the true diseases.

Faced with a single deviant red blood count, just what do all of the implications of interpretation mean to the practicing physician? There are a series of precautions to be followed in every case unless clinical signs are so absolute as to make suspicion fruitless. If this be the case, the laboratory work probably should not have been done in the first place.

In evaluation, begin by examining the validity of the count itself. Remember that enumeration of erythrocytes is subject to extremes of error; be careful of offering any interpretation within the range of these extremes. For example, should a healthy-appearing young lady report to your office and, upon a single count, show 3.9 million red blood cells, remember the possibility that she may have an entirely normal count. The error may not be in her bodily processes but in the test itself.

In general, the hemoglobin determination varies with and is a check upon the red blood count. There are exceptions in certain types of anemia but these are rare in practice. A distinctly lowered count with a distinctly lowered hemoglobin roughly in proportion should raise the suspicion of anemia. It is by no means conclusive proof.

At such a time remember that both hemoglobin determination and red blood count measure the amount of hemoglobin and the number of red cells in a specific unit of blood. No hint is given as to alterations in the total number of red blood cells or as to the total amount of fluid elements in the blood.

There are times when physiologic mechanisms may operate to lower the relative number of cells per milliliter without actually lowering the total red cell content. At such times treatment for anemia is useless. One should never accept the findings of a blood count without at least enumerating the possible physiologic conditions that might account for the change.

The same thing applies, of course, to the increased blood count. The increased blood count has an occasional utilitarian function not related to diagnosis of polycythemia vera. It can be an excellent indicator of conditions causing hemoconcentration and may serve to allow prognosis on a more firm footing than physical findings will permit.

In the first few hours following a severe burn the case can often be followed rather accurately by repeated blood counts. After three or four hours there appears evidence of red cell destruction and the blood picture may change sufficiently that the method loses its accuracy. The red blood count and similar (and better) tests are likely to show the existence of hemoconcentration before the evidence is incontestable on physical examination. One should be observant of such changes.

Another example: In cases of early cardiac decompensation a hemoconcentration is often one of the early findings, with a gradual increase in the red blood count as failure progresses. This can provide excellent auxiliary information as to the status of the decompensation.

One of the most useless things in clinical medicine is the attempt to follow the course of a minor anemia by utilizing repeated red blood counts. Let us take as an example the case of Mrs. A, a housewife, who comes to the doctor complaining of tiredness, chronic exhaustion, and a typical chain of symptoms which inevitably lead one to the diagnosis of psychoneurosis, anxiety type. As a precaution the blood count is taken and reported as 3.92 million. Mrs. A is immediately placed on treatment for anemia by her physician. She is told to return in two weeks for a second red count. In the interim the treatment will probably help her symptoms because of its psychotherapeutic implications. The second count is reported as 4.16 million and Mrs. A is told that she is getting better, a fact which the physician firmly believes. Now the whole case assumes the aspect of a comedy. The difference between 3.92 and 4.16 million is well within the standard error of the test. Two blood counts taken 30 seconds apart or even two counts on the same specimen of blood might have shown this much difference. There is at least a 50 per cent chance that any improvement has taken place in the counting chamber, not in the patient.

Mrs. A, of course, was rather well managed from a temporary psychotherapeutic standpoint and unquestionably her physician was able to help her. But if he believes for one instant that there is any proof that (a) the patient had any anemia to begin with or (b) this anemia has improved, he is mistaken in the extreme.

It cannot be emphasized too strongly that minor deviations from the normal may be deviations in the laboratory, not in the patient.

Indications

There seems, in actuality, no clear-cut indication for the red blood count. Other tests give more accurate results in diagnosis of the anemias and are easier to perform. The hemoglobin determination and the hematocrit are both superior tests and both require less time on the part of the technician.

On the other hand, we are bound by custom. The erythrocyte enumeration has for many years occupied a place of unchallenged honor in our hierarchy of laboratory tests. It will unquestionably continue for several decades to be used when more efficient procedures are available.

The principal indication for any such test is to determine the existence of an anemia. Within the limitations imposed by its probable error, the red count will do this well. It is not of great use in following the course of an anemia. A simple smear stained for reticulocytes is superior.

Several important ratios are calculated by using the red blood count as one factor. For this reason it may be necessary as a part of the examination. These ratios will be discussed later.

There is one advantage that, while not subject to expression in exact scientific terminology, nonetheless, is present. This is the only test in its field that offers a look at the erythrocytes themselves. The experienced physician can gain much information from the study of unstained blood. See page 111.

Discussion

I believe that the red blood count is a test which will gradually lose much of its popularity as physicians come to appreciate the fact that there are other and better ways of determining the presence of the anemias. A hematocrit determination will give the proportion of cellular and fluid elements in the blood with greater accuracy and with considerably less energy expended on the part of the technician than will the red blood count.

The hemoglobin estimation is also of more benefit than the count. Anemias can be followed with greater assurance by estimating reticulocyte percentages, which give a very accurate means of proving the response to treatment.

However, being bound by custom, the patient and the physician both have become thoroughly indoctrinated in the usage of the erythrocyte count and will probably continue to demand that it be done for a great many years. Certainly the test has been and is blessed with some adequacy. It provides good information and can be extremely valuable to the practitioner if it is interpreted conservatively. On the other hand, if one forgets the inherent errors in the count and, in addition, fails to take into consideration various changes induced by variations in the fluid elements of blood, difficulties will continue to arise.

The two greatest errors in practice which occur as a result of mistakes in the red blood count are probably (1) the physiologic blood dilution that happens in pregnancy and is often accepted by the physician as a disease, and (2) minor deviations downward in the count, which are often given impossible interpretations by the unwary. These minor changes are often used to regulate treatment when the inaccuracy of the procedure is such that this is not possible.

WHITE BLOOD CELL COUNT

In this section we shall consider only the total enumeration of white blood cells. The differential count and its implications will be discussed, beginning on page 120.

Technique

The technique for white blood cell counting is very similar to that for the red cells and subject to the same mistakes. Since the pipette used for the white blood count has a bore somewhat larger than that for the red count, it usually cannot be filled by capillary attraction. To fill it properly one must use suction through the rubber tube accompanying the pipette. It is a good trick to put a needle adapter on one end of the rubber tube and to use a hypodermic needle through which to apply suction. This allows greater control. An apparatus prepared this way looks like this:

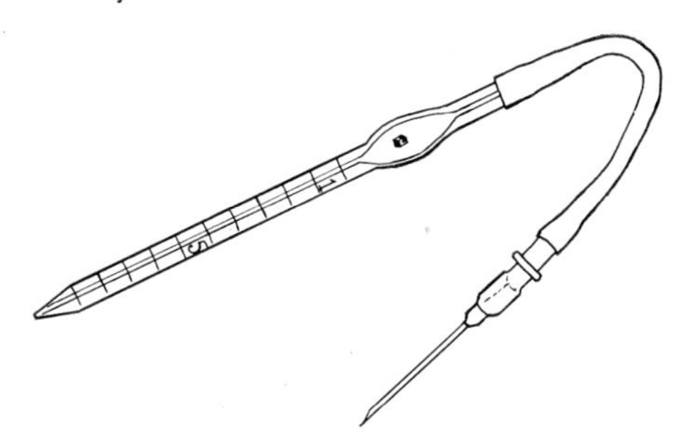

The blood is drawn up to the 0.5 mark on the pipette which is then filled to the 11 mark with diluting fluid, using all the precautions already mentioned in the section on erythrocyte counting. A good diluting fluid is as follows:

Glacial acetic acid	1.0 ml.
Aqueous gentian violet, 1%	1.0 ml.
Distilled water, q.s. ad.	100.0 ml.

This solution will impart a slight stain to the nuclei of the white cells, which makes proper identification much easier. The solution should be filtered every week or two to prevent accumulation of yeasts and molds which are occasionally mistaken for white blood cells.

The counting chamber is charged exactly as for red cells and with the same precautions. One then counts the leukocytes in the four corner areas of the slide like this:

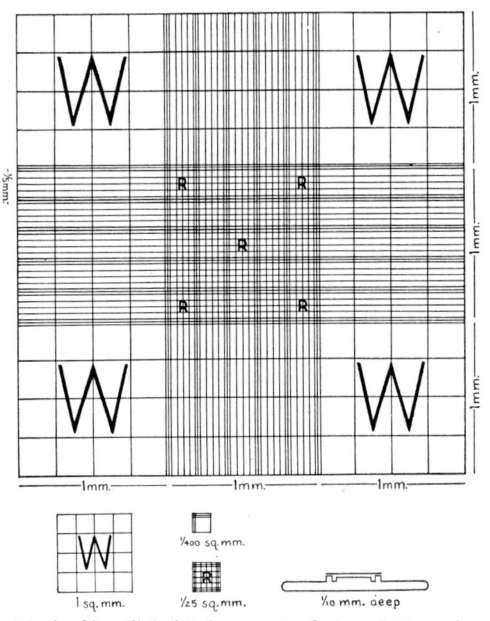

(Gradwohl: *Clinical Laboratory Methods and Diagnosis,* 1956, *The C. V. Mosby Co.*)

The total number of leukocytes counted in all four corner squares is then divided by two. Add two zeros to the sum thus obtained for the final figure.

Errors

Since the sample taken for counting white blood cells is proportionately larger than that for red blood cells, there is less chance for error in the leukocyte enumeration. Certain "weak points" are present, however, and must be considered.

Occasionally the acetic acid solution fails to destroy completely the red cells and one sees shadowy remnants of these cells in the counting chamber. Unless the count is carefully done, the red cell remnants may at times be mistaken for white corpuscles, which will result in a spuriously high count. Yeasts and molds may also be mistaken for white cells. They will grow in the acid diluent and may give difficulty unless this fluid is filtered regularly.

Maldistribution of the fluid in the counting chamber, improper mixing, clotting of the blood in the pipette before diluting, and other sources of error mentioned under the red blood cell count apply equally to the leukocyte determination. The test must be scrupulously and accurately done if it is to be of value.

The white blood count probably has an inherent error of 5 to 8 per cent. The average total error, allowing for human frailty, will be from 10 to 15 per cent. Since interpretation generally does not depend upon determination of this narrow difference, the error is often insignificant. Even so, it is important to realize that a 15,000 leukocyte count followed two hours later by a 16,000 count is within the range of error of the test and, therefore, not utilizable for making predictions. On the other hand, a 12,000 count followed by a 16,000 count shows a significant change.

Interpretation

When interpreted in the light of known facts, the white blood count can be a good test and of great help to the practitioner. As in all other tests one must take into account possible physiologic variations before reading too much of significance into the results.

Of great importance is the wide range of normal. Total leukocyte counts are somewhat higher in children. The normal range under the age of 14 may be taken as from 6,000 to 12,000. In adults normal counts show an average of 5,000 to 10,000, but may rise as high as 12,000 at some times without indicating abnormality.

For some reason which we do not understand with entire clarity, the white blood count in a normal person is related to the adequacy of nutrition. It falls in the undernourished subject and tends to reach its higher normal levels as nutrition progressively improves. Because of this there is some validity in using the white blood count as an index of nutritive adequacy. This is true only in the individual who shows no evidence of disease.

There are hourly variations in the white blood count of the normal individual, and there exists a distinct rise throughout the day until midafternoon, when the count may reach 10,000 to 12,000 without indicating pathology.

An increase in the number of leukocytes may be caused by physiologic reaction to a number of stimuli which are not usually considered noxious. Among them are a cold bath, muscular exercise, nervous tension, and pain itself. The latter concept is an interesting one. It seems to have been proved beyond question that sudden onset of severe pain can cause a marked rise in the leukocyte count. One report mentions a total count of 30,000. If no detrimental stimuli other than pain develop, this count diminishes rapidly, returning to normal within a matter of hours. One should always remember this possibility in considering the leukocyte count in a case that is bizarre clinically.

Pathologic reasons for increase include infection, breakdown of tissue such as that seen in burns or following severe trauma, and foreign substances in the tissues. In connection with this we should remember that blood itself is a foreign substance when extravascular and that bleeding, both into a viscus and into the tissues themselves, may cause an increase in the total white blood count.

The most common pathologic cause, surprisingly enough, is probably the everyday bruise. If there is enough extravasation of blood and crushing of tissue there will be a rise in the leukocyte count. I have seen a number of counts in the 18,000 to 20,000 range resulting from what appeared to be trivial bruising. Before depending too much on the white blood count one should think of such a possibility.

Probably the next most common cause of an increased count is acute infection. It sounds ridiculous to say this but one must remember that the leukocyte count does not indicate where the infection is. In the presence of one known infection the count is of little help in revealing whether a second infectious process is present. Here is an example:

We have seen many cases of bacterial enteritis (or food poisoning or intestinal flu) in which, during the course of the disease, there was a question as to whether or not the appendix might be involved. More than once an intelligent physician has suggested that we get a blood count to see if the patient had appendicitis. The patient already had one known infection so we could be almost positive that he had an elevated blood count *from the enteritis*. There would be no reason therefore to get a blood count in such a case unless for quantitative estimate, and there are so many, many factors that enter into the white blood count response to infection that an attempt to quantify would be dangerous.

In the presence of a known infection the white blood count will almost always be increased. It makes no difference whether the infection be in the intestinal wall, the appendix, the throat, or the rectum. We must never forget this fact in interpreting the increased leukocyte count.

Custom has decreed, at least to the laity, that the white blood count be considered the necessary diagnostic tool in pinpointing cases of appendicitis. It may be useful occasionally, although I would call it the least important part of the total findings. Nonetheless, it should always be done if possible. Remember that it only indicates the presence of some infectious or tissue-destructive process. It does not show whether or not the appendix is involved.

To recapitulate: One must be wary of reading into the white blood count report a specificity which it does not have. Changes in the count, to be significant, must show a deviation of more than 10 per cent from the first count. Finally it must be remembered that the count is not solely an indicator of infection. Increased counts are seen with chemical insult to the tissues and trauma. They may even follow emotional disarrangements.

In the noninfectious cases with increased leukocyte count the differential enumeration of white cells will be helpful. It is discussed, beginning on page 120.

Decrease in the number of leukocytes is usually an indicator of pathology. In certain cases it may be useful for differentiation. For example, most of the secondary anemias are accompanied by a relative leukocytosis. Pernicious anemia, on the other hand, usually shows a leukopenia proportional to the decrease in red cells. This point should be remembered, for it may often be the first indication that points to pernicious anemia.

A fall in the total count usually indicates depression of the entire group of blood-forming elements. It is probably due either to toxicity or to inadequate nutrition. Such a fall in the count in the presence of a normal differential is seldom indicative of danger to the patient. It is only when the granulocytes disappear selectively that danger becomes rapidly manifest.

Various diseases are listed in almost every textbook as being the cause of leukopenia. We have not found this confirmed often enough to be used as a diagnostic point. There is a difference between a leukopenia and a lack of leukocytosis. Many writers, when they speak of leukopenia, actually seem to mean that there is no leukocytosis. For example, certain types of virus pneumonia as differentiated from pneumococcal pneumonia may show a normal or only slightly elevated white blood count. Very few show a white blood count below 5,000.

When the physical findings would lead one to expect a leukocytosis, and it is not present in the laboratory report, one should become suspicious of this group of diseases which purportedly cause leukopenia.

A particular indicator that caution should be used is the equivocal white blood count. If such a result is reported, one should rely solely on the clinical findings and ignore the count. Another determination should be ordered.

We hear a great deal about the infection that is so severe it quite overwhelms bodily defenses and proceeds apace with no leukocyte response. Such cases do occur rarely. It is obvious the patient is so desperately ill that the white blood count becomes of small diagnostic import. In such a case the white blood count should not be allowed to confuse the picture and the clinical findings should be taken as truth. Such an absence of leukocyte response is seldom seen in patients who have much chance of recovery.

Indications

Any infectious process of sufficient seriousness to warrant careful appraisal is an indication for a white blood count. Even more important is its use in following the bodily response to infectious processes which are extended in time. Periodic enumeration of leukocytes is extremely valuable in such cases.

To utilize the leukocyte count as an indicator of nutrition is poor judgment. While it is just that, so many other factors enter in that the test has little other than academic value. In practice, clinical appraisal is far more accurate.

Suspected aberrations in white cell formation, such as leukemia, are often picked up on white blood count but are positively diagnosed by means of smear.

Basically, the white blood count is a means of following the course of an infection that is of sufficient seriousness to be watched carefully by the physician.

Discussion

The white blood count is one of the simplest and best tests that the small laboratory can do. It offers some information as to the status of nutrition in a normal patient and is a means of estimating the presence of tissue insult from either bacteria, trauma, or chemicals. If interpreted conservatively and in the light of known facts, the test can be of great value.

Like most tests, it is used far too often. Sometimes we act as if the indication for a white blood count might be any approximately human organism that seems alive and has the pelf to pay for it. One need not mention that such overuse is unwise.

I conceive the basic purpose of the test to be a confirmation of a clinical impression, *if confirmation is needed*, and a means of follow-up.

The presence of an infection is not per se an indication for a white blood count, for most infections can be diagnosed and treated adequately without it. Neither should the test be used as a "fishing expedition" to see what it might pick up. Cases of diagnostic desperation may be an exception to this. The test will provide information about certain things, but to use it without careful clinical appraisal of the case first is bordering upon the improper.

We must always remember the inherent error of the count and the physiologic changes which have been mentioned above.

If they are forgotten, embarrassing mistakes will occur.

PLATELET COUNTS

The platelet count is principally useful in establishing the presence or absence of thrombocytopenic purpura. It has other occasional uses but, in the small office, will find its greatest value in the diagnosis of this rare disease.

Technique

There are extremely accurate methods for enumeration of platelets but they are so cumbersome that they are not properly a procedure for the office laboratory. This one allows a good estimation:

Begin by examining carefully the glassware to be used and recleaning it if there is any doubt that it is perfectly clean. Platelets adhere to foreign surfaces and dirty glassware will result in a major lowering of the final count.

The patient is instructed to wash her hands vigorously with warm, soapy water and the finger to be used is cleaned immediately thereafter with alcohol and ether, after which it is allowed to dry in the air for a few seconds.

Many diluting fluids are available but that of Guy and Leake is as satisfactory as any for the small laboratory. The formula is as follows:

Crystal violet	0.01	Gm.
Sodium oxylate	1.6	Gm.
Formalin, 40 per cent solution	6.0	ml.
Distilled water	94.0	ml.

The fluid is filtered and stored in ordinary laboratory glass-stoppered bottles. It is best kept in the refrigerator; the unused portion should be discarded every six months and a new supply made up. When only a few tests are done, one fourth the specified quantity may be made every six months.

Use the pipette for diluting red blood cells and draw the diluting fluid to the 1 mark. Next make a stab wound on the lateral side of the cleaned finger tip. Using a clean surgical sponge or a bit of facial tissue, gently sponge away the first drop of blood extruded. Now draw blood to the 0.5 mark in the pipette already prepared. At this stage there will be blood from the tip to the 0.5 mark on the pipette and a column of diluting fluid above the blood. Quickly wipe the excess blood from the tip of the pipette and draw diluting fluid to the 101 mark. The filled pipette is shaken *immediately* and steadily for two minutes, after which the counting chamber is filled exactly as for a blood count. Put the chamber on the stage of the microscope and allow it to set undisturbed for three to five minutes before counting is begun. Do not wait longer than five minutes.

Count the platelets under the high dry lens exactly as you would count red blood cells. Total the number counted in the five squares, like this:

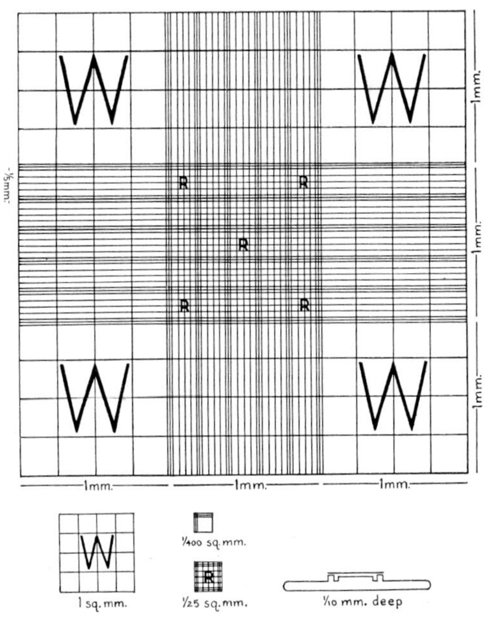

(Gradwohl: Clinical Laboratory Methods and Diagnosis, 1956, The C. V. Mosby Co.)

and add four zeros. A convenient way of reporting is to ignore the last three zeros. Thus, if 22 platelets were counted in the five squares, the actual count would be 220,000. It may be reported as 220 M.

To be sure of adequate control, blood from a normal person may be secured and counted at the same time as blood from the patient. Once a month, when the technician has time, it is a good idea to run a blank, using the diluting solution only in the counting chamber. If any structures that might be confused with platelets are seen, the fluid should be filtered or, better, discarded.

Errors

In counting the platelets one is dealing with structures whose normal destination is fragmentation and disintegration. For this reason errors are frequent and one usually obtains lower counts than are actually present.

Rarely a contaminated diluting fluid may result in a count higher than is actually present. This can be obviated by regular checks of the diluting fluid and by often running a normal control blood with the pathologic blood. Even more rarely, fragments of red or white cells may be mistaken for platelets, but experience at counting will check this.

Two errors which result in lowering the count are very common. The first is contamination of the blood with tissue fluids which cause active disintegration of the platelets. The finger must not be squeezed either before the puncture (this results in mobilization of tissue fluids as well as venous hyperemia) or after the puncture. Stick deep enough so that the blood will flow freely. The second error is dirty glassware. A few trivial particles of dust or any foreign substance will entrap many thousands of platelets, with resultant spurious values for the final count.

The lobe of the ear is not desirable for obtaining blood for the platelet count nor is blood from venipuncture as ordinarily done. The ear is often covered with fine hairs which hold many platelets, and literally millions may collect along the sides of the needle and syringe in venipuncture.

The normal values for human adults is reported as 250,000, with a standard deviation of more than 50,000.

Interpretation

We assume much and know little about the function of the platelets. Agglutination and liberation of thromboplastin are two functions of which we are relatively sure.

At the site of injury platelets agglutinate into a mass much like a log jam in a river, additional platelets being enmeshed as they come along. This forms the so-called "white clot" which is seen in intravascular thrombosis. Either extreme stasis (phlebothrombosis) or a foreign particle such as a bacterium (thrombophlebitis) may initiate the process. Such "white clots" are formed upon contact with tissue fluids and serve to initiate the sealing process when a vessel is injured.

As the clots disintegrate, thromboplastin is liberated and the process of coagulation is begun. By no means are platelets the only tissues containing thromboplastin. Clotting can and does occur in their complete absence, but adequate clot retraction is not present when the count is below 70,000. Persistent counts below this level are a warning that severe bleeding may (not will) occur.

Interpretation of the platelet count is made difficult by many factors. To begin with, the procedure of enumerating them is subject to gross error. Even when the technique is as nearly flawless as possible, a single platelet count should not be taken as absolutely indicative of pathology. It has been our routine to do successive counts for three days before accepting a count for diagnostic purposes.

Observations of the peripheral blood in situ have indicated that platelets are not constant in number. Over a period of several seconds only a few platelets will be seen and then a burst of them will literally bring thousands into view. Again, visualize the river as an example. At times it may be filled with floating debris and again for relatively long periods of time only occasional bits may float on the surface. Apparently this is so with thrombocytes. If it is true, a single count taken at a time when the area is relatively free of these bodies may give spuriously low values. Since many capillaries are cut in a single stab wound, we get a fair cross section of the platelet count of peripheral blood. Chance plays too large a part for us to say it is always accurate.

Certain physiologic variations occur which may be confusing if one does not remember their existence. Newborn babies show a platelet count of as low as 150,000 normally. This gradually rises, striking normal adult levels at approximately the age of 3 months.

Tremendous daily variations take place. In the resting adult the count may change as much as 10 per cent in two or three hours. In the active patient exercise may add as much as 25 per cent to the count in a period of minutes.

Of particular importance is the sudden great decrease just before menstruation. The count often drops to about 125 M. There is a gradual climb after the second day of flow and normal levels are usually approached by the time bleeding ceases.

The platelets, insofar as we know, are broken off from the cytoplasm of the megakaryocytes in the bone marrow. It would seem reasonable, therefore, to assume that diseases that affect the marrow would also affect the platelet count.

In general, one may say that those diseases characterized by leukopenia may also show a thrombocytopenia, and those diseases associated with leukocytosis may also show thrombocytosis. This is of little use in clinical office practice, for it indicates only a generalized reaction of the bone marrow.

When chronic blood loss is present there is first an excess formation of thrombocytes and then, as the marrow "fails to keep up" with the loss, a thrombocytopenia. Sometimes leukemia shows a thrombocytopenia, possibly because the megakaryocytes are literally engulfed by the exuberant and aberrant leukocytes. Aplastic anemia, for obvious reasons, shows diminution of the platelets.

These factors are reasonably obvious. The obtuse condition is the disease in question, thrombocytopenic purpura. In this entity the myeloid elements all seem normal. There is an ample supply of megakaryocytes. In fact, they are often increased. No increase in splenic destruction of platelets has ever been proved.

The most satisfactory theory is that thrombocytic purpura represents widespread vascular damage centered mainly in the capillaries. What we are seeing, then, represents a secondary finding. The platelets are literally "used up" in patching millions of tiny holes in the capillary bed. This, of itself, furthers the hemorrhagic condition by making insufficient material available to stop the slight bleeding induced by trivial trauma or by physiologic processes such as menstruation. Knowing the susceptibility of the vascular bed to injury by allergic and toxic processes, this theory makes easy the understanding of the role of drugs, burns, and some infections in causation.

If these theories are true we can separate the thrombocytopenias into actual and relative. In actual thrombocytopenia there is a depression of the entire marrow. The relative cases—principally thrombocytopenic purpura—are those in which the platelets are simply used up.

Unfortunately, things are not this simple. Beyond any question there is some connection between the spleen and the disease since splenectomy has been seemingly curative or beneficial in about one third of cases. So have the cortisone series of drugs.

This suggests an interesting conjecture. The reticuloendothelial system, of which the spleen is a part, seems particularly liable to injury by the quasi-allergic and ill-defined group called collagen diseases and their near relatives. This group responds well to cortisone. Could it not be that thrombocytopenic purpura is a reactive disease belonging to this group? Be that as it may, reported thrombocytopenia is an indication of one of three things in this order of frequency:

1. Mistaken count.
2. Bone marrow damage or overload (chronic hemorrhage).
3. Thrombocytopenic purpura.

Indications

The platelet count is not a frequent procedure in the office laboratory. It is indicated in any purpuric state not immediately explained by the evidence at hand. Rarely in cases of unexplained splenic enlargement the count may be of some significance.

General Discussion

The platelet count is not a good test. Very seldom should any great reliance be placed upon one result obtained in the office laboratory unless completely supported by historical and clinical signs. A minimum of three daily determinations, averaging the results, lends some dependability.

One must guard rigorously against the error of assuming that a low platelet count indicates a hemorrhagic tendency. It actually indicates that vascular insults, *if initiated*, will not be corrected with normal dispatch.

Platelet counts are subject to such great variations that they cannot be used to follow the progress of thrombocytopenic purpura except in a general way. Small changes, even changes of as much as 50,000, may be due to an error in the count and not a change in the patient.

SPINAL FLUID CELL COUNT

Spinal fluid is usually obtained by entering the dura mater between the fourth and fifth lumbar vertebrae like this:

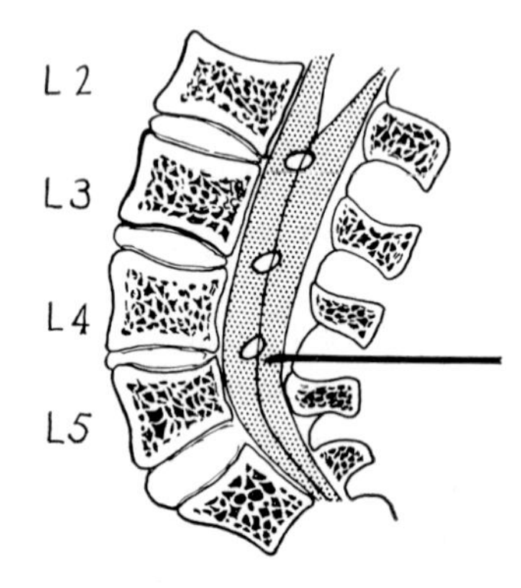

After anesthetizing the skin in the midline, just below the fourth spinous process, insert the spinal needle about one-half inch below the lower border like this:

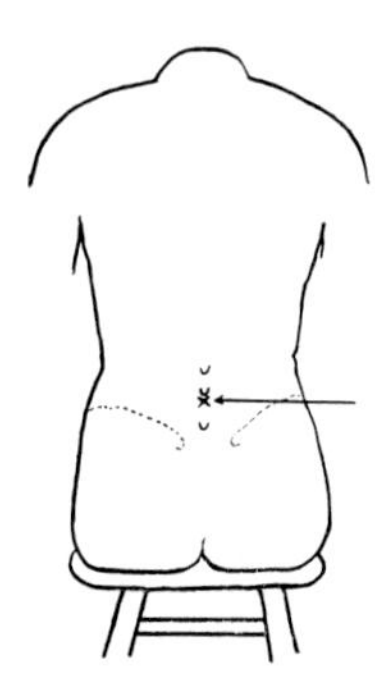

Notice the tract to be followed by the needle. With the patient sitting on a stool "arching his back" toward you, the needle is inserted in a horizontal plane about parallel with the floor. If the patient is lying in bed, the needle is inserted at an angle of about 10 degrees cephalad.

This matter of positioning is really the most important point in doing a spinal tap. It is also the point at which most errors are made. Take your time and try to visualize the tract through which the needle will go. Do not insert the needle until you are as nearly certain as you can be that it has a clear way to the dura.

When the dura is perforated one has the sensation of penetrating a heavy sheet of paper with the needle. When this is felt the obturator should be withdrawn and several drops of spinal fluid allowed to exit. The first fluid may be bloody and must be discarded because fresh blood interferes with the tests to be done subsequently.

Expression of a maximum of ten drops of fluid should result in distinct clearing of the red coloration. If this does not occur and if the fluid remains a homogenous bloody color, you may assume that the blood was in the spinal fluid before the tap. This is not true if there has been much poking about with the needle before spinal fluid is withdrawn. In such a case there are several possibilities.

First, the tap may be repeated higher. This is not a recommended procedure in the office. It is better to defer the tap for forty-eight hours or more, unless an acute emergency exists. Hospitalization will be indicated and further procedures can be done at that time.

If you feel it is necessary to gain what information is available immediately, put a drop of fluid under the microscope and observe the red blood cells. Those from the tap have the characteristic appearance of normal cells. Those that have been in the spinal fluid for an hour or more have begun to break up and fragment. Bizarre shapes and sizes are common. This finding is not an absolute indication.

Spinal fluid that has contained blood for some time is xanthochromic. Actually it looks like urine. Surprisingly, the discoloration is not an absolute indicator of previous bleeding into the fluid, for there are cases in which the fluid was xanthochromic and no lesion could be found on autopsy. For practical purposes it indicates bleeding.

Assuming that the tap is satisfactory, notice the pressure under which the fluid is exuded. Normally it drips from the needle at 60 to 80 drops a minute (compare it with your own or the patient's pulse rate). An increase to 100 drops is not significant. A steady trickle or a spurt from the needle is an indication of increased pressure. Usually manometric pressure determinations are not an office procedure and, in the average case, are not necessary. The principal matter of interest is whether or not the pressure is increased and, if it is, a rough estimation of the degree of increase.

If the flow is slower than normal, have the patient close his mouth, hold his nose, and blow. This is a way of performing the Queckenstedt test without the services of an assistant. The flow of spinal fluid should quicken immediately. If it does not, assume that there is a block to normal fluid circulation and hospitalize the patient for further study.

It is seldom necessary, and never a good idea, to withdraw more than 5 to 6 ml. of spinal fluid in the office. By careful utilization this will be all that is needed.

When the needle is withdrawn observe the puncture site for a few seconds. If there is bleeding or escape of fluid, make pressure over the puncture site with an alcohol sponge. No dressing is needed, but patients usually feel better if an adhesive strip is applied.

To do a tap in a very young child, have your office nurse hold the child like this:

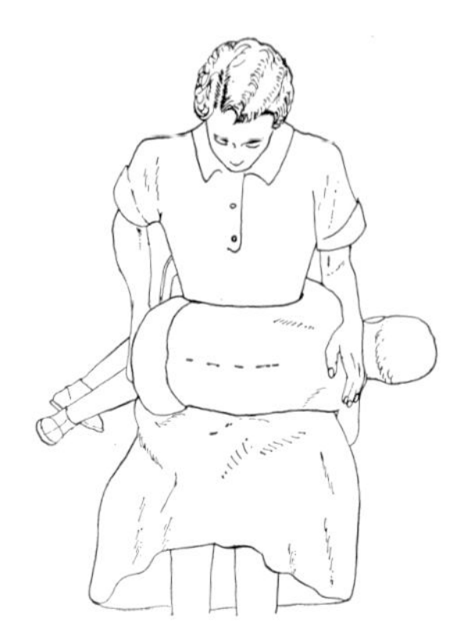

Use a 2- or 2½-inch 20-guage needle attached to a 2 ml. syringe for the tap and control the exit of fluid with the syringe. In the newborn infant it may be exceedingly difficult to withdraw more than a few drops of fluid, for infants have a considerably smaller amount in proportion than adults.

Cells in the fluid are counted like this: Use ordinary white blood count diluting fluid to which has been added a few drops of methylene blue stain. Draw this diluting fluid up to the mark 1 on the white blood cell pipette and fill to the mark 11 with fresh spinal fluid. If the spinal fluid is more than one-half hour old, cellular degeneration will have begun and results will be spurious.

Be particularly cautious to shake the pipette well and then fill the counting chamber. Count the cells in the four corner squares exactly as is done for a white blood count. Total the number of cells in all four areas and multiply by 2.5. The result is the number of cells per cubic millimeter of spinal fluid.

Errors

The actual counting procedure is subject to little error. If it is done carelessly one may mistake red cells that are not completely destroyed for white cells and obtain a count higher than is actually present.

If one tries to do a count on a grossly bloody tap, the white cells from the extraneous blood will give a false high count. Examination of fluid more than one-half hour old may result in a lowered count. It is imperative that the fluid be examined while fresh.

Errors in obtaining the fluid are legion. They will be discussed in detail in the complete section on the spinal fluid, beginning on page 176.

Interpretation

To begin with, one must realize that there is a shift in normal levels of spinal cells. The newborn infant often has 30 to 40 white cells per cubic millimeter of spinal fluid, even in the absence of intracranial injury. A few red cells, usually ranging from 2 to 4 per millimeter, may also be found in the fluid of a normal newborn infant. These disappear within a few days.

As many as 30 white cells per millimeter may presist until the child reaches 1 year of age. Until the age of 4 the normal count may range as high as 20. After the first five years of life anything over 10 is considered abnormal.

Only lymphocytes or monocytes are found in the normal fluid. Rarely a polymorphonuclear leukocyte may be seen without significance, but if there are enough of these leukocytes to allow calculation of percentage, abnormality is present.

Increase of the spinal fluid cell count is indicative of an irritative, inflammatory, or infectious process. It has no specificity whatsoever, and diagnosis beyond the three general processes just mentioned is impossible by count alone.

In the presence of nonpyogenic inflammation the cells are lymphocytes. There is one exception. During the acute invasive stage of a nonpyogenic process there may be a preponderance of polymorphonuclear cells, but this lasts only a few days. In general, such a count is indicative of virus, spirochetal, tuberculous, or fungous inflammations. Polio and encephalitis show such counts after the acute invasive phase.

Rarely a lymphatic leukemia will show all signs of meningeal irritation and upon examination will reveal a high lymphocyte count in the spinal fluid. Examination of peripheral blood and the systemic symptomatology serve to make diagnosis clear.

An increased count with polymorphonuclear leukocytes predominating has three possible interpretations. It can indicate the invasive stage of a nonpyogenic infection, an acute pyogenic process, or irritation of the meninges from a near-by pyogenic process.

The acute infections of the meningeal areas are prone to produce high counts of 300 cells and above. Often the fluid is milky in appearance and may show signs of increased viscosity. Such fluids are seen in infections with the meningococcus, pneumococcus, staphylococcus, and streptococcus, and the influenza bacillus.

Low polymorphonuclear counts in the 10-to-100 group are more often seen as irritative phenomena. They indicate a meningeal irritation usually due to abutment of a pyogenic focus to the meningeal area. Typical examples are severe mastoid disease and brain abscess.

Needless to say, none of these counts are absolute criteria but they will hold good in a majority of cases. As an example, let us trace the count in a typical case of poliomyelitis.

By the time signs of meningeal irritation are present, there will be an increased count, often predominantly polymorphonuclears. It usually is in the area of 100 cells per cubic millimeter. Within twenty-four to forty-eight hours the process has usually invaded maximally, and the count, which may be either higher or lower, is now made up predominantly of lymphocytes.

Certainly only one office count will be done on any polio patient (if there are any polio patients in the next few years), but it will depend entirely on the stage of the central nervous system disease whether the count be predominantly lymphocytic or neutrophilic.

The level of the spinal fluid cell count is not a predictive device. It may very well reflect the present response of body defenses and thereby indirectly indicate the immediate severity of the process. But it cannot predict with any accuracy what will happen in the next few hours or days. To use it for such purposes is to court difficulty.

Indications

In the adult there are only three acceptable indications for the spinal fluid cell count:

1. When a careful history and physical examination show unequivocal signs of meningeal irritation. If the signs are not definite enough to arouse positive suspicion, there is no indication for immediate spinal tap.

2. When detailed history and neurologic examination indicate the presence of neurologic disease or tumor. Here it must be pointed out vigorously that the spinal puncture is not a means of differentiating neurologic disease from psychoneurosis. The psychoneurotic patient does not have acceptable neurologic signs, and the disease should be diagnosed on a positive, not an eliminative, basis.

3. To obtain what information is possible when spinal fluid is withdrawn for a serologic test for syphilis.

In infants and very young children the picture is somewhat different. Meningeal infections are much more difficult to diagnose and probably are of more serious import in such patients. When the patient is less than 1 year of age, such minor signs as fullness of the anterior fontanel, periods of drowsiness alternating with extreme irritability in the presence of fever, and nonresponse of an infectious process to treatment are indications for spinal tap.

Probably it could be said that the procedure is done too seldom in very young children and too often in adults.

General Discussion

The spinal fluid cell count is an acceptable office procedure if used conservatively. Actually, in adults it serves more as a confirmation than as a means of diagnosis. The ancillary procedures done on spinal fluid are more important diagnostically.

In children under 8 months of age the importance of the procedure can scarcely be overstressed. This does not mean that every sick child should have a spinal tap. But perhaps one of every one hundred patients with an acute infection that is not diagnosed at once should be tapped.

As a differentiating factor the count has some small value. Other tests on the fluid are worth more for this purpose.

CHAPTER TWO

The Routine Urinalysis

The dominant characteristic of the normal kidney is its ability to change the composition of the urine to meet various body exigencies. The routine urinalysis, surprisingly, gives little direct information on this point. Essentially it is a "spot check" for abnormalities in urinary composition. When unusual constituents are found this is an indication for further study and not a means of making a diagnosis.

Lower urinary tract lesions are more accurately pointed out by the routine urinalysis than are lesions of the upper tract. Even so, the test seldom allows specific diagnosis. It may, however, be useful in confirming a clinical impression.

Even with these severe limitations in mind the fact remains that the test is an excellent one. It is one of the few laboratory procedures that experts say should be done on most new patients whether or not the symptoms and physical findings indicate urinary tract disease.

Collection of the specimen is of some importance. Since pathologic ingredients are not always present at all times, it is more accurate to examine a mixed twenty-four-hour urine sample. For practical purposes this is impossible. The next best thing is to examine a specimen of the first urine voided in the morning, which usually represents a four- to eight-hour formation period.

Urine should be examined as quickly after voiding as possible, for decomposition soon begins. At times the advantage of this fresh examination may outweigh advantages of the longer period of collection obtained in the early morning specimen. This is particularly true in the examination for cells and bacteria.

A good method of securing a satisfactory specimen is to give the patient a 6-ounce, wide-mouth bottle (capped ointment jars may be secured from the druggist) to which has been added eight drops of 40 per cent formalin solution. Be sure the lid is firmly in place and instruct the patient to keep it so. Have him add a small quantity of urine to the jar at 2 P.M. and before retiring, and fill it upon arising. In this way a fair cross-section of twenty-four-hour production can be obtained.

If more than eight drops of formalin are added the drug may cause positive reactions for sugar and albumin.

Always remember the possibility of vaginal contamination in females. Even girls

Many of the pathologic and physiologic processes discussed in this chapter are deliberately oversimplified to reach a working hypothesis. I cannot recommend too strongly that the physician, after establishing this working hypothesis, go to the standard and advanced texts for a more complete understanding.

of 3 and 4 years of age may extrude enough cells from the vaginal tract to cause confusion. Instruct the patients to wash thoroughly between the labia with soap and water, rinse all soap away with clear water, and dry before securing a specimen. Even in the presence of a marked discharge an uncontaminated specimen may be secured if this procedure is carefully followed.

In the routine office urinalysis one should examine for color, transparency, pH, specific gravity, albumin, and sugar.

COLOR

The normal yellow color is due to the urochrome pigments and accessory substances which occur in minute traces. Their formation involves chemistry far too complex to be entered into here.

Technique

No technique is involved. Simply observe the urine in a clear container.

Errors

Surprisingly enough, it is very difficult to convey orally or in writing the subtle color changes to which the urine is subject. Also it seems nearly impossible to convince the average technician that urinary color is worth describing accurately. One of my associates once put a little purple dye in a specimen and sent it to the laboratory. The report came back "yellow."

Custom has given us a set of meaningless words which we use in describing urinary color. "Straw" is an example. The only way to avoid these descriptive errors is for the physician himself to look at the urine.

Interpretation

Within the range of normal variation much indirect information can be obtained. In general, the coloration reflects the state of hydration. The fevers with their increased water loss are productive of deep reddish brown urine of high concentration. This is the "strong" urine so often mentioned by patients and usually indicates excellent kidney function under a severe handicap. Urine of normal specific gravity or dilute urine with seemingly normal kidney function can usually be taken as definite evidence that no prolonged febrile disease or severe water loss has been present.

While there is nothing positive about this small point it can be of exceeding value in the office examination. For example: A woman comes to the office complaining of severe nausea and vomiting of early pregnancy and states that she "hasn't been able to keep a thing—even water—on her stomach for three days." The urine is of a normal light yellow color. You have a clue. The lady is undoubtedly overalarmed and the severe nausea and vomiting she describes is probably, in actuality, a mild nausea that causes sharp limitation of appetite.

We live in an age that decrees terror to be the fashion. Utter trivia that would be ignored by any well-balanced person are built up in the minds of many patients into terrifying disease. Never overlook the value of the office laboratory and x-ray in demonstrating how much is fear and how much is disease in any case presented to you.

Abnormal constituents may greatly change the color of the urine. Blood pigment, either in or out of red cells, gives characteristic changes. In barely perceptible concentration it blunts the normal yellow of the urine to a deep tannish gray that looks like coal smoke. As the concentration increases, the urine assumes a tobacco color and then progresses through red to frank bloodiness.

Certain pigments may look much like blood and may be mistaken for it. In the newborn infant, uric acid crystals may leave a pink stain on the diapers for a few days. The characteristic of this is that it is pink while hemoglobin is not. The red or brown stains of blood should never be confused with this.

Several drugs that are frequently used may give coloration that can be confused with hemoglobin. Notable are cascara and senna in alkaline urine. A test for hemoglobin will settle the matter. It is described in the next chapter.

Deep brown, intense yellow, blue, and green solutions are almost always due to ingestion of drugs. For practical purposes there are no physiologic alterations that will produce these colors.

When bile is present the urine assumes a yellowish brown color and, when shaken, the foam appears yellow instead of white. After standing for a time, biliverdin may appear and give the urine a dirty green color. If, when shaken, the foam appears yellow, a sample of the urine should be set aside in an open test tube and allowed to remain overnight.

Bilirubin, the pigment responsible for color changes when bile is present in the urine, is formed from the breakdown of hemoglobin. In the normal process the reticuloendothelial cells probably engulf and certainly act upon worn-out, trapped, or injured red blood cells to release the hemoglobin.

The reticuloendothelial system is of such great size that it is rarely possible to overload it with damaged cells. Only in the case of massive intravascular hemolysis or release of myohemoglobin does it seem that a greater burden is placed on these remarkable cells than they can carry. In such cases free hemoglobin appears in the urine. Needless to say, such patients are not office problems.

In the ordinary course of events the reticuloendothelial cells withdraw iron from the hemoglobin molecule, probably in the form of an iron-protein complex. The remaining molecule consists of bilirubin attached to an unidentified protein. This bilirubin-protein complex is released into the blood stream and is ultimately acted upon by liver cells. The liver acts to separate the protein and bilirubin, excreting the latter in the bile and preserving the protein for ultimate re-use. In cases of liver damage the protein-bilirubin complex may increase in the blood stream, literally being dammed up behind the poorly functioning hepatic cells. Such cases are characterized by clinical jaundice, bilirubin-protein complex in the urine, and the indirect van den Bergh reaction. They are more rare than the next category to be discussed.

Often we see an accumulation of bile pigments in the blood when both reticuloendothelial cells and liver cells are functioning properly. This happens when there is a blockage to the excretion of bile between the liver cell and the duodenum, usually stone or carcinoma. In such cases bilirubin alone accumulates in the blood stream and appears in the urine. The van den Bergh reaction is direct.

Urine of a very light, pale greenish color should make one think of diabetes.

TRANSPARENCY

Normal fresh urine is so transparent that ordinary newspaper type can be read through several inches in a specimen bottle. The presence of particulate material, such as cells, crystals, or casts, will so refract the light rays that this is not possible and the lines of type become blurred and indistinct. This is the best test available to determine transparency.

Technique

Simply tear a bit of one column from a newspaper and hold it against the specimen bottle and try to read it through the urine. Another useful means of examination is to tack a sheet of black art paper to the laboratory wall and hold a test tube of urine in front of the paper for examination. This is best done in a moderately strong, indirect light. We use a flashlight to afford illumination. The light should be held at a 45-degree angle with the plane of vision.

Errors

Urine checked for transparency should be examined while fresh. After the urine stands for a few hours there normally appears a faint cloud of cellular debris and mucus which usually settles to the bottom of the specimen container. This is usually of little or no significance but may serve to confuse results if not understood.

Interpretation

Lessening of urinary transparency is not necessarily an indication of pathology. It does indicate that particulate material exists in the urine. Crystals, blood, pus, and bacteria are the most common foregin components, but there is no way to tell by this examination which is present.

Actually, the test is of very little use except as a general indicator.

REACTION

The kidney is one of the principal acid-base regulators of the body. Its function as such ranks among the most important biochemical processes of life itself. Unfortunately, so many factors unrelated to this specific function operate to change the pH of the urine that the test is of indicative value only.

Normally the twenty-four-hour specimen is slightly acidic in reaction, the pH averaging about 6.2. Spot checks taken throughout the day show a range from 5 to 7.5, the alkalinity becoming most pronounced after large meals and the acidity more evident after exercise.

Acid-base regulation may be oversimplified and represented by a single chemical formula:

$$H^+ + HCO_3 \rightleftarrows H_2CO_3 \rightleftarrows H_2O + CO_2$$

Addition of H^+ will drive the reaction to the right, requiring excretion of CO_2 (lungs) or H^+ (kidney) to re-establish normal equilibrium. By measuring the renal excretion of H^+ we may gather some degree of information as to the status of this chemical equilibrium in the body.

Technique

Nitrazine* paper is the most readily available means of getting a reasonable estimate of urinary pH. It is dipped in the urine and compared with the chart which is furnished with each bottle.

Errors

During the first hour or two after voiding, urine may increase in acidity. This is of little significance and seldom affects the test enough to be taken into consideration. After urine has been standing several hours (in or out of the bladder) there is a decomposition of urea, with release of free ammonia and consequent alkalinization.

To check for this error if you believe it to be present, dip a piece of litmus paper into the urine. If free ammonia is present the paper will turn blue. Now gently heat the litmus paper above a Bunsen flame. The ammonia will be evaporated and driven off and the paper will assume once again its pink color. Another way to check is to hold a bit of pink litmus in the vapor above boiling urine. The paper will turn blue if ammonia is present.

Interpretation

Consistent and marked acidity may be due to various body processes that cause an in-

*E. R. Squibb & Sons.

crease in H^+ in the body fluids, i.e., acidosis. Severe infections, diabetes, loss of base as in vomiting and diarrhea are the examples most frequently seen.

Acute or chronic dehydration with a reduced quantity of urine makes for increased acidity. This, of course, only means that the kidney attempts to excrete a normal amount of H^+ in a greatly reduced amount of urine, thereby increasing the urinary acidity without an increase in the total H^+ excreted. Such urine is very irritating and may, of itself, be the cause of frequency and burning. This is particularly true in children.

Methanol poisoning may usually be diagnosed by the simple expedient of taking the urinary pH if a suspicious history is elicited. The methyl alcohol is oxidized to formic acid and the pH will be excessively low.

Certain urinary tract infections occur only in the presence of acid urine. The most common is invasion by *Bacillus coli* which is responsible for more than 40 per cent of all urinary tract infections. During the course of treatment alkalinizing agents are often used and the patient may be instructed in the use of nitrazine paper and asked to determine the pH of his urine three times daily in order to ascertain that alkalinity is being maintained.

Persistently alkaline urine seldom occurs except in the presence of urinary tract infection. *Proteus vulgaris* is the most frequent offender, but it must be remembered that several of the common urinary tract pathogens are capable of splitting urea, with consequent formation of ammonia and alkalinization of the urine.

Discussion

In cases of more or less extreme acidosis the urinary pH determination is of little value. Clinical symptoms so far outweigh the single finding of a lowered pH that the test assumes little practical worth.

In the presence of urinary infection the determination is of the utmost utility. Often therapy is guided as much by the reaction of the urine as by the more detailed bacteriologic studies. The most frequent error in these cases is not to test the urine sufficiently often to be certain that drugs are maintaining the desired acidity or alkalinity. A minimum of three daily tests (which can be done by the patient) is necessary.

SPECIFIC GRAVITY

The specific gravity of the urine is a method of measuring the solids dissolved in the urine. The more concentrated a specimen is, i.e., the more solids it carries in solution, the higher the specific gravity.

Diseased kidneys are often unable to concentrate urine to the extent that a normal kidney can and the specific gravity gives a clue to this. Particularly is the finding valuable if the physician takes a few minutes to inquire about fluid intake in the twelve hours preceding the test.

In man, glomerular filtration is remarkably constant. It is reabsorption in the tubules that varies water output. This tubular reabsorption may be divided into two phases: (1) The resorption which occurs in the tubules and when glucose and other solutes are selectively taken up from the intratubular fluid and passed back into the blood stream. The changes that occur in osmotic pressures operate to cause return of water also until intratubular and intravascular osmotic pressures equalize. (2) The distal tubule resorbs water actively under control of the antidiuretic hormone of the pituitary pars nervosa.

Normally the fluid entering the distal tubule has a specific gravity of 1.010. To change this requires active work on the part of the tubule cells. When the tubules are diseased, they cannot function adequately.

There are, therefore, two common pathologic reasons why urinary specific gravity may remain constant around 1.010. The most common would be disease of kidney cells; the least common (actually, excessively rare) would be disease affecting the secretion of posterior pituitary hormone.

Technique

A sample of urine is placed in a clean urinometer, the float added, and the specific gravity read from the scale.

Errors

Slight errors may be caused by temperature changes but these are nearly insignificant. The most frequent source of error is a dirty urinometer. After every use the instrument should be washed in tap water and dried.

One should never accept a single reading as diagnostic. Even repeated readings, unless conditions of fluid intake are controlled, can be deceiving.

Interpretation

In the diseases that affect the kidney, concentrating ability tends to be lowered gradually until the specific gravity becomes fixed around 1.010. When the specific gravity is either higher or lower than this figure, it implies that the renal cells are doing active work to concentrate or dilute the urine.

A single finding of 1.010 means nothing unless there is a clear-cut history of lowered fluid intake during the twelve hours immediately preceding. It is rare for the first specimen of morning urine to have such a low specific gravity; therefore this finding is significant if present.

Specific gravity of below 1.010 is most often seen in the psychoneurotic patient with the nervous tendency to drink much water or coffee. Less often it is an indication of diabetes insipidus. Some authors have stated that specific gravity is lower than 1.010 in some forms of nephritis, but the reasons for this, if it does occur, are not clear.

Pathologically increased specific gravity, on the other hand, is most often due to diabetes mellitus. A history of polyuria along with pale urine of high specific gravity is almost pathognomonic of the disease.

In the presence of fevers or other dehydrating disease, the specific gravity may be raised, but this, in actuality, is an indication of good kidney function rather than a sign of disease.

Discussion

As in most other tests encompassed in the routine urinalysis, the determination of specific gravity is more of an indicator than a positive diagnostic factor. Properly used it can be of great assistance. As an example, take this case:

A 60-year-old man with hypertension and some known kidney damage reports to the office in midsummer at 11:30 A.M. A specimen is secured and the specific gravity reported as 1.012. Upon questioning, the patient states he had a cup of coffee and two glasses of water for breakfast. He urinated upon reaching the office and has taken no fluids since. As a matter of fact, he reports himself thirsty at the moment.

Chances are great that it is time to do a concentration and dilution test, for the specific gravity should have been more than 1.012 under the circumstances. It is only when subjected to such interpretation that the specific gravity is of great value.

ALBUMIN

Picture, if you will, an ordinary kitchen wire strainer with most holes between the wires of normal size and an occasional hole the size of a cigarette in cross section. Fill the wire strainer with a solvent that contains, among other things, raisins. When the strainer is shaken an occasional raisin will escape through the larger holes, but most of them will remain in the strainer.

Such is the relation of the glomerulus, as the strainer, to the albumin molecule, as the raisin. Normally a few molecules of albumin leak through, but the number is very small.

To carry the illustration further, picture a toy steam shovel, below the strainer capable of picking up one raisin at a time and putting it back in the box. So long as only an occasional raisin escapes, the toy steam shovel can see that all are picked up and put back in the box. If too many escape of if the shovel slows down or is broken, it will not be able to keep up and raisins will accumulate. Such is the function of the tubule in resorbing albumin.

There are three points of possible damage: the strainer may be attacked and ruined so that it will let literally thousands of raisins through and make it impossible for the shovel to keep up; the shovel may be engaged in other work and not have "energy" to do the primary assignment and pick up raisins, too; or the shovel may break down or slow down.

By considering this little example carefully, one significant fact about proteinuria will immediately come to light. Proteinuria may occur without an actual breakdown (i.e., disease) of the system. Anything that slows down the shovel or keeps it busy doing other work will allow raisins to escape.

The analogy with tubular epithelium is exact.

By no means is the discovery of albumin in a single urine sample significant of severe disease. Inconstant, episodic proteinuria may occur with stress, either physiologic or psychologic. It is seen sometimes as a postural phenomenon, albumin being present when the patient stands erect and disappearing when he reclines.

Albumin is a constituent of pus cells, red blood cells, epithelial cells, etc. When these structures are present in the urine, a positive test is often obtained. When this is the suspected cause, a microscopic examination usually settles the question. If the microscope does not convince the physician, a sample of the urine may be centrifuged for five minutes, the supernatant liquid carefully pipetted off and tested for albumin.

Technique

Begin by determining the pH of the specimen. If it is greater than 6.5, add a drop or two of concentrated acetic acid. Then place 5 ml. in a test tube and gently heat over a Bunsen flame until the urine is nearly to the boiling point. A white, cloudy precipitate will form in albuminous urine.

If a positive test is obtained, acidify another specimen in a separate test tube and filter to remove mucin. Heat the filtrate. Should the white cloud again form, the test for albumin is positive. To be absolutely certain, add another two drops of glacial acetic acid to the cloudy specimen and shake gently. If nothing happens, chances are overwhelming that the precipitate is albumin.

Errors

The most common error is to assume that any precipitate which forms upon heating is albumin. Once we calculated the chances that a precipitate would be albumin by surveying one hundred cases in which heat clouded urine. In sixty-one of the one hundred the precipitate gave more definitive signs of being albumin. In thirty-nine it promptly dissolved or disappeared upon application of one of the above procedures.

Errors in interpretation are almost as common as errors in the test itself. They will be discussed in detail in the next section.

Interpretation

In young children the renal epithelium seems to be more sensitive to minor insult than is the case in older persons. For this reason one should be exceedingly careful not to base diagnosis or prognosis upon the single isolated finding of a trace of albumin in the urine.

When confronted with such a patient, it is always wise to obtain daily specimens for several days unless the history and physical examination elicit positive evidence that the kidney is not the site of disease. Even in such a case two additional specimens should be examined at three-day intervals, despite the negative history and physical examination.

Even in the adult the renal epithelium evinces a decided susceptibility to noxious influences. The fevers and extreme toxicity from either disease or nonfatal poisonings often permit the escape of protein into the urine. The mechanism is probably dual. The tubular cells are both busy and somewhat slowed by the toxic reaction. They fail to resorb the albumin which normally escapes through the glomerulus and a trace or more of protein appears in the urine. No great significance should be attached to this.

When an adult appears with mild albuminuria and there are no findings, either historical or physical, confirming the presence of renal disease, one must be exceedingly careful, for chances are better than 40 per cent that the finding is incidental rather than evidence of pathology.

Specimens taken at weekly intervals for several weeks will serve to demonstrate whether or not the loss of albumin is consistent or only an isolated finding. If it appears more or less consistently, one should think of early kidney impairment, without physical findings or orthostatic albuminuria.

If one suspects a postural factor, have the patient urinate just before retiring and preserve the specimen. Then, immediately upon arising, another specimen should be secured. If postural factors are operative the specimen obtained before retiring will usually contain albumin, while the one voided immediately upon arising will not. The test is even more effective if the patient is asked to arise briefly about midnight, urinate, and discard the urine.

Unfortunately we do not know too much about the early onset of the more serious kidney diseases. It would seem that a certain number of patients who show episodes of transient and apparently innocuous albuminuria will later develop frank nephritic disease. The number who will do so has never been established exactly but it is greater than would be expected from chance. For this reason any patient who shows albuminuria, even transient and in the absence of other symptoms, should have urinalyses at three- or six-month intervals for several years.

In our own practice we have found it wise to teach such patients to test their own urine and to request that they report to us if albumin appears. Of course, it is needless to say that we always retest.

The nephrotic syndrome is characterized, in part, by extreme loss of plasma protein, largely albumin, in the urine. When such urine is tested it often solidifies into a jelly-like mass in the test tube upon application of heat. This is by no means a positive diagnostic factor but in actuality is seldom seen in other conditions.

Most researchers feel now that this loss is due to glomerular damage. If the example stated earlier in this chapter be accurate, only glomerular damage could release enough albumin to show more than a small amount in the urine.

In summary, there are three possible causes for albuminuria:

1. Cellular matter in the urine. The microscope will clarify this issue. When

cellular matter is present it is most often due to infection or trauma, such as that caused by stones.

2. Deficient tubular resorption. This is the most frequent cause of the minor albuminuria. It is more often due to toxic interference with tubular cells than to severe disease involving these same cells.

3. Glomerular damage. So far as we know, the "leakage rate" of albumin does not greatly increase under minor insult. Probably (but by no means certainly) there is some degree of permanent damage to glomeruli when proteinuria is due to increased glomerular filtration.

From what little we know of kidney disease it would seem that damage most frequently affects the nephron more or less as a unit, only rarely becoming apparent in one particular part to the exclusion of all others. The primary concept which is of interest in daily practice is that minor albuminurias, transient and of short duration, may result from minor insults that have no known relationship to the long-term and ultimately fatal diseases of the kidney. Particularly is this true in children.

SUGARS

The glomerular filtrate is essentially blood plasma with only a small bit of the protein. In other words, the glomerular filter retains only cellular elements and most of the protein molecules. Sugar molecules pass freely through the filter, and the carbohydrate in the filtrate is, in essentiality, the same as that in plasma.

Kidney tubules resorb all but a small amount of sugar and the residue which appears in the urine is far too little to be detected by ordinary tests.

The capacity for tubular resorption of carbohydrate seems to vary with the individual. Some patients can reabsorb large amounts and, therefore, have a high renal threshold for sugar. Others spill sugar in the urine when the filtrate contains relatively little. In general, the renal threshold averages 160 mg. per cent. It has been reported as low as 120 and as high as 250 in older subjects.

The presence of sugar in the urine brings two possibilities to mind:

1. Escape of abnormally large amounts of sugar through the glomerulus into the filtrate. This implies no disease of the glomerulus but rather a greatly increased plasma level.

2. Interference with tubular resorption.

The converse of the first of these facts is a point to remember. If the intact glomerulus allows a maximal amount of sugar to escape, then the possibility exists that the diseased and sclerotic glomerulus will retain many of the carbohydrate molecules. When this occurs the reabsorptive powers of the tubules continue to be exerted maximally. The final result is a major rise in renal threshold to sugar, often to as much as 250 mg. per cent or more. When there is such a rise, a frank diabetes may occur without sugar in the urine.

Technique

Benedict's test is the most commonly used. The reagent can be purchased commercially or prepared. The formula is as follows:

Copper sulfate	17.3
Potassium citrate	173.00
Anhydrous sodium carbonate	100.0
Water q.s. ad.	1,000.00

Be sure to dissolve the sodium carbonate and potassium citrate in 800 ml. of water without adding other ingredients. In 100 ml., dissolve the copper salt and add the resulting solution slowly to the first. Add water to complete the 1,000 ml. volume.

Approximately 5 ml. (3/4 inch in the average test tube) are added to several test tubes and they are kept in a hot-water bath.

When a specimen of urine is to be tested, 10 drops are added to one of the test tubes, and it is replaced in the water bath while other examinations are completed.

When time to complete the examination for sugar arrives, the tube is removed from the water bath and heated in a Bunsen flame. Reports are made as follows:

Trace	Light green, no precipitate
1+	Yellow green with flocculate
2+	Yellow with precipitate
3+	Orange with heavy precipitate
4+	Brick red with heavy precipitate

Errors

Mucin in urine may yield a carbohydrate which will give a false positive reaction. This seldom happens, for application of intense heat over a period of time is usually necessary, but it is a good possibility to keep in mind when a specimen that contains many mucous threads is presented for examination. The specimen may be acidified with glacial acetic acid and filtered to remove the mucin.

When present, albumin acts in the opposite way. It may interfere with proper precipitation in a positive specimen. It may be removed by acidifying, boiling, and filtering before performing the Benedict test.

In pregnancy, lactose frequently occurs in the urine. This is most common in the last two trimesters and the two months after delivery in the nursing mother. It may occur after miscarriage. It has no significance, but it will give a positive test.

When a positive test for sugar is obtained during or immediately after pregnancy or miscarriage, no diagnosis should be made. Lactose should be tested for in such cases. Rubner's test is the most satisfactory.

Put 10 ml. of the suspected urine in a test tube and add 2 Gm. of lead acetate. Shake well and filter. Heat the filtrate to boiling and add 1 ml. of strong ammonia. If sugar is present the solution will turn red and a precipitate will form. Glucose gives a yellow precipitate, lactose a red precipitate.

Interpretation

To reiterate, there are two possible sources of urine glucose. The least likely is a deficiency in tubular resorption of filtered glucose. This sometimes occurs as an inborn error of metabolism but more often occurs in certain toxic reactions as a transient and not particularly significant phenomenon. It is also found in certain types of poisoning, but these cases are not often seen or studied in the office.

The most frequent disarrangement is that involving an increase in blood sugar. The result is that more sugar is filtered than the tubules can resorb and the excess appears in the urine. Anything that will increase blood sugar to the requisite levels will cause glucosuria. By no means does a positive test prove the presence of diabetes. It proves that *something* elevated the blood sugar.

An example of nondiabetic glucosuria may be found in the typical hyperglycemia of fright. College students faced with a long and difficult examination or soldiers under extreme battle conditions may show sugar in the urine. Some people give a positive test after a large carbohydrate meal, and it is well known that certain neurologic mechanisms and endocrine imbalances may cause profound alterations in blood sugar levels.

A more complete discussion of blood sugar control will be found on page 77. From the standpoint of urine testing, the important thing to remember is that, while an increased blood sugar may be indicated, there is no information as to why the blood sugar is increased.

No greater error can be made than to assume that a single positive urine sugar means diabetes. It does mean that further investigation is in order.

I have mentioned previously the danger of misinterpreting the positive urine sugar test in pregnant women. In the vast majority of cases this represents lactose which is of no significance.

The kidney in a child seems much more susceptible to minor insult than is true in the adult. Small children with relatively minor gastrointestinal or infectious disease often show a temporary glycosuria.

CASTS

In spite of the fact that casts have been observed and studied for several hundred years, we cannot explain their formation or give anything like an accurate estimate of their exact significance. Casts are molds of the distal tubule or collecting system formed from precipitated proteins. Exactly why the proteins should precipitate in these situations we do not know.

There is little doubt that this coagulation of plasma proteins which have "leaked out" into the tubules has pathologic significance. We do not know whether one cast signifies involvement of a single nephron when most nephrons are normal or whether it represents chance coagulation in the presence of generalized injury. To use a more pungent example: Does it represent one dog howling with pain in the presence of 500 normal dogs or does it indicate 501 dogs in pain, only one hurting enough to yelp? Present belief is that an occasional cast in the urine is probably due to purely localized insult and has little significance. Showers of casts, on the other hand, may be of the utmost diagnostic import.

The fact should not be overlooked that casts themselves may sometimes act as obstructing agents and result in major kidney damage. No distinct proof has ever been offered, but physicians well versed in the pathology of the kidney have speculated extensively upon this point. The sequence of events would be something like this: Minor damage allows the escape of proteins into the lumen of the tubule. This damage is probably to the glomerulus because deficient tubular resorption of normally filtered proteins would not allow sufficient albumin or globulin in the tubular lumen to form a coagulum. For some reason which we cannot explain, a cast is formed. Pressure is built up back of the cast, which tends to expel it. There probably is some dilatation of the tubule by this pressure.

In many instances the cast is expelled and appears in the urine. In others, the cast may be "jammed at the turn" in a tubule and stubbornly refuse to be dislodged. When this occurs, back pressure soon nullifies any function of the nephron which is as effectively removed from the useful ranks as if it had been extirpated. We do not know whether this is a frequent or a rare occurrence. The purpose in writing about it is to suggest that the physician remember the possibility when confronted with a urine containing many casts.

Cellular products and pigments may be found in the substance of casts. Formerly, great significance was attached to the presence of these products, and extensive schemes were devised for the classification of casts according to the cells, pigments, or recognizable chemicals contained. Time has made it apparent that such extensive classifications are not useful in daily practice. When cells appear in casts it simply means that cells were present in the tubule at the time the cast was formed. Some inferences can be drawn by the type of cells. Renal epithelium, red blood cells, and white blood cells have obvious significance.

Granulation of casts seems to be related directly to the conditions of acidity under which they were formed. For that reason it has little significance. The appearance of heme pigments, on the other hand, is of serious import.

Technique

There is no reason to look for casts in urine not examined while fresh. Particularly is this true if the urine gives an alkaline reaction. The structures have a great tendency to dissolve with the passage of time and the examination of fresh urine is the only way to be certain as to their presence.

The urine is centrifuged and a drop of the sediment placed on a microscopic slide and covered with a cover glass. The low-power objective is used and the condenser stopped down until the light is greatly dimmed. A good criterion of proper lighting is to stop the light down until white blood cells look like this:

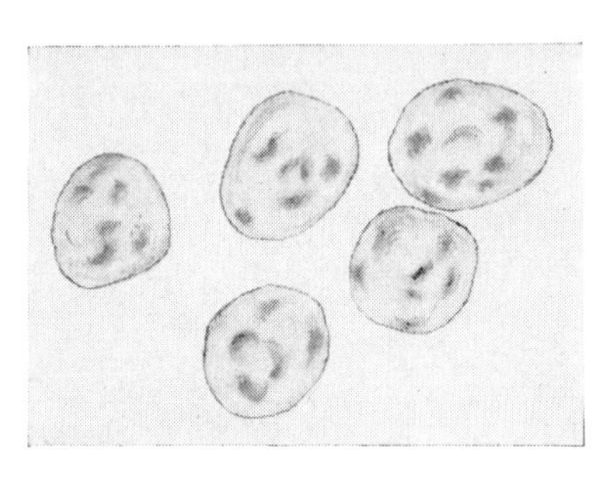

Even in this light, casts must be looked for carefully. They vary from approximately twice the diameter of a white blood cell to ten or more times the diameter. There are times when it is difficult to be certain and one may take advantage of the cylindrical shape of the casts to be positive. Use an ordinary household sewing needle that has been mounted in a matchstick, like this:

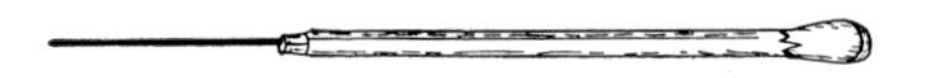

The needle point is placed on the cover glass and used to move it slightly on the slide. This causes the casts to roll and often gives good proof of their identity. At least it proves they are cylindrical.

Rarely one may wish to stain casts, although this is seldom necessary. Iodine is taken up by casts, and a drop of Lugol's solution placed at the edge of a cover glass and allowed a minute to diffuse will produce adequate staining. India ink applied by the same process will allow the casts to stand out as white against a brown or black background.

Errors

There are two structures seen frequently in the urine which may be mistaken for casts:

1. Mucous threads. These usually exhibit longitudinal striations which casts never do. They are tapering, the ends often coming to a point or splitting and curling back upon themselves. And they are often longer than casts. The long edges of a cast are clear-cut and well defined, while those of a mucous thread are indistinct and hazy.

2. Crystals. These may form around a mucous thread and appear very much like casts. Rarely crystals orient themselves into castlike groups. This is a matter of chance and has little significance. In most instances careful examination will serve to differentiate the crystalline structure, but if one is in doubt after careful examination, refer back to the pH of the urine and change it. If the urine was acid, add a drop of 1 per cent NaOH at the edge of the cover glass; if alkaline, add a drop of 1 per cent acetic acid. The crystals will disappear within minutes. Casts may dissolve, too, but it takes them an hour or more.

Interpretation

The fact that casts are present indicates that kidney pathology is present. There is no known normal condition in which sufficient protein to allow coagulation is found in the tubules. Unfortunately, it is possible to draw no other inference from the presence of casts. How much pathology, whether or not an irreversible process has occurred, or exactly what the process is is not predictable.

The content of casts may give some clue as to what is going on. A hyaline cast or granular cast (they are the same thing, the granules having been brought out by conditions of precipitation) is the most commonly seen of all types. Apparently it can occur in any insult to the kidney, even trivial ones.

Despite this there are two important inferences that may be drawn from hyaline casts. If they are present on repeated examinations, even in small numbers, one is justified in assuming that detrimental processes continue to operate in the kidney. This is an indication to take further diagnostic steps without delay. It is wise to remember that the failing kidneys of elderly people frequently show the continued presence of casts. It is doubtful whether such a finding in an otherwise healthy man of 75 or 80 offers much indication for further study.

Perhaps you will permit me to interject a personal thought here. There exists no excuse for running up a large laboratory bill on patients who are approaching dissolution in very old age or from hopeless disease. The laboratory is a means to add useful information to that supplied by our senses for patients who may be helped to achieve a healthy, lengthened life. It should never be used as a device to extract money from the dying. There are no scientific, moral, or medical indications for extensive laboratory work on the patient obviously doomed to die.

To return to the subject at hand, the second inference may be drawn if the hyaline (or granular) casts are of great width. Normally, casts do not form in the collecting tubules because the urinary stream is flowing faster and under greater pressure in this location. When renal failure is imminent the dribbling flow of urine in these collecting ducts may be so slow that protein precipitation occurs. The casts so formed are short and wide, at least the width of ten to twelve white blood cells. Caution should be used in making this interpretation. Usually, when such casts occur, clinical signs of renal shutdown are apparent. When they appear in the absence of clinical signs, a good maxim is, "Be ready but say nothing."

What are known as "coarsely granular casts" actually may be one of two different things. Often degenerated cells are responsible for large granules. When this is so, no special significance can be attached to the casts unless the type of cell be known. At other times the coarse granules represent deposits of lipid. There is no ready means of identification between the two types available to the office laboratory. For this reason no exact diagnostic significance should be attached to the coarsely granulated cast.

Casts containing reddish brown pigment are often important. They occur almost exclusively in the group of clinical syndromes which are known as lower nephron nephrosis. They may be seen in quantity in the urine before the clinical disease is clear-cut. Patients with such diseases, of course, must be cared for in the hospital.

Cellular matter appearing in casts indicates what cells were free in the renal tubule at the time the casts were formed. White and red blood cells usually appear free in the urine when they are found in casts, but their presence in the cast is indicative of their origin, which may be an important point in diagnosis.

In case one cannot be sure what type of cell is contained in casts under examination, a drop of dilute acetic acid should be placed at the edge of the cover glass and allowed to diffuse. This will clear the cytoplasm and bring the nucleus out so that identification becomes easy.

Perhaps the most important structure seen in such casts is the renal epithelial cell. When such cells come away in sheets so they are embedded in the surface of casts, one may impute the presence of severe renal disease. The typical renal cell looks like this:

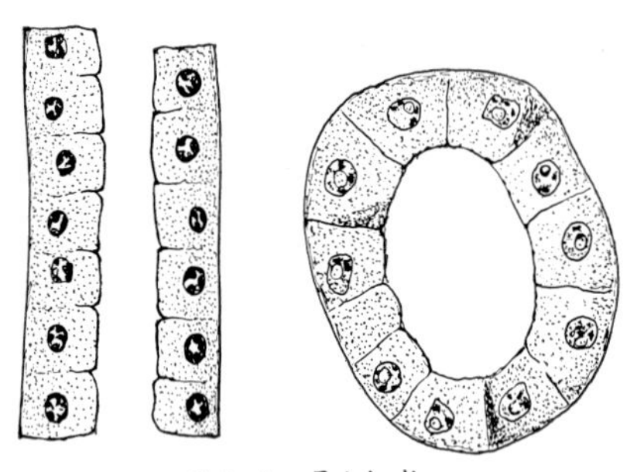

Tubular Epithelium

and the cellular cast containing renal epithelium, like this:

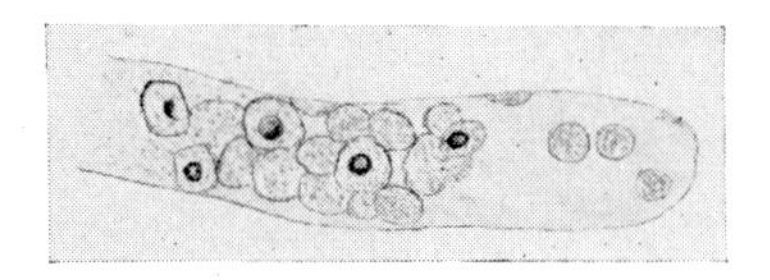

Such casts in large numbers indicate that the patient should be hospitalized.

RED BLOOD CELLS

Erythrocytes in the urine usually, but not always, indicate the presence of some serious lesion in the urinary tract. There is some evidence to show that transient minor lesions and even nervous tension may result in hematuria. Certainly such cases are rare (with one exception) and one should assume the presence of a serious lesion when hematuria appears.

The exception is hematuria in young infants. Kidney insults of the most trivial nature will often cause erythrocytes in the urine for several weeks. There are no records of gross hematuria of long-time duration from minor pathology, although this is possible. For this reason it is of the utmost importance to be very conservative in interpreting hematuria in infants.

Another point of importance is that all hematuria is relative. In the normal individual there is loss of several million red blood cells in the urine each day. Ordinarily this is such a small number compared to the daily volume of urine that only an occasional low-power field will contain one or two red blood cells. This is true even in centrifuged urine.

It is possible, however, that several red cells may appear in a single field due to this normal loss. In such cases a grave error may be made if only one microscopic field is examined. Surprisingly enough this is not a rare mistake. It has happened more than once in my own laboratory.

The common sources of red cells in urine are as follows:

1. Vaginal contamination at or near the menses or in the presence of a bloody discharge. An example would be the woman with trichomonad infestation and a pink discharge. There will be sufficient blood in the discharge to reveal many red blood cells per high-power field in the urine if there is vaginal contamination.

2. Generalized hyperemia of the kidney. The pathologic processes which may cause this are legion. The important point to remember is that any insult resulting in sustained hyperemia can, and usually does, cause erythrocytes to appear in the urine. The same is true of bladder hyperemia.

3. Necrosis. Necrotic areas anywhere in the urinary tract may cause blood to appear in the urine. Malignant tumors and the granulomatous diseases are most often the cause.

4. Defective glomeruli. Any of the diseases which attack the filter may so ruin it that red blood cells escape.

5. Defective tubules. Much more rarely, tubular disease may be responsible for the escape of erythrocytes.

6. Trauma. The urinary tract is highly vascularized. Any kind of scratch usually bleeds. By far the most common of all lesions causing hematuria is the scratching of mucous membranes by urinary stones.

7. Blood dyscrasias. This is rarely seen in office practice although urinary bleeding is very common when the blood dyscrasias are present.

Technique

The urine should be examined primarily in the uncentrifuged state. Seldom will urinary bleeding occur in such slight amount that it is undetectable in uncentrifuged urine. As a matter of fact, the best way to differentiate normal red cell loss from pathologic bleeding is to check the freshly voided urine without treatment of any kind. If several blood cells are found per high-power field, there can be little doubt that hematuria exists.

Identification of red blood cells in freshly voided urine offers no difficulty at all. They appear exactly as seen in unstained blood in any circumstance. When the urine is of high specific gravity, the cells may be crenated and look like this:

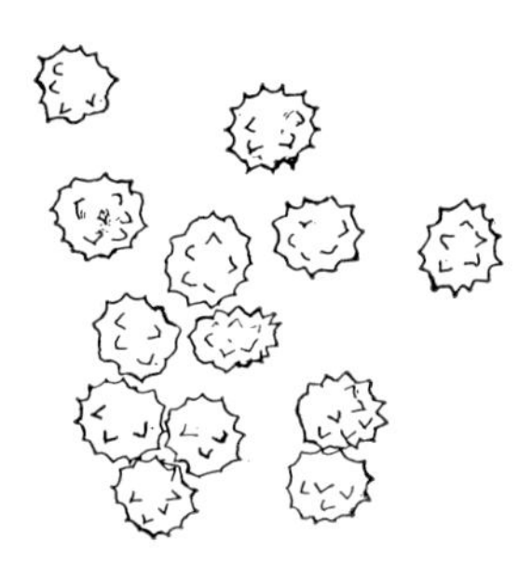

Crenated cells are gradually fragmented, becoming so broken up that identification is impossible. This happens only in urine that has not been examined while fresh, for the fragmentation requires several hours to occur. The opposite, of course, occurs in very dilute urines, the cells absorbing water and enlarging. Seldom, if ever, is this process virile enough to break up the erythrocytes or render them unidentifiable.

In certain urines, hemoglobin is dissolved out of erythrocytes, leaving "shadow cells." These actually are seen as an outline of the red blood cell and may assume bizarre shapes and sizes. They look like this:

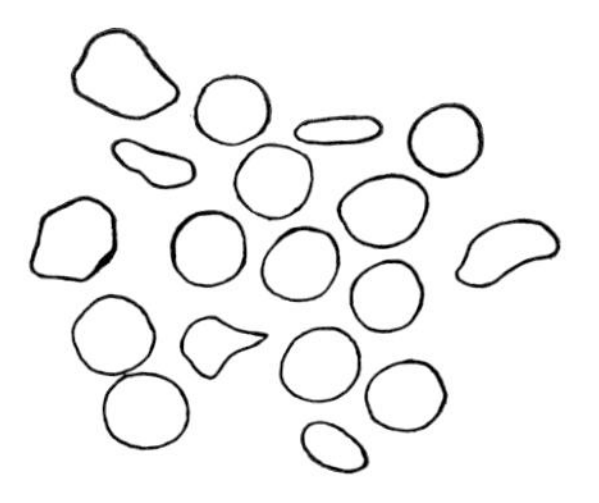

Their significance is the same as red cells.

Errors

The most common error in the office laboratory is to confuse red and white blood cells during an examination under the low power of the microscope. Usually examination with the high-power dry lens will serve to differentiate the two. If you still cannot be sure, add a drop of dilute acetic acid at one side of the cover glass and let stand a few minutes before re-examining. The acetic acid will clear the cytoplasm of the white blood cells and make the nucleus clearly visible.

Too much interpretive importance can be placed upon the finding of red blood cells in the urine. In the usual case, pathology is indicated, but the presence of erythrocytes throws no light on where the process is located or upon its seriousness. The old saw that painless hematuria is cancer until proved otherwise is needlessly alarming. In at least four of every five cases "otherwise" is easily proved.

Hematuria is an indication for further careful study and the physician should never forget that the most important part of this study is a detailed history. Various procedures, such as cytoscopy and roentgenography, are useful adjuncts only.

Interpretation

Since there are no direct and specific inferences that may be drawn from the presence of erythrocytes in the urine, little in the way of interpretation is possible. The balance of probability is that a lesion of some importance exists in the tract. To go further than this is to court error.

When there is a known disease such as nephritis, the significance of hematuria is greatly changed.

One may estimate the status and progress of the disease with fair accuracy by even crude measurements of red blood cell loss. Repeated urinalyses which report the average number of red blood cells in ten high-power fields selected at random will give a clue to progress and status of the disease. A constant hematuria with gradually increasing numbers of erythrocytes bespeaks a bad prognosis.

In hypertensive patients who are beginning the terminal phase involving kidney damage, the same prognostic significance may be inferred. Remember, in such cases, that the slowly progressive hypertension with gradually increasing renal involvement may go along for several years showing a constant hematuria before explosive and fatal complications occur.

Children, particularly under 5 years of age, may show a few blood cells in the urine for weeks at a time when no other evidence of pathology exists. Our only explanation is a rather weak one—that the youthful renal cells are more susceptible to noxious influence than older cells. This must be true, yet it follows the same specious reasoning we use when we say that most people who are buried are dead. We can offer no reasonable explanation. It may be that we are simply failing to demonstrate existing pathology in such cases. For this reason it is unwise to assign any import (or lack of it) to the presence of a few blood cells in the urine of children. Such a finding is an indication for careful observation but not for alarm, unless other unequivocal evidence of disease is present.

Rarely hemoglobin or related pigments appear in the urine when red blood cells are absent. This is usually of serious import and such patients are seldom seen as office problems. Ordinary Hematest tablets, which are obtainable at any surgical supply, may be used to make the determination.

WHITE BLOOD CELLS

White blood cells in the urine represent an exudative process brought on by inflammation or necrosis. Since there are always "minor repairs" going on in the tract, one would expect the usual specimen to contain an occasional white blood cell, which it does. Again we have the problem of a relative and not absolute finding. A few pus cells are normal; many pus cells represent pathology. Somewhere between these extremes is a dividing line but we cannot place it exactly.

For example, six pus cells per high-power field are found upon routine urinalysis in a patient who has no urinary tract symptoms. Is infection present? Not necessarily, for the cells may represent exudate from a tiny area of necrosis and repair which is insignificant from the standpoint of illness.

On the other hand, the same urinary findings in the presence of definite symptomatology may be of the utmost significance. The laboratory serves to substantiate your diagnosis.

Pus corpuscles, when their number is borderline, are of importance only when clinical or historical evidence is also present. As is true of all dogmatic statements, there are exceptions. The principal one is in regard to infants. Moderately severe urinary infections may occur during the first year of life when little clinical evidence exists.

The most common sources of pyuria and an estimate of relative importance may be tabulated as follows:

1. The nephron. Seldom subject to infection, but the necrotic and inflammatory changes of the nephritides often result in the appearance of leukocytes in the urine. Other findings so greatly overshadow this one that it is not of great importance.

2. The kidney pelvis. A frequent seat of infection and stones.

3. The ureter. Often the site of stones, with subsequent inflammatory changes. Not too often the seat of primary infection except in pregnancy, when hydroureter, with consequent stagnation of urine, is seen in as many as 80 per cent of cases. Infection of noticeable degree occurs in about 5 per cent.

4. The bladder. The most common seat of urinary infection.

5. Male genital tract. Infections of the prostate, seminal vesicles, even the epididymis, may result in pyuria.

6. Skene's glands. May produce enough pus in the female to cause pyuria.

7. Urethritis. Most often gonococcal in the female and about 50 per cent gonococcal in the male.

Technique

Pus cells degenerate and disappear in urine that has been kept in the laboratory or a specimen bottle for several hours. If at all possible the specimen should be examined while fresh. If not, a preservative may be added as specified at the beginning of this chapter.

In the ordinary case where pyuria is suspected it is not necessary to centrifuge the urine before doing a microscopic examination. If symptoms are such that one suspects infection, there will ordinarily be enough pus cells present in the fresh specimen to allow diagnosis from direct examination.

The opposite is true for the routine urinalysis. Here, the sediment after centrifugation should be examined.

Rarely will it be difficult to be sure one is seeing pus cells. Differentiation from some types of epithelial cells and even from artifacts is not always easy. Use a drop of dilute acetic acid placed at the edge of the cover glass to make differentiation easy.

Errors

Errors in diagnosing pyuria are rare. The most frequent error is the one that is most often totally unsuspected by physicians. As mentioned, white cells degenerate when urine is allowed to stand several hours before it is examined. Frequently errors are made when this fact is not taken into account. Particularly is this true when the pyuria is moderate.

Another frequent error often made when the urine is allowed to stand is the confusing of albumin from fragmented white cells with true albuminuria. In fresh urine, cells may be centrifuged to the bottom or filtered off and the remaining fluid tested for albumin content. After one or two hours enough cells are fragmented so that a positive test for albumin may be obtained under all circumstances.

Vaginal contamination is a frequent source of difficulty. It is possible to obtain a specimen almost free of contamination but the routine is exacting. Have the patient observe the following routine:

1. Wash the external genitalia with soap and water, being careful to wash the vaginal opening deep between the labia. Dry thoroughly.

2. Pull apart the labia, both major and minor, while urinating into the specimen jar so that the urine exits from the urethra in a stream and does not run over the labia.

As a practical point, most women will think this over and then remark that they need three hands to accomplish it. Suggest that they close both "lids" on the commode, place a paper towel on the top lid and set the specimen jar on this. Both hands are then left free.

Interpretation

Borderline cases that show slight pyuria should be diagnosed by other means and no significance at all placed on equivocal or inconstant urinary findings. This is probably the most important single factor to remember in interpreting pyuria.

Microscopic examination rarely gives any clue to the location of the inflammatory or necrotic lesion responsible for the white blood cells. The one important exception is the urine which has many free white blood cells along with casts containing leukocytes. In this instance one may be relatively certain that the individual nephrons contain pus cells. Other portions of the tract may be affected as well.

It is also important to recognize the fact that *inflammatory* changes are at the root of the exudation. Infection may or may not be present. In the great majority of cases there is infection, but if one assumes that pyuria always indicates infection, a mistake will occur sooner or later and may be embarrassing.

General Comment

The routine urinalysis is one of the most important tests done in the office laboratory. The information to be gained far exceeds that usually obtained. One reason is the tendency of the usual technician to routinize the determination and to report findings in stereotyped phrases that soon grow to mean nothing. Another reason is failure on the part of the physician to interpret results in the light of facts known about the patient. For example, a specific gravity of 1.010 means nothing if the patient has had two cups of coffee and several glasses of water two or three hours before voiding. On the other hand, a specific gravity of 1.010 in a patient who has taken little fluid during the preceding six hours may be of the utmost significance—particularly on a hot summer day. Such interpretation in the light of actual conditions under which the test is done is the basis of successful and worthwhile results.

Actually, it is my tendency to abhor any "routine" test, for this usually degenerates ultimately into a means of extracting money from the patient and little else. Tests done on every patient often make the record look good and accomplish nothing. On the other hand, a urinalysis, even when not seemingly indicated, may offer some surprising information.

I should warn you that this opinion is exactly contrary to the opinions of most medical leaders, but I believe firmly that the urinalysis should *not* be a routine procedure done in the office laboratory. Here is what influenced that decision:

We suspected that the procedure might be an undue financial burden without justification as a routine test. One time we checked 1,000 cases, selected at random from our files, noting wherein a routine urinalysis was done. In only one case was a totally unsuspected disease discovered, and the fact that the case was unsuspected was my fault. It was the case of a diabetic with a clear-cut familial history and I had simply failed to inquire about familial diabetes. In the 1,000 charts there were forty-odd cases of a positive urinalysis, but in each of these either historical or physical findings clearly indicated the need of a urinalysis.

For ease in figuring let us say that there were fifty people in the group that needed a urinalysis and in each case the indication was clear-cut according to the history and physical findings. In 950 cases there was no indication and nothing was gained. Since we charged $1.50 for a urinalysis, this represented a monetary loss of $1,425 to our patients, *without one single patient* benefiting therefrom.

After these findings we abandoned the "routine" urinalysis and used the test only under three circumstances:

1. When clear-cut suspicion of genitourinary disease or diabetes existed.

2. In the process of working up an obscure case.

3. To follow known disease.

This worked out very well. The final conclusion at which we arrived was this: The test is among the best and simplest we have, but it can become a ritual rather than a test if allowed to do so.

May I emphasize that the above view is diametrically opposed to the view held by most medical experts. One word of advice about this directed to the young physician: Let neither a dissenter such as myself nor the men wiser than I, who hold opposite opinions, sway you. Try an analysis of cases in your own practice and decide for yourself.

CHAPTER THREE

Special Urine Examinations

In more than 95 per cent of the cases the routine urinalysis as discussed in the last chapter will provide all the information needed regarding the urine. There are, however, a few tests of sterling value which are seldom used but which are of the utmost importance when needed. In this chapter they will be mentioned in the order of their importance as shown by the number of times they have been used.

KETONE BODIES

The ketone bodies (acetoacetic acid, beta-hydroxybutyric acid, and acetone) are not abnormal constituents of the human body. They are readily metabolized in some tissues and, in the process, are broken down into carbon dioxide and water.

We do not know what specific mechanism regulates the amount of ketone bodies in the blood, nor do we know what establishes how much shall be utilized. We do know that they are present in almost inverse ratio to carbohydrate utilization. When ample amounts of carbohydrate are present, only trivial amounts of the ketone substances appear in the blood.

On the other hand, when carbohydrates are not present (starvation) or are not used (diabetes), the amount of ketone bodies is increased. The compounds are produced in the liver as a part of the metabolism of fat. How the liver is stimulated to produce more, we do not know.

The presence of the ketone bodies as metabolites is actually desirable in certain circumstances. They represent an attempt to preserve nutrition through accessory methods when the main method is blocked. It is only the side effects of these compounds which are peculiarly dangerous.

Each is a relatively strong organic acid, and when the ketone bodies are present in quantity, profound disturbances of the acid-base mechanism result. Severe acidosis can usually be inferred to be present when these compounds appear in the urine.

Several authors make the statement that acidosis per se is seldom or ever fatal, which is probably quite true. It is the underlying mechanism which causes the acidosis that is deadly. For practical purposes this is begging the question. When carbohydrate utilization is so disturbed that ketone bodies appear in the urine, one either does something to secure return to normalcy or expects the possibility of a fatal outcome.

The most important concept to keep in mind is that the presence of ketone bodies in the urine indicates a metabolic disturbance of serious import. Carbohydrates are not being properly utilized and the remarkable compensatory mechanisms of the body are shifting to supply these breakdown products of fat for metabolic purposes. The acidosis that occurs is an "accident," for the fat breakdown products are strong organic acids.

True acidosis can occur with no relationship to the ketone bodies.

Technique

There are several tests for each of the ketone bodies. For practical purposes commercial Acetest tablets, which can be secured at any surgical supply house, are entirely adequate and consume less of the technician's valuable time. Complete directions for use are printed on every box.

Errors

There are no grave errors to which the test itself is subject. Most errors are in the field of interpretation.

Interpretation

Ketonuria does not always have the same significance in children that it does in adults. A convincing explanation is the following:

Children have a higher metabolic rate than adults, and the younger they are, the higher the metabolic rate tends to be. Quite naturally this high and sustained metabolic rate requires constancy of food intake, as well as a proportionately greater amount of food. As a matter of fact, the infantile digestive tract must work nearly full time to supply a sufficient quantity of nutrient material. For this reason even a minor interruption of carbohydrate intake may result in a rapid increase in circulating ketone bodies, with their consequent appearance in the urine. This may occur with much greater rapidity than is usually seen in the adult. It also resolves with greater speed.

In the field of pure speculation there is some reason to suppose that the so-called "absorption of toxins" in the severe infections of childhood may bear some relation to the utilization of the ketone bodies. Certainly this is only a part of the cause of symptoms, but this "acid intoxication" is worthy of thought.

Be that as it may, the appearance of ketone bodies in the urine has a practical significance almost in direct proportion to the age of the individual. Infants may show a trace of acetone when only a trivial interruption of carbohydrate metabolism occurs. When a positive test is obtained in adults, a much more serious metabolic disturbance is indicated.

Again, the important point to realize is that the disturbance is basically metabolic in nature and that pH changes are entirely secondary. For practical therapeutic control one must realize that no quantity of alkaline solutions injected or ingested will have more than supportive action unless utilizable carbohydrates are supplied.

Our own experience with ketonuria has been, in some respects, directly opposite to those reported in most of the literature. By far the greater number of cases showing a trace of acetone in the urine are the result of carbohydrate deprivation. Usually this is seen in small children who have not been eating due to an infection. Only rarely does one of our diabetic patients get far enough out of control to exhibit ketonuria.

Most often, in diabetic patients actual ketosis seems to occur when there is some deficiency in nutrition or insulin dosage, but this is readily explainable and usually even predictable. Most reports in the literature are from medical centers, while our figures come from a representative office practice. I assume other office practices would show comparative findings.

URINARY CHLORIDES

Normal urine contains from 10 to 15 Gm. of chlorides daily, mostly in the form of sodium chloride. This excretion is changed in many pathologic conditions, but alterations in urinary chlorides are not specific and the diagnostic value of testing for these changes approaches nil.

On the other hand, the test has a definite value in office practice. Many of our treatment routines call for a sharp reduction in salt intake, and often our patients do not achieve an adequate reduction even though they try. Testing the urinary chlorides is an excellent way to detect this.

Technique

First test the urine for albumin and cellular debris by heating. If a precipitate forms, filter and reboil the filtrate. If a second precipitate should form, filter once more. Next add two or three drops of strong nitric acid and then a few drops of 10 per cent silver nitrate. If chlorides are present in normal strength, a heavy, curdy precipitate of silver chloride is formed. If salt restriction has been adequate, the solution will become milky, but no precipitate will be thrown down.

Errors

Errors are practically unknown. Occasionally one may forget to acidify the urine with nitric acid and a precipitate of phosphates will form.

Interpretation

Since this is a simple and rough test, there are no entwining ramifications of interpretation. Either there is a heavy precipitate, which indicates a normal chloride intake, or a milky fluid, which points to major diminution of intake. Of course, there are all gradations between these points, but one may take the point of obvious precipitation as a good dividing line.

In regard to this test a word of caution about practical public relations is not out of line. Some patients look upon this as a snoopy way of checking up on them, and I can see their viewpoint. To avoid such feelings tell the patient when putting him on a low salt diet that there is a simple test to determine whether he has reduced his intake enough to be beneficial. Then when he returns he will be as interested as the physician in seeing what results have been achieved.

An intelligent patient can do this test for himself at home and thereby regulate his diet. Be sure to tell him not to do the test if a precipitate forms when the urine is first boiled.

BILE

On page 39 there is a brief discussion of the mechanism by which bile pigments enter the urine. For the sake of additional clarification and simplification this is another résumé seen from a slightly different aspect.

Bilirubin is normally formed by the breakdown of red blood cells. The reticulo-endothelial system throughout the body is capable of destroying erythrocytes which are degenerating or have escaped from the vascular system. When this is done, the reticulo-endothelial system acts to split off iron from the hemoglobin molecule. The remaining compound enters the blood stream as a bilirubin-protein complex. This complex probably represents adsorption of the bilirubin molecule by the plasma proteins. In the liver the hepatic cells act to split away the bilirubin from the protein molecule upon which it is absorbed.

If the factors be the correct ones, we may then say that there are two possible "causes" of bilirubin free in the blood stream:

1. Damage to liver cells which slows down their action upon the bilirubin-protein complex and results in accumulation of this complex in the blood.

2. Obstruction to the biliary secretion which causes resorption of the bilirubin and its accumulation in the blood.

It will be apparent immediately that obstruction of the biliary tract and disease of the liver cells are the two entities most likely to cause sufficient bilirubin in the blood to allow its excretion in the urine.

There is one other possible condition that rarely causes such excretion in urine, but it is almost never seen in office practice. In the event of severe intravascular hemolysis, the reticulo-endothelial system may feed so much bilirubin into the blood stream that the liver cells cannot excrete it as fast as received. This implies no disorder of function in the liver cells; they are simply outnumbered by reticulo-endothelial cells and cannot keep up.

Technique

Yellow, concentrated nitric acid is the only reagent needed. Place a clear glass bottle of nitric acid on the shelf and expose it to light. It will gradually turn yellow.

Pour a little urine on a piece of heavy filter paper (a blotter will do) and immediately apply one drop of the concentrated acid on the paper. Bile pigment is oxidized rapidly by the acid and the play of colors is characteristic. A green color is first seen, which may rapidly turn to a deep, shining violet—a positive test for bile.

Errors

Blue or red coloration is seen in the presence of indican or urobilin. The technician should be cautioned that it is not the presence of color but the particular colors green and violet that are significant. If one cannot be certain from the play of colors, follow this routine:

Mix 1 ml. of a solution of lime water with 5 ml. of urine and shake. Filter the resultant solution and apply a drop of acid to the filter paper upon which the precipitate is deposited. The precipitate is a bilirubin-calcium complex, while other substances that might have interfered have remained in solution.

Interpretation

The test is of most value in confirming suspected early cases of liver and bile duct disease. In the far-advanced case, when jaundice is present, one may safely assume that bile is present in the urine and the test therefore has no real value. Even in early obstructive disease of the bile ducts the test is usually greatly overshadowed by clinical findings.

In our own laboratory we have found that the principal value of the determination is in the confirmation of early hepatic disease which is suspected clinically. Often a hepatitis may be suspected several days before unequivocal clinical evidence appears. In such cases testing the urine for bile has distinct value.

One must always remember that the test offers no evidence as to whether there is obstruction of biliary outflow or damage to the cellular elements of the liver. This decision must be made on the basis of clinical evidencc or other tests.

HEMOGLOBIN

The glomerular filter is of such size that it will pass molecules with a molecular weight of less than about 70,000. The hemoglobin molecule has a molecular weight approaching 68,000. For this reason, when hemoglobin appears free in the blood stream, it is rapidly filtered into the urine.

The conditions then that may show hemoglobinuria are as follows:

1. Intravascular hemolysis
2. Trauma with resultant appearance of myohemoglobin
3. Bleeding and hemolysis in the urinary tract

In office practice all three are exceedingly rare. Most people with intravascular hemolysis or trauma of sufficient intensity to cause myohemoglobinuria are ill indeed and are hospital problems.

Chemical tests for hemoglobin in the urine will detect the pigment whether it be in or out of red blood cells. Rarely, such tests may be useful for determining hematuria, but the microscope is more reliable. Hemoglobinuria is readily detected.

Technique

Hematest tablets, which may be purchased through any surgical supply house and often through local drugstores, are the most satisfactory means of testing in the small laboratory.

Errors

Errors in the test are practically unknown. It has been reported in the literature that large quantities of vitamin C in the urine will interfere with tests for hemoglobin. I have not noticed this effect in working with a small laboratory, but occasionally it may be present.

Interpretation

In actual clinical work this test is not often used. Rarely, a patient with a moderately severe trauma may be brought to the office. One may wish to know whether the injury is severe enough to have released quantities of myohemoglobin. Testing the urine will answer that question, but to be certain one must do both a microscopic test to eliminate the presence of erythrocytes, and the chemical test.

Rarely one sees structures in the urine which appear to be red blood cells but it is difficult to be certain. In such cases the chemical test is very useful.

Hemoglobinuria may be found in several rare conditions that cause hemolysis of red cells in the vascular system: snake bite, severe malaria, mushroom poisoning, and the so-called "paroxysmal hemolytic" diseases. In none of these does diagnosis rest upon the finding.

BENCE JONES PROTEIN

Bence Jones proteins are a group of abnormal, or at least unusual, proteins of low molecular weight that appear in the urine most often in the presence of neoplastic blood disease. In rare instances the Bence Jones proteins have been found in the presence of other disease (and even in normal persons), but for practical purposes their presence points to neoplastic disease.

Multiple myeloma shows these substances in almost all cases. A small percentage of chronic leukemia cases may also be characterized by Bence Jones protein.

Much is conjectured but little is known about the source of these compounds. When, why, or where they are formed has not been clearly proved. The assumption that they are made by neoplastic cells because of changes in cell metabolism is tempting but not subject to proof. Because of this lack of knowledge it is not possible to offer exact interpretation when they are found. All our interpretative efforts must be based on empiric observation.

Technique

Bence Jones proteins are not often suspected but are most often discovered while doing a routine urinalysis. When the urine is slightly acidified and heated during performance of the test for albumin, one notices the appearance of a precipitate almost immediately upon application of heat.

When this is apparent place 5 to 10 ml. of urine in a test tube, put a laboratory thermometer in the tube so that the bulb is in the urine, and place the test tube in the water bath. If Bence Jones protein is present a precipitate will begin to form at a point little above body temperature, 40 to 45° C.

By the time the temperature is in the vicinity of 60° C., the precipitate will have reached maximum density and will begin to dissolve as the temperature approaches boiling. By 90° C. most of the precipitate will have re-entered the solution. These changes are repeated in reverse as the urine cools.

Errors

The most frequent error is the confusing of Bence Jones proteins with albumin. There are two readily appreciable differences. Albumin requires a much higher temperature for coagulation and, once having formed a coagulum, only slowly passes back into solution.

If there is doubt, strong nitric acid should be added to a 5 ml. portion of the urine. A precipitate will form if Bence Jones protein is present. It will dissolve upon boiling and reappear upon cooling the specimen.

Should albumin be present also, it will interfere with these tests. A filter should be prepared and heated by filtering a small sample of boiling water. The urine sample should then be brought to a boil and filtered in the hot filter. This will remove the albumin but not the Bence Jones protein.

Interpretation

For many years the presence of Bence Jones proteins was taken as a specific indicator of multiple myeloma. It has been found, however, in many diseases. For practical purposes of office diagnosis you may assume that chronic leukemia or multiple myeloma is present when the Bence Jones proteins are detected. The test is not diagnostic but only indicative. When positive, it is imperative that these two diseases be ruled out by careful clinical examination.

DIAZO REACTION

The aged and venerable diazo reaction has fallen into disrepute and is seldom used. This is probably because we know so little about it. Nonetheless, in an occasional case it may be of the utmost value.

Technique

The standard diazo reagent of Ehrlich (which is the same as that used for the van den Bergh test) may be made as follows:

Solution 1

Sulfanilic acid	1.0
Concentrated HCl	10.0
Water	200.0

Solution 2

Sodium nitrite	0.5
Water	100.0

These solutions should be stored in separate bottles, and the final reagent, which is a combination of the two, made up for the test.

Place 5 ml. of solution 1 and one drop of solution 2 in a test tube and add 5 ml. of urine. Mix by inverting and then add 1 ml. of strong ammonia solution so that this overlays the mixture of urine and reagent. A purple ring will form at the area of contact if the test is positive.

Next shake the tube well and notice the color imparted to the foam. Yellow or orange foam may occur but means nothing. Only when the foam is red, ranging from a deep crimson to a light pink, is the test positive.

Errors

The most frequent error is to misinterpret, as positive, tests which show colored foam that is not red or pink. Any other color means nothing.

Bile in the urine will interfere with the test but is very seldom seen in conditions in which the diazo reaction is used.

Indications

The indications for the diazo reaction are as follows:

1. Diagnosis of measles
2. Prognosis in pulmonary tuberculosis
3. Typhoid fever

Interpretation

Measles may occasionally be difficult to diagnose, particularly after immune globin has been given. Allergic rashes sometimes are confusing, and, rarely, German measles may be hard to differentiate.

The diazo reaction is usually positive about the time the rash appears and remains positive for three to five days. Since it does not occur in the other conditions mentioned and since it is easy to perform the test, it may be useful in diagnosis.

In the diagnosis of tuberculosis the diazo reaction has no significance whatever. When it becomes positive and remains consistently so, a serious prognosis is indicated. Actually, the utility of the reaction is slight in office practice, but it can sometimes be used to help form a prognosis in an occasional case.

The diazo reaction becomes positive about the end of the first week in typhoid fever and remains so for about two weeks. It is not positive in the other enteric fevers, particularly when the urine is diluted 1:20 or 1:30 with water before running the test.

Comment

The diazo reaction is one of the older tests that is seldom used today. Even so, it is a handy test to remember and will sometimes be of great help in clearing up a puzzling case. In our own laboratory it has been particularly useful in the diagnosis of early and questionable cases of measles.

BROMIDES

Not infrequently patients take large quantities of bromide-containing nostrums over a period of several months. Occasionally one may be unable to get a clear history and may wish to know whether or not bromides are being excreted in the urine.

Use dilute sulfuric acid to acidify 5 ml. of the urine in a test tube and then add three or four drops of fuming nitric acid and 2 ml. of chloroform. If bromides are present, the chloroform, which settles to the bottom of the test tube, assumes a dull yellow color.

PHENOL

Large quantities of phenol, even a sufficient amount to cause severe toxic reactions, may be absorbed from ointments applied to abraded or burned surfaces. If this is a possibility, test the urine as follows:

Add hydrochloric acid to a sample of the urine until it becomes highly acid. Distill several milliliters into a test tube and add 10 per cent ferric chloride, drop by drop. A deep blue color indicates the presence of phenol.

CHAPTER FOUR

Kidney Function Tests

The kidney function tests are among the most practical tests available to us. They indicate not only whether or not the kidney is damaged, but also the approximate extent.

In interpreting each of the tests, one fact must be kept in mind: no function is a static thing related only to the amount of organic damage sustained by the functioning organ. Instead, it is a dynamic equilibrium made up of thousands of forces. As such, it may change profoundly from week to week and from day to day. The function tests measure depression of function from a theoretical ideal and from this is inferred the degree of impairment.

Generally the tests are accurate enough to allow good assessment of the amount of damage that has occurred, but not always.

It is possible to divide the kidney function tests into three groups. Each group is then considered to test a specific part of the nephron: the glomerulus, the proximal convoluted tubule, and the distal tubule. While it seems that this would be a technicality in clinical practice, it is actually helpful. Our knowledge of kidney disease is steadily increasing, and with each step forward, functional tests of the different areas of the nephron become of increasing value. In this chapter we will consider two tests for each of the groups: glomerular function, proximal tubule function, and distal tubule function.

ADDIS COUNT

The Addis count is not directly a measure of kidney function. It is included among the function tests because the final inferences to be drawn are essentially the same as those obtained from the true function tests.

Any bleeding from the urinary tract can be measured quantitatively by the count of erythrocytes in a twelve- to twenty-four-hour specimen. In actual usage the Addis procedure finds its principal indication in conditions wherein the red cells escape from damaged glomeruli.

In the normal person red cells escape into the urine constantly. A twelve-hour urine specimen from healthy adults will contain 500,000 to one million erythrocytes. Just why these cells escape is a matter of conjecture. Perhaps localized damage to a few glomeruli allows the constant loss of cells. Since children normally show a smaller loss of red blood cells than adults do, this local damage theory is a distinct possibility.

It would seem probable from the results of pathologic studies that most cells are lost from the glomeruli. In acute inflammatory disease involving the tubules one might expect a loss of some blood cells through diapedesis and this undoubtedly occurs, but this is not of principal clinical importance.

In acute glomerulonephritis, inflammatory changes in the glomeruli result in constant loss of erythrocytes through the damaged membranes. This loss is roughly proportionate to two things: the number of glomeruli involved and the intensity of the involvement.

When glomerulonephritis becomes chronic a more exact relationship exists, for the two possible variables both point in the same direction. Constant hematuria with stable or slightly increasing Addis counts point to severe glomerular damage and offer a bad prognosis. Bursts of hematuria at frequent intervals point to further episodes of damage and also indicate a bad prognosis.

Cases of vascular hypertension with slowly increasing Addis counts usually indicate an approaching termination because of renal damage and/or generalized vascular degeneration.

Technique

Actual counting of the cells is a relatively simple laboratory procedure. The difficulty comes in collection of a proper specimen. It is usually best to give the patient exact written directions for the collection of urine to be followed at home.

Usually a twelve-hour specimen collected during the night is ample, although some authorities insist that twenty-four-hour samples be used. Begin by furnishing the patient a wide-mouthed one-liter jar. Actually we get one-gallon pickle jars from local restaurants. Before giving it to him, wash the jar thoroughly with soap and water, rinse, and dry. Then pour about 100 ml. of 10 per cent formaldehyde solution in the jar and shake thoroughly. Empty the jar and put the lid on tightly at once. Enough formaldehyde will cling to the glass walls to act as a preservative.

In the case of a female patient, instruct her in the technique of obtaining an uncontaminated specimen as detailed on page 38.

At exactly 7:30 P.M. the patient is to urinate and empty the bladder completely. This urine is not to be saved. Then all urine passed from this time throughout the night is to be passed directly into the prepared bottle. At 7:30 A.M., twelve hours after the test began, the patient is to empty the bladder completely, passing the urine into the jar. The jar should then be capped and brought to the office.

In the office the jar is gently inverted a number of times to mix the contents, and exactly 10 ml. of urine are transferred by means of a pipette to a centrifuge tube. This is thoroughly spun down, taking at least three minutes, preferably five minutes, in the centrifuge. While this is being done, measure the total volume of urine in the specimen jar. Of course, add 10 ml. to the total.

Take the test tube from the centrifuge, and, using a pipette, remove 9 ml. of the supernatant fluid so that there remains in the centrifuge tube 1 ml. of urine containing the sediment from 10 ml.

Add to this sediment 4 ml. of normal saline and mix thoroughly by repeated but gentle inversion. Use a blood cell pipette (either white or red) to fill a standard counting chamber with the resulting solution. Count all of the red cells in each of the nine big squares, i.e., the entire enclosed ruled area of the counting chamber. Do this at least a half dozen times and average the results.

This average number of red cells per counting chamber is the key to the test. Calculate as follows:

Let x = total of red blood cells in the specimen.

Let n = average number of red blood cells per chamber.

Let v = total urine volume in milliliters.

Then: $x = n \times 20 \times v$

Errors

The Addis count is not at all accurate. For one thing, repeated measurements of small quantities cannot be done accurately in the office laboratory. One, however, seeks an estimate, not a determination of research accuracy. This inherent error in the test can be discarded, but not forgotten, for practical purposes.

The most frequent gross error is in the collection of the specimen. Patients must be carefully instructed in the methods of collection and will do better if given explicit written schedules. I have found it valuable to have the patient keep notes on the exact time of urination and whether it was discarded or saved. Usually he is asked to note on our instruction sheet exactly what he did.

Office errors in the count are simply due to carelessness. Most often mathematical mistakes creep in. You would be surprised at the number of doctors and medical personnel who multiply seven by three and get sixteen.

Interpretation

In ordinary office practice the Addis count has little utility unless you are relatively certain that you are dealing with glomerulonephritis or hypertensive vascular disease. Other entities are more easily followed using different procedures.

When glomerulonephritis or hypertensive disease is present you may assume that the red blood cells found in the urine occur as a result of glomerular damage. Therefore, the Addis count gives a fairly accurate picture of glomerular condition. A serious error often committed is to assume further that the count gives an estimate of the amount of irreversible damage. Such is not so. The reparative processes of the human body are usually far greater than even doctors of wide experience believe them to be. Even a marked rise in the Addis count may disappear completely, and repeated tests as time goes on may show no evidence of kidney disease.

A single Addis count, no matter what the result, has little use. Obvious hematuria will be picked up by other methods and a single increased Addis count is difficult to interpret. The count is of inestimable value in following a case of chronic nephritis or hypertensive vascular disease.

Normal values range from one-half to one million erythrocytes per twelve hours. A slight increase to 1.2 million or so has no clinical significance. Actual interpretation is more easily illustrated by example. This is a typical clinical record, much abridged:

June, 1946. The patient is a 46-year-old man, seemingly in good health. Diagnosis for the last four years; chronic nephritis. Urine shows a trace of albumin. No casts. Blood pressure, 168/92, nonprotein nitrogen, 26 mg. per cent, Addis count 1.35 million. Clinically negative.

January, 1947. "Just don't feel good." No essential change in clinical findings. Addis count, 1.6 million. (Note: *This is within the range of possible error of the test. Not particularly significant.*)

September, 1947. "Feel some better but no pep." Albuminuria, 1 plus. Addis count, 2.24 million. (Note: *This is significant. Steady rise indicates a bad prognosis but is not sufficiently certain to warrant discussion with patient.*)

January, 1948. "Feel terrible." Some puffiness around eyes. Albuminuria, 1 plus; hyaline casts. Blood pressure, 170/100. Addis count, 1.2 million. (Note: *Something is wrong here. In case of doubt, believe the patient, not the test. Count rechecked. Was 3.2 million and technician accidentally wrote 1.2 million.*)

February, 1948. Patient looks very ill but seems cheerful about the whole thing. Albumin, 2 plus; Addis count, 5.42 million. Prognosis now definitely bad. Had frank discussion with patient.

April, 1948. "Well, Doc, I came in to die." Patient definitely approaching terminal stage. Albumin, 1 plus; Addis count, 10.3 million. Obvious clinical signs. Nonprotein nitrogen, 54 mg. per cent.

May, 1948. Patient died.

You cannot help but notice that the Addis count was the most reliable single test used in this case. It was prognostically significant long before other tests became so and before clinical evidence was available.

Of course, it does not always work out this way, and no doctor is justified in telling a patient of his approaching dissolution on the basis of Addis counts alone. On the other hand, this is the best test we have with which to follow such patients.

I usually explain to my patients somewhat as follows: "This test is the best test we have to show whether or not a patient is going to get well, but it is not perfect. We see some of these cases that look almost hopeless from the standpoint of the test but the patients recover completely."*

UREA CLEARANCE

Urea clearance is another test that, in essentiality, measures glomerular function. Urea is one of the three principal end products of protein metabolism, the other two being carbon dioxide and water. Insofar as we know, it is purely a waste product and has no function. It freely passes the glomerular membranes.

Urea is extremely soluble in water as much as 100 grams entering into solution in 100 ml. of water. Such high solubility makes it inevitable that urea will, if possible, follow water; i.e., when water is resorbed it will "go along" in solution if cellular membranes permit. Apparently they permit to some degree. Approximately 40 per cent of the urea which escapes through the glomeruli re-enters the blood stream as the water is absorbed in the tubules.

Since over 90 per cent of the water is resorbed and is accompanied by only 40 per cent of the urea, there must be some kind of inefficient barrier to the transport of urea through the renal cells. Of course, this is exactly what we would expect from the cell membranes. The surprising thing is how great the inefficiency of the barrier is.

The actual resorption rate of urea does not stay entirely constant. It varies greatly with the rate of urine formation and with other complex chemical functions. For practical purposes it may be assumed to be a constant 40 per cent when the rate of urine formation is greater than 2 ml. per minute.

The concept of "clearance" is not difficult to understand, but it implies something that just is not true. For example, if the blood contains 10 mg. of urea per milliliter and the kidneys excrete 100 mg. of urea per minute, then the kidneys are said to "clear" 10 ml. of blood per minute, i.e., all urea in 10 ml. of blood per minute represents the glomerular flow. This is based on the interesting concept that all fluid elements are removed from the blood as they pass through the glomerular tuft and the dry cells are left to roll down the vessels enclosed in a cloud of protein "dust," which accompanies them until some fluid is resorbed. (I admit this is a bit overstated.)

Actually, when we speak of clearance we mean not how much blood *is* cleared of urea, but how much, theoretically, could be if complete filtration occurred.

Impairment of glomerular filtration is accurately reflected by the clearance rate. This

*I hope you will pardon a slight but perhaps valuable digression here. I learned the trick of "we see some of these cases" from a very fine old physician. He never allowed himself to be badgered into giving an exact prognosis unless he could do so with certainty. Instead, he would give the prognosis he thought true and then *always* add, "But we see some of these cases . . ." and go on from there. It is a good trick to remember. By using it you can be truthful and satisfy patients without getting yourself in the position of having made a false prediction.

is a particularly useful test in chronic nephritis.

Technique

Have the patient report to the laboratory at 8:50 A.M., after having eaten a full breakfast but no coffee. Upon arising he should drink two large glasses of water and another two glasses should be taken with breakfast. As soon as he arrives at the office another glass of water should be given.

At exactly 9:00 have the patient void, being certain to empty the bladder completely. At this time, withdraw 5 ml. of venous blood and place it gently in a clean oxylated tube. Have the patient drink another glass of water and then instruct him to report back to the office at 9:45 A.M. Caution the patient specifically not to urinate in the ensuing time. Also instruct him to have no coffee or coke, and that in the unlikely event he should want either, he may have another glass of water. At exactly 10 o'clock have the patient empty his bladder and save the entire specimen. He is then finished with his part of the test.

First determine the blood urea. It is much more simple to determine the blood urea nitrogen which, of course, bears an exact relationship to urea. One then checks urea nitrogen of urine and uses the urea nitrogen figures in lieu of the total urea concentration.

In discussing chemical determinations throughout this book, I have assumed that the practitioner either owns or is willing to purchase a small photoelectric colorimeter. Total cost for the colorimeter, glassware, and reagents is less than $300, and that much will be saved in a few months.

A complete book of instructions is furnished with each instrument, so it would be needless duplication to include in this book the same instructions to be found in the colorimeter manual.

Do the blood urea nitrogen exactly as instructed.

Dilute a sample of the urine with ten times its volume of physiologic saline solution and do the same test. If the concentration is still too great to get a reading, take 1 ml. of the final solution (after Nessler's reagent has been added and just before the solution is to be read in the colorimeter) and add it to 10 ml. of physiologic saline. Read this solution in the colorimeter and multiply the result by 100.

To calculate the clearance, first make sure that the total specimen voided during the one-hour period is more than 120 ml. If urine formation is less than this, profound inaccuracies will be found. While it is possible to calculate clearance by using special formulas when the volume is less than 120 ml., we have usually found it easier and much more reliable to repeat the test.

If total excretion is more than 120 ml., calculate the clearance like this:

U = urine urea nitrogen expressed in milligrams per 100 ml. (300)

B = blood urea nitrogen expressed in milligrams per 100 ml. (10)

V = volume flow expressed in milliliters per minute. (2)

$$\text{Clearance} = \frac{U \times V}{B} =$$

$$\frac{300 \times 2}{10} = \frac{600}{10} = 60$$

Normal values for young and middle-aged adults may be taken as anything above 50. For persons over 65 years, any figure above 40 should probably be taken as normal.

Calculated in children the test is not so accurate as it is in adults. In office practice it is only rarely that we see a child who needs such determinations. If the physician will remember that the inherent error of the test is greater in children, he will find it possible to use the methods herein detailed with reasonably accurate results.

Many physicians prefer to express the final values obtained as per cent of normal. If the urine formation is over 2 ml. per minute, the average clearance is taken as 75 ml. per minute and the actual figure resulting from the test expressed in terms of its percentage relationship to 75. If, for example, the figure obtained from the calculation is 50, then urea clearance is 66.66 per cent.

Errors

The main errors to which the test is subject are those common to all exacting chemical determinations. Probably the most frequent point of difficulty is in making the protein-free blood filtrate. Precipitation must be complete, and unless the reagents are of proper strength and the procedures followed with great exactitude, errors may occur.

When properly done, even considering the limitations of the average office laboratory, the chemical determinations are probably accurate within ± 2 per cent.

Interpretation

Urea clearance is an extremely sensitive test of glomerular filtration rate. If anything, it is too sensitive. Minor kidney insults, even those resulting only in temporary cloudy swelling of the renal cells, can profoundly alter urea clearance. For that reason only gross or prolonged changes can be taken to be of major significance.

Ordinarily any adult who has a clearance of 50 or over may be taken as being within normal range. Depressions to 20 or less are not unknown in severe glomerulonephritis and the depression seems to parallel closely the degree of functional impairment but *not* the degree of permanent organic impairment.

Older people usually have somewhat less clearance. A minimum of 40 may be considered normal in people 65 years or more.

One must remember that when we speak of impairment we mean specifically diminution of the glomerular function.

Comment

The urea clearance test is an excellent one and may be of the greatest utility in establishing the status of glomerular disease or in following its course. Despite this, it is not often indicated in the office laboratory. The average busy practice will not use the procedure more than twenty-five to fifty times a year.

It is important to realize that there is no indication for such a procedure in the aged and obviously terminal nephritic patient. It is mainly of use to establish glomerular function in younger individuals in whom there is some hope for prolongation of life and comfort.

PHENOLSULFONPHTHALEIN TEST

Phenolsulfonphthalein is a purple dye in alkaline solutions and colorless in acid solutions. For this reason it has been used for an indicator in some titrations. When injected into the body, either intravenously or intramuscularly, it is an inert chemical.

When injected intramuscularly it is rapidly absorbed into the blood stream. A portion of the dye (perhaps 10 to 20 per cent) is removed from the circulation by the liver. The rest is excreted by the kidneys. This excretory function is an active process, the cells of the proximal tubules selectively picking the chemical out of the blood stream and excreting it into the lumen of the tubule.

Since phenolsulfonphthalein is not a large molecule, there has been, for some years, a problem as to why only small amounts pass the glomerular filter. Recent work has indicated that the dye, while in the blood stream, is loosely linked to the serum albumin. The linkage is strong enough to prevent filtration at the glomerulus.

The foregoing explanation makes it perfectly clear why the test may be considered almost exclusively a measure of proximal tubule function. It is the best, least expensive, and easiest test we have to delineate this function.

Technique

No special preparation of the patient is needed, although for some years we have asked the patient to report to the clinic at 9 A.M. without breakfast. This is probably an excellent example of a doctor following custom whether there is reason for it or not.

When the patient arrives for the test instruct him to drink two large glasses of water. Immediately thereafter, inject intravenously 1 ml. of a standard solution of phenolsulfonphthalein containing 6.0 mg. The ampules on the market contain slightly more than 1 ml. To be precise, it is well to use a tuberculin syringe and measure as nearly 1 ml. as is possible.

One caution is in order: on a hot, humid day it may be necessary to have the patient drink four or five glasses of water before starting the test and then one glass every fifteen minutes.

At fifteen-minute intervals following the injection have the patient urinate into a specimen bottle; treat the urine as instructed in the booklet issued with the photocolorimeter. Each fifteen-minute specimen should be diluted to the full 1,000 ml. and tested for percentage of dye excreted.

At the end of one hour, four specimens should have been secured. Now give the patient another glass of water to drink, after which instruct him to wait. Exactly two hours after injection of the dye have him once again empty the bladder. The specimen should then be tested.

We report the results on a little homemade, mimeographed slip like this:

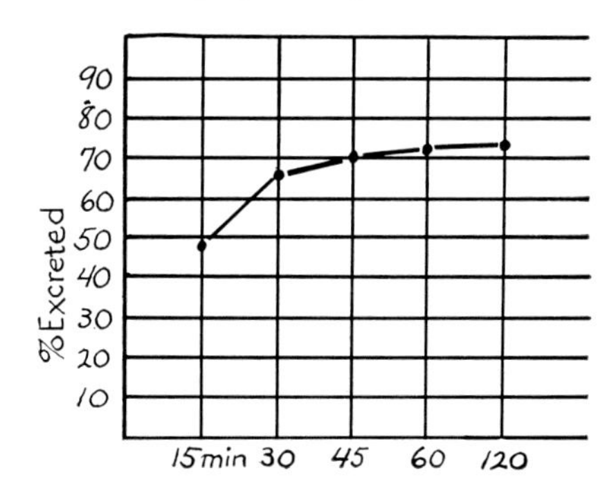

After becoming familiar with this method of reporting, the physician can merely glance at the shape and height of the curve and obtain a total view of the meaning of the test. Incidentally, obvious errors in technique show up readily, too.

Errors

Perhaps the most frequent error is to inject the entire content of an ampule and thereby give too much dye. This, of course, gives a spuriously high result.

Next in the frequency is the error of attempting to test a patient who is producing too little urine for accurate determination. At least one glass of water must be taken before the test is begun. On a hot day three or four are often needed. I do not like to count the test as adequate unless at least 20 ml. of urine are voided for each fifteen-minute period.

Another error that completely invalidates the test is to run it in the presence of severe circulatory changes. When the blood is moving sluggishly past the tubule cells, they have no chance to pick up the dye and excrete it at normal rate. It just is not there for them. Under such circumstances a normal kidney may seem to be greatly impaired when tested. Always know the circulatory status before testing a patient.

Interpretation

There are several conditions that may enter into interpretation which have little or nothing to do with the condition of cells in the proximal tubules. One of them is the condition of the circulation as mentioned under errors.

Another, which is much less apparent clinically, is the condition of the liver. Normally the liver removes a portion of the dye from the blood stream. When liver cells are damaged they do not remove dye and the kidneys have a proportionately greater amount on which to work. Consequently there is a renal excretion greater than would be expected. A good example of this is the increased excretion of phenolsulfonphthalein in people with cirrhosis. Those who have permanently depressed function from hepatitis also show this.

Still another extraneous condition affecting the excretion of phenosulfonphthalein is the level of blood proteins. Injection of 6 mg. of the dye binds most molecules to protein molecules in the blood. Apparently in normal blood there are not enough "exposed linkage sites" to bind all of the dye. The dye not bound to protein is readily filtered out by the glomerulus.

When blood proteins are lowered (as in severe nephrosis) there are even fewer linkage sites available, and an increasing amount of dye is filtered out. This, of course, increases the concentration of phenolsulfonphthalein in the urine and gives false high values for the test.

Actually these are rare circumstances which might be seen in the average office once every four or five years. They are mentioned only because of the confusion that may arise when such a case appears. They should be retained in the recesses of one's mind.

Now let us turn our attention to the normal graphs of excretion and their abnormal changes. A perfectly normal result looks like this:

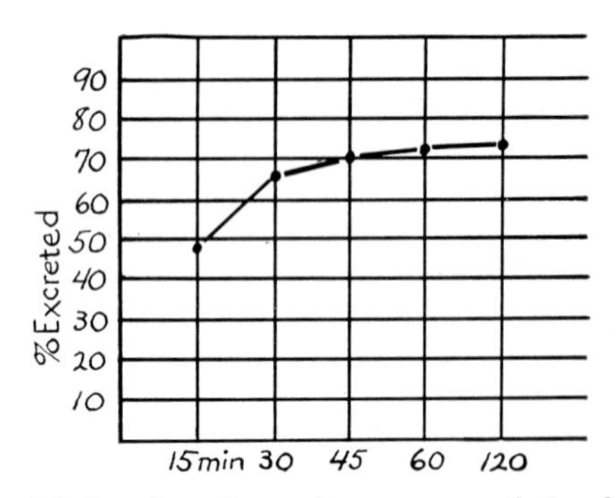

Notice that about 48 per cent of the dye is excreted in the first fifteen minutes and that successively smaller portions are excreted during each time period thereafter. In mild insufficiency of the proximal tubule cells the peak excretion usually shifts to the second period and the total output is less. The chart looks like this:

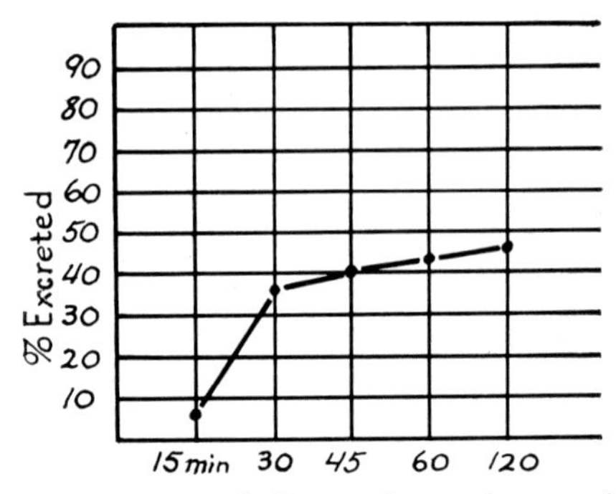

In severe renal disease the peak excretion shifts to the third period and the final total is much lowered. The chart looks like this:

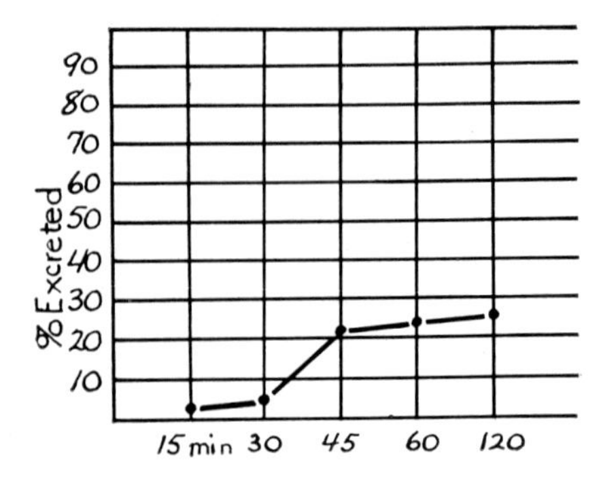

When there is general impairment of kidney function due to infection where in actual organic damage is evanescent, there are often signs of a "slow-down" without actual decrease in total function. In such a case the amount excreted in two hours is normal but the peak excretion is delayed. The graph looks like this:

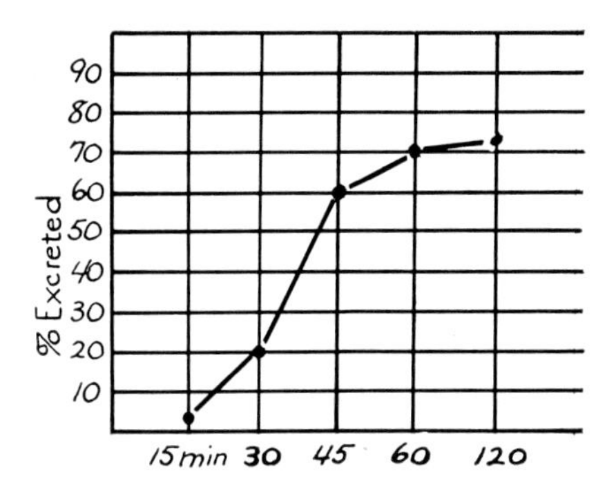

In cases exhibiting slowed circulation or extensive loss of functional kidney tissue, the curve remains normal in shape but the total excretion is lessened. Such a chart looks like this:

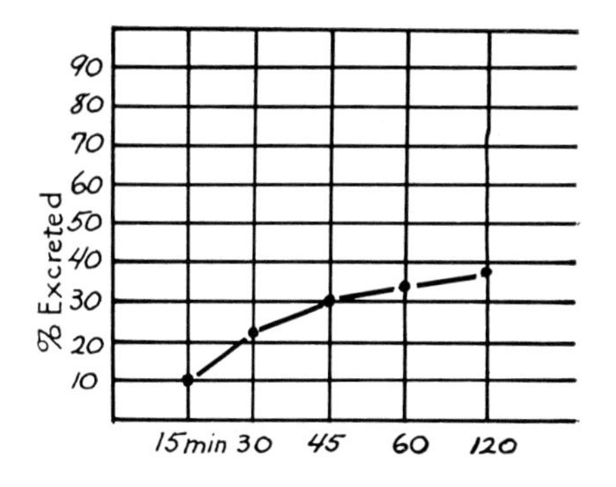

I know you will agree with me that this makes a nice, simple way to diagnose kidney disease. Other than the fact that it will not work, it is nearly perfect.

Seriously, the phenolsulfonphthalein test is one of the best tests we have to delineate renal function so long as we realize the sharp limitations to which it is subject. Probably the most important restriction is the one least often taken into account by the physician. It is this:

The test reflects accurately the functional state of the proximal tubule cells, but this functional state by no means parallels organic changes. Take a mechanical example: Suppose we have a new automobile with a perfect engine except that it is badly out of time. The car will not run. The "PSP test" on such a car would indicate a badly damaged motor when, as a matter of fact, no damage at all exists. All that is needed is an adjustment of the timing mechanism.

Now suppose we have an old engine with the bearings just about worn out, yet not so far impaired but that it runs perfectly. The "PSP test" on such an engine might show only the limitations of function expected with age, whereas, in actuality, the engine is about ready to fall apart.

Since organic damage and functional damage usually bear some direct relationship, we seldom see such gross deviations in practice. But one must remember that the phenolsulfonphthalein test tells only the functional part of the story.

One concept of glomerulonephritis which has been very useful to me, although by no means completely accurate scientifically, is the idea of disease "descending the nephron." If it is possible to conceive the process as one which begins in the glomerulus and gradually spreads distalward, the various tests become of greater utility. The first signs are those to be expected from attack upon the glomerulus. Often the phenolsulfonphthalein is not greatly helpful in this early stage.

As the process spreads to the proximal tubules, the phenolsulfonphthalein test becomes positive and, finally, when the distal tubule is attacked, specific gravity tests become positive. Again, this is not proved scientifically. It does work out clinically.

RADIOLOGIC TESTS

While radiology is seldom used solely to measure renal function, it may be valuable in such measurements. Under ordinary circumstances it is not wise to attempt intravenous radiography in patients with acute nephritic infections or severely damaged kidneys. However, diagnosis by x-ray examination is often made on patients with minor or chronic damage.

Of the two common substances used in intravenous urography, one, Neo-Ipax, is excreted almost entirely by glomerular filtration. The other, Diodrast, is excreted by tubular secretion. A much more complete discussion of these drugs will be found in the x-ray section of this book.

Three factors enter into the rate of excretion. Concentration of the drug, which varies with the size of the patient and the dose, is largely under the control of the physician. The speed of renal blood flow can be estimated from an evaluation of the general circulation. The last factor, functional condition of the kidney cells, can be determined from results of the test.

The intensity of the renal shadow depends entirely upon the amount of drug in the renal pelvis. Because of the vast difference in configuration of the kidney pelvis in individuals and even between opposite kidneys in the same individual, no precise scientific measurements of shadow density are possible.

Because of these things the test does not meet the criterion of a true scientific determination. Be that as it may, a great deal of valuable information can be obtained from certain practical observations.

Technique

The complete technique for intravenous urography will be found beginning on page 293.

Errors

Many of the technical errors to which the procedure is subject are discussed in the section mentioned above. One common error in interpretation happens so frequently that it should be mentioned here.

To do good excretory urography with adequate visualization it is necessary to compress the ureters with abdominal pads. When properly applied the pads allow only minute quantities of the dye to escape and pass into the bladder. Occasionally a pad will slip out of place and allow the dye and urine in one kidney pelvis to run into the bladder. When this happens one kidney will show a great deal more radiopacity than the other. One immediately assumes that the kidney exhibiting the poor shadow is not functioning well. *Be sure* to examine the bladder shadow before making such an assumption. If the bladder is full of radiopaque substance, one of the pads has slipped and the test is worthless.

Interpretation

Normal kidneys show good concentration of the radiopaque material in the pelvis within five minutes after injection. At this stage the shadows may not be of equal density, but no significance can be attached to minor inequalities.

If neither kidney shows more than a trace of dye after five minutes, one should think first of circulatory impairment, although this fact should have been known long before any urographic procedure was attempted. The second possibility is that of severely damaged kidneys, but this, too, should have been known without using the x-ray.

If concentration at five minutes seems considerably less than one would normally expect, one should make arrangements to extend the period of the test, taking films at thirty minutes, one hour, and even at two hours, if necessary. A characteristic of moderate nephron damage is that the dye appears much more slowly than normal but does appear. Ultimately, using compression of the ureter, good concentration is obtained.

The time taken to secure concentration of the radiopaque substance is a rough measure of the degree of functional kidney impairment. Normal kidneys show good concentration within fifteen to twenty-five minutes. Mild functional impairment is so close to this that no diagnostic determinations are possible.

Good concentration at forty-five minutes to one hour indicates moderate impairment, and good concentration delayed as much as two hours is indicative of severely limited function. Rarely, the drug is eliminated so slowly that several days elapse before the blood is cleared. In such cases x-ray should never be used.

When a single kidney fails to eliminate the opaque substance, one should think first of some obstruction to the outflow tract with loss of kidney function from back pressure. This is a much more frequent happening than many of us realize. It is seen particularly often in elderly persons.

So far as I know there is no such thing as a unilateral glomerulonephritis or hypertensive arteriolar disease involving a single kidney. There are cases, however, wherein one kidney seems to suffer more functional impairment than the other.

Such cases show marked disparity in concentration of radiopaque substances in the two kidney pelves. A difference at five minutes is of little significance, but a disparity easily seen in the twenty- to twenty-five-minute film strongly indicates functional damage in the kidney showing poor excretory powers. Remember always that it is strongly indicative but not proof-positive. Only rarely are all the nephrons in both kidneys called into function. We do not know the mechanism that chooses which units will function and which will not. Certainly it is possible that pure chance might dictate during any single five- or ten-minute period the functioning of one kidney to a greater extent than the other.

Time should serve to clear up the question. In our own practice we tend to take the result of one radiologic examination as indicative but not as positive.

CONCENTRATION AND DILUTION

The fluid that passes from the glomeruli is exactly the same as the intravascular fluid, with two exceptions. Cells are held back by the filter as are the larger protein molecules. Apparently anything with a molecular weight of less than 70,000 freely passes through. This means that only plasma proteins and cellular elements are retained. Otherwise the fluid filtered out is exactly the same as that in the vessels. The chloride, sugar, urea, and other chemicals are found in the same concentration as in the blood.

The specific gravity of blood without its cells and proteins is 1.010. Quite naturally we would expect the glomerular filtrate to have the same specific gravity. It does. As the fluid passes down the tubules, passive diffusion of substances may change the specific gravity slightly so that glomerular filtrate excreted, subject only to the processes of diffusion, has a specific gravity ranging from 1.008 to 1.012.

To give the fluid either a higher or lower specific gravity requires that substances be actively put in or taken out of the filtrate or that water be added or removed. The function of the tubule cells is to do just that. Certain substances are added to the filtrate (excretion) and certain substances are removed (resorption). Water is actively resorbed but, so far as we know, the tubule cells are not able to put water into the filtrate.

It takes active work to do these various things. Just as a sick man finds it difficult or impossible to do exhausting work, so a sick tubular cell cannot work well. It is upon this apparent fact that the concentration and dilution tests are based.

We simply put the cells in position where they have to do much work and see if they do it. If not, we assume they are sick or damaged.

The main increase in the specific gravity occurs in the distal tubule where water is resorbed actively, thereby "dehydrating" the filtrate and increasing its content of solids. If the cells of the distal tubule are not able to work properly, there is no possibility of concentrating the urine to a great degree.

Technique

Many methods have been proposed for the test. We have adopted a greatly simplified method designed to give all essential information in a twenty-four-hour period. Give the patient a complete explanation of the purposes of the test and caution him to take fluid of any kind only as directed. For the morning of the first day instruct him to take a big glass of water (an iced tea glass) at 9 A.M. and at each hour thereafter until 2 o'clock in the afternoon. In the hot summertime, we sometimes ask that the patient take such a glassful every thirty minutes.

Instruct the patient to urinate as necessary and to discard the urine. Request that between 2 and 3 o'clock in the afternoon he pass a specimen into a four-ounce bottle (wide-mouthed) which is given to him for this purpose. This specimen is to be tightly corked and saved.

Further instruct the patient that after 3 o'clock in the afternoon no fluids of any kind are to be taken until the test is completed the next morning. Caution him especially about soups and other liquids with meals. The next morning he is to urinate upon rising and discard the urine, after which no fluids of any kind are to be taken until he is able to urinate again. Usually this is possible by 9 o'clock in the morning. Inform the patient that as soon as a specimen bottle is filled he may drink as much fluid as he wants.

The two bottles are to be brought to the office and tested for specific gravity.

Errors

The test is so simple that errors in making the determinations are practically unknown. Occasionally a patient will take some fluid during the concentration test but this is not a frequent happening. We have all seen patients who seem mentally incapable of appreciating the purposes of such a test and will try to "sneak by" without fulfilling the conditions.

Years of increasing experience teach us to ignore such a test result and to use clinical findings as the basis for further treatment.

In extremely cold weather the diuresis induced in the first part of the test may continue for twenty-four hours or more. When such seems possible, do the concentration test first and the dilution test the following day.

Interpretation

The dilute urine should show a specific gravity below 1.006 and the concentrated specimen above 1.020. In young and middle-aged subjects maximal concentration should approach 1.030, but there seems to be a gradual loss of concentrating power with age so that, after the age of 60, a maximal concentration of 1.020 is not grossly abnormal.

If the specific gravity of the concentrated specimen is less than 1.020, we assume there is some impairment of the tubule cells that prevents proper resorption of water. With increasing injury to the cells the concentrating power is further and further impaired until, in the final stages, glomerular filtrate is excreted essentially unconcentrated. When this has happened the specific gravity of the urine is "fixed," i.e., remains at approximately 1.010. Kidneys in such a condition are often capable of sustaining life for a long period of time if no emergency occurs which requires increased renal function. If such an emergency should occur, death is almost certain.

Failure to form dilute urine is much more rare than failure to concentrate but has essentially the same meaning.

MOSENTHAL TEST

The Mosenthal test is an older procedure which has been abandoned in many clinics. Even so, it is the best single method we have to measure the most important function of the kidneys, which is adaptability.

The other renal function tests are essentially "spot checks" of function either under normal conditions or under induced strain. Only this test gives us a good idea of daily kidney function under the conditions occurring in ordinary life. For this reason the Mosenthal test is one of the most valuable tests that can be performed in the office laboratory.

The urine exhibits marked changes during the day as the kidneys are forced to accommodate to bodily conditions in a state of flux. In the Mosenthal procedure one measures these changes in the urine under conditions roughly specified.

Technique

No particular restrictions are placed on the patient's activities. Instruct him to go about his affairs as much in the usual way as is possible, eating full meals of the type ordinarily taken at 8 A.M., noon, and 5 P.M. Caution him to take no food or liquid at any time other than at mealtime.

Furnish the patient with six urine specimen bottles and a liter flask. Request that he empty his bladder completely into a separate bottle every two hours, beginning at 10 A.M. and continuing until 8 P.M. These bottles need not be labeled as to the time at which the urine was passed.

Tell the patient that all urine after the 8 P.M. specimen should be passed into the liter flask, this flask to hold all urine excreted between 8:01 P.M. and 8 A.M. During this period he is to take no fluids.

All specimen bottles and the flask are to be brought to the laboratory. The specific gravity volume of each sample is then taken and recorded.

Errors

The samples must be taken at exactly the time specified. If the dietary rules are followed and the times are exact there is no reason for error in the test.

Interpretation

For ease in interpretation it is best to have the Mosenthal report on a standard form which can be typed in the laboratory. A good form is this one:

Patient__________________ Date__________
Address__________________ No.__________

Day Vol.________ Night Vol.________ Ratio__*__
Day Spec. 1______
2______ Max. day S. G.____*____
3______
4______ Min. day S. G.________
5______
6______ Difference____*____

The three critical points in the report are marked with an asterisk. The day/night ratio should be at least 2:1. In people who are entirely normal, the day urine is often three times as much as the night urine. If it is not, one suspects that a diuresis is occurring or that partial fixation of specific gravity is imminent.

Maximum specific gravity during the daytime should be at least 1.018. If it is not, one suspects inability to concentrate. Even more important is the difference between the maximal and minimal specific gravity. If it does not exceed eight points, a lack of adaptability on the part of the kidney is inferred.

Because it evaluates kidney function under relatively normal conditions, the Mosenthal test is one of the most valuable tests we have. It should never be neglected.

GENERAL COMMENT

The tests we have mentioned in this chapter are ideally suited to the office laboratory. By proper use, along with careful physical and historical evaluation, almost any ambulant case of renal disease can be followed in the office as well as it can be done in the hospital.

If you will allow the intrusion of a few personal reflections, I should like to tell you of my own belief about such cases and the part played by the office laboratory and x-ray.

When I first graduated from medical school I frequently hospitalized such patients "for study." It took several years to reach the perfectly obvious conclusion that only one thing was being achieved. We were running up big hospital bills and, on the average, getting assembly-line tests which could have been done better and at less cost in the office.

Now only rarely do I hospitalize such people. Judicious use of rest and ambulant or home therapy achieves just as much as hospital therapy and at a much reduced cost. As time goes by I become more and more convinced that the office laboratory and x-ray, wisely and conservatively used, is a better answer than hospitalization. This is so in many cases which are hospitalized.

If the doctor will take time to know the physiology behind these tests and the pathology to be inferred from the results, the office laboratory can do all that is required.

Of the tests mentioned in this chapter, two stand out as simple and worthy of particular attention. The Mosenthal, with its evaluation of kidney adaptability, is essentially a concentration and dilution test adapted to everyday life circumstances. It is very sensitive to serious renal disease. The phenolsulfonphthalein is another test worthy of note.

CHAPTER FIVE

Blood Chemistry

This chapter is written on the supposition that the physician either has or is willing to buy a photocolorimeter. The introduction of standard models of the instrument more than a decade ago has rendered needless much of the complicated apparatus and many long, difficult techniques formerly associated with blood chemistry.

Even though the technician may have only a little experience in chemistry one can still get results of sufficient accuracy for clinical work. Fortunately the cost is low, an excellent instrument and all accessory reagents and apparatus being obtainable for $300 or less. In a busy practice this amount can be saved (in terms of time) in less than a year.

For many years I have used the Leitz instrument and, therefore, cannot speak authoritatively of any other. I do know that colleagues who have other makes seem equally well satisfied.

Several hundred chemical procedures for blood are in common use today. A great majority of these are needed only in rare cases or for hospitalized patients. So that the instructions and interpretations may be kept simple, brief, and clear, I have selected the tests most frequently used for inclusion. The tests herein described will cover 99 per cent of the cases seen in the office.

BLOOD SUGAR

While nothing teleologic is implied in this statement, body metabolic processes are directed toward one final goal—the sparing of protein. In situations of desperation and in maintenance of life, the animal organism will utilize its own proteins as a means of nutrition. Except in such situations the main energy requirements are supplied principally by the carbohydrates and secondarily by fats.

When glucose is absorbed from the intestinal tract it may take three possible routes in the body:

1. It may be utilized directly by body tissues.

2. The muscles and certain other tissues are capable of storing this glucose in the form of glycogen so that a small residue of energy-producing material is available in the individual cells. A certain per cent of glucose absorbed is used for this purpose.

3. Glucose may be taken up by the liver and stored. In this way it is made available within minutes to meet various body needs. It has been estimated that the liver contains enough glucose to supply a metabolic requirement for five to twenty-four hours if no other glucose is available from any other source.

Absorbed glucose will take one of these three pathways.

The blood sugar is a dynamic equilibrium maintained by processes which are incompletely understood. There are three possible sources of the blood sugar. The first of course, is, direct absorption from the intestinal tract. The second is release into the blood stream from stores in the liver, and the third is the manufacture of new sugars by the liver itself. By drawing from these three sources as needed, the regulatory mechanism tends to keep blood sugar within relatively constant limits.

This regulatory mechanism is not perfect. Certain occasions may arise in the normal course of events when it fails to maintain an entirely or even relatively stable blood sugar. The most common such event is a heavy carbohydrate meal. Apparently, intestinal cells will absorb sugar so long as any is available. The blood sugar concentration makes little, if any, difference.

In the event that large quantities of carbohydrates are ingested, they may be absorbed into the blood stream quicker than they can be utilized or stored. In such a case the normal blood sugar, ranging from 80 to 120 mg. per cent, may rise to as much as 150 to 160 mg. per cent and sometimes even more.

It has been known for years that blood sugar responds to stress and is increased by the secretion or injection of epinephrine. This may be at least a partial explanation for the occasional case of well-proved psychogenic diabetes.

Classically we have been taught that insulin is the main regulator of blood sugar levels and that its influence is related to utilization of the sugar in the blood stream. More recent investigations have proved this only partially true.

There is no agreement as to the action of insulin in the human body, but two schools of thought stand out as paramount. One school maintains that insulin is concerned with passage of sugar through the cell membrane and another that insulin and a pituitary hormone are antagonistic in the control of certain chemical reactions necessary for the utilization of sugar. If such is the case (insulin producing the "utilization" reaction and the pituitary hormone tending to stop it), the abscence of insulin then lets the pituitary antagonists have full sway. Neither of these theories is proved but both are interesting as possible etiologic factors involved in blood sugar changes.

Regardless of the specific action of insulin the old theory that carbohydrate is not used in the abscence of insulin can be disproved from facts that have been known for at least 100 years.

The cerebral tissues and, in particular, the brain cells seem to derive most of their nutrition from carbohydrates. If this be so, and it seems well proved, then diminution in the amount of insulin would result in immediate impairment of brain cell nutrition and the obvious changes to be expected. This does not happen in diabetes. It has been suggested, but not proved, that brain cells and possibly other tissues are peculiar in that they do not require insulin to allow their use of carbohydrates.

Be all these things as they may, one must face the practical point in the office laboratory that increases in blood sugar can be counteracted in the vast majority of cases by administration of insulin. Therefore, for these practical purposes we shall consider that insulin has a direct bearing on carbohydrate utilization. Let me emphasize that from the research standpoint this may or may not be so. From the purely practical standpoint in daily practice it is the only possible way to consider the situation.

In this section we will consider that hyperglycemia represents a deficiency in insulin unless it can be proved to be temporary and the exact method of its induction explained.

Hypoglycemia, on the other hand, seldom is the result of oversecretion of insulin. This, of course, can and does occur in patients with certain pancreatic tumors, but in office practice such patients are seen perhaps once in ten years.

If one can imagine such a thing, the blood-sugar-regulating mechanism tends to follow established patterns. Many people in our present generation tend to take in large quantities of carbohydrates with each meal. Particularly is this true of people who indulge in alcoholic beverages. When such a person is absorbing large quantities of carbohydrates, the liver is storing most of it as glycogen and the pancreas is secreting quantities of insulin. Within an hour or so most of the sugar is absorbed from the intestine and the blood sugar begins to drop. Since there is a supply of insulin greater than normal in the circulating blood, this drop is rapid. As this drop progresses one would expect the liver to begin supplying glucose to increase the blood sugar. But the liver is not a perfect mechanism and there is a lag between lowering of blood sugar and the breakdown of glycogen to build it up once again. This lag may be demonstrated by serial determinations of the blood glucose.

After a large carbohydrate meal the liver stops breaking down glycogen and putting it into the blood stream because there is already too much sugar in the blood. After about on hour this heightened blood sugar has been removed, both by utilization and by being stored in the liver. Then the lag comes into play. It is time to add sugar to the blood but it takes from thirty minutes to an hour for the liver to do this. During the period in which this is being accomplished, there may be a marked hypoglycemia. Represented as a curve, it looks like this:

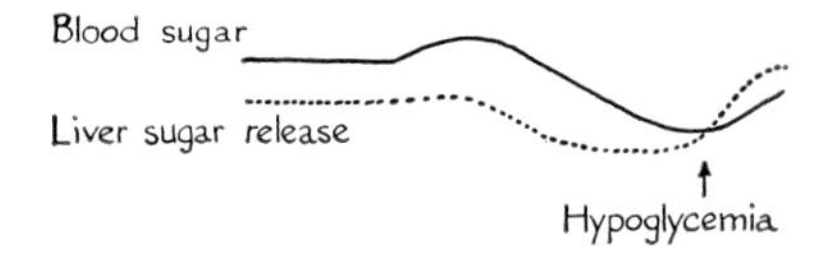

Such dietarily induced changes are becoming much more frequent. While this probably has no great medical significance, it has seemed in my practice to be most frequent in teen-agers and young married people.

Other hypoglycemias are related to pituitary changes, thyroid changes, and adrenal function. These are actually so rarely seen in practice and so much in the province of the highly skilled internist that they need not be considered here.

Technique

Instruct the patient to eat his usual lunch and to eat supper not later than 11 P.M. Caution him to eat approximately his customary meal.

The patient should be told that upon arising on the morning of the test he is to have a cup of black coffee, and specify that it be without any sort of sweetening agent. He should then report to the clinic, where a blood specimen is obtained.

Specific technique to be followed is explicit in the instruction book with the colorimeter and need not be detailed here.

Errors

Other than the usual errors of chemical manipulation, which includes dirty equipment, unstandardized reagents, and careless measurements, the test is practically error-free. Any cautious, careful technician who will follow directions can furnish blood sugar determinations with a margin of error of less than 10 per cent.

Interpretation

The blood sugar test is seldom done in the abscence of a previous finding of sugar in the urine. There are certain conditions in which glycosuria occurs but in which blood sugar is normal.

In the normal kidney, sugar diffuses freely through the glomerular membrane and is reabsorbed by the proximal tubules. The tubular cells do have a maximum absorptive power beyond which they cannot go. Ordinarily, until the blood sugar rises above 150 mg. per cent, the tubule cells can absorb all that passes through the glomerular membrane, and urinary tests for sugar are therefore negative. When the blood sugar rises sufficiently so that a greater quantity is filtered than the tubular cells can absorb, then sugar appears in the urine, and the blood sugar is said to have advanced above the renal threshold. This renal threshold is not a static thing. It varies greatly from individual to individual and apparently may at times vary in the same person. Certain diseases may profoundly effect the kidney's handling of sugar.

An example is the case of true diabetes in an aged person with glomerular changes. Filtration may be so retarded that even with a blood sugar of 250 mg. per cent or more only a small quantity of sugar gets through the filter into the proximal tubes. Often this quantity is so small that it is readily resorbed by the tubular cells and no urinary sugar may appear in spite of a blood sugar obviously within diabetic levels.

It is not rare to see an individual with a renal threshold somewhat lower than average. Such a person may have a true threshold level of 125 mg. per cent. When such occurs, sugar may be found in the urine after any meal in which moderate or large quantities of carbohydrates are ingested. Sugar is not found in the urine when the patient is fasting. There are no changes in the blood sugar.

Such cases must be rigorously differentiated from renal glycosuria which is excessively rare. True renal glycosuria appears to be a hereditary metabolic defect in which the patient is incapable of reabsorbing sugars to the fullest possible extent and, therefore, sugar appears in the urine at any and all times, regardless of the level of blood sugar. As mentioned, such cases are extreme rarities.

To repeat, persons with a relatively low renal threshold are, however, not rare. One sees a number of people who show postprandial glycosuria with perfectly normal blood sugar pictures. *These persons are not diabetics.* They simply have a low renal threshold.

As a matter of fact, almost anyone can absorb sugar in such quantity that the blood sugar level rises above his renal threshold. This alimentary glycosuria disappears relatively rapidly after meals, and the fasting blood sugar is perfectly normal.

We do not know all about the mechanisms that regulate blood sugar. While we were taught for years that the blood sugar is essentially a stable dynamic equilibrium with minor fluctuations only, the truth seems to be that major fluctuations are possible and not entirely explainable on the basis of our present knowledge. For example, we have known that stress conditions raise blood sugar, but it has been taught that this rise is slight and transient. As a matter of fact, blood sugar may rise as much as 60 to 70 points and remain there for many hours under conditions of extreme stress. Such persons, of course, show sugar in the urine and an increased blood sugar.

There is much speculation about the relationship of this particular condition to diabetes. Is there such a thing as "stress diabetes"? I do not know, but an occasional case of apparently proved diabetes mellitus has responded to psychotherapy. Most cases however, certainly seem to be on an organic metabolic basis. On the other hand, since we do not know the answer to this problem, it is decidedly dangerous to assume that stress plays no part in the origin of the disease.

All these things add up to one warning which every doctor should observe: There is no final and complete diagnostic meaning to be applied to a single test of blood sugar. Under proper circumstances with supporting history and physical examination, one may assume that a heightened fasting blood sugar means diabetes mellitus until proved otherwise. But unless one keeps well in mind that a certain number of cases are proved otherwise, errors are sure to result.

In our own small clinic we assume that persons showing a blood sugar level between 140 and 180 are either diabetics or are likely to become so and that those showing a fasting blood sugar level of over 180 are almost certainly diabetic. We ordinarily do not, however, establish an extensive routine until we have investigated the case thoroughly historically and until blood sugar tolerance tests are done on patients in which there exists the slightest question.

The sugar tolerance test is a simple procedure which establishes not only the fasting blood glucose level, but also the ability of the body to handle a sudden influx of sugar. The true diabetic patient, of course, does not handle this well. Blood sugar levels rise to a greater extent than they do in a normal person and remain elevated for a longer period of time than in the normal person.

For at least forty-eight hours before the test is performed have the patient take a diet of ample or slightly excess carbohydrates. On the morning of the test he is to have no breakfast at all. He may have one cup of black coffee. Upon reporting to the office, usually at 9 o'clock, a sample of blood is drawn, and immediately thereafter the patient is given 100 Gm. of glucose in water. This is a nauseating mixture which may be made to taste somewhat better by the addition of lemon juice.

Additional blood samples should be drawn at one, two, and three hours after ingestion of the carbohydrates. Typical curves look like this:

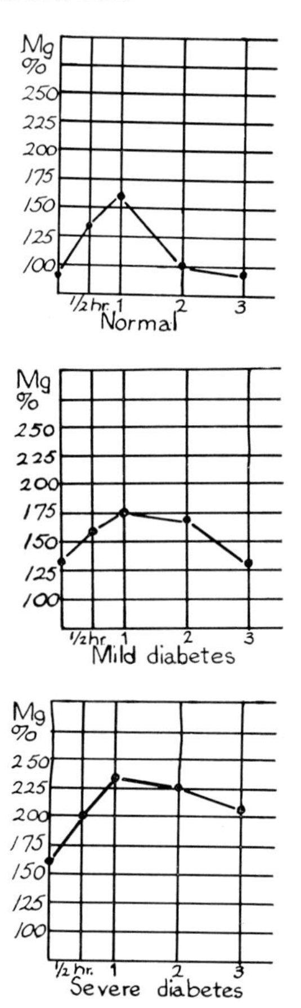

Hypoglycemia is usually a transient phenomenon and is somewhat difficult to detect in the office laboratory. To do this, however, take a careful history and make arrangements with the patient to report immediately upon the onset of weakness, sweating, and other typical symptoms.

The causes are actually legion but the most frequent cause seen in office practice is injudicious diet, which has been mentioned previously in this section. To summarize briefly, when large quantities of carbohydrates are ingested, they are absorbed somewhat more quickly than the body can handle them, and the blood sugar rises. This rise in blood sugar stops the process of glycogen breakdown in the liver, and the formation of glycogen for storage purposes is enhanced.

Within an hour or so most of the absorbed sugar is stored in the form of glycogen and it is necessary for some of this material to be broken down to supply sugar as it is utilized in the blood. Unfortunately, there is a time lag in this breakdown process and it may be from thirty minutes to an hour after it is initiated before an ample amount is supplied to keep the blood sugar up to usual levels. During this time lag a hypoglycemia occurs.

Such patients are usually thought to be psychoneurotics, but a careful history involving the timing of the attacks and an adequate dietary history will make one suspicious of the typical postprandial hypoglycemia syndrome. If this is suspected the patient may be instructed to take a high carbohydrate luncheon at 12 o'clock and report to the office at 1:15 or 1:30 P.M. No test of blood sugar is made until onset of symptoms, but blood is withdrawn immediately if the patient complains of weakness. The usual level in such conditions will range from 60 to 80 mg. per cent.

While one such finding reasonably well proves what the condition is, the diagnosis should never be taken as final until one has a chance to observe how the patient responds to dietary changes, notably a high protein diet.

Liver disease, deficiency of anterior pituitary hormones, and hypothyroidism are among the glandular conditions which may cause hypoglycemia, but the symptomatology is usually so apparent that the blood sugar test is only an accessory determination which is seldom used.

HEMOGLOBIN DETERMINATIONS

In order to understand the exact significance of the hemoglobin determination, one must review the red cell cycle as it occurs in the human body. The following is a much abridged and greatly simplified picture of what happens:

The human body is apparently able to synthesize all portions of the hemoglobin molecule by utilizing material commonly obtained in the diet. So far as we know, a person eating anything approaching a normal diet can form hemoglobin if iron is present.

To state this another way, the ordinary protein building blocks which are present in the body and which are taken in with 90 per cent of the ingested foodstuffs can be altered to form the hemoglobin molecule if iron is present. This obviously would indicate that the ingestion and absorption of iron can be a critical point. It is.

The intestinal mucosa contains a substance which has great affinity for iron. However, the intestinal mucosa is also one of the storage depots for iron and will not absorb any unless its stores are depleted. To use a crude example one might say that each cell has an iron hook upon which a molecule may be stored. If iron is needed in the blood it may be released from this hook into the blood. Then the hook is empty and can catch another iron molecule from the lumen of the gut. If the hook is full, i.e., has an iron molecule hanging on it, the iron in the lumen will not be absorbed, no matter how much is present.

Maximal body iron stores are a little over one-half gram. Because of this selective absorption and relatively small amount of storage it is interesting to speculate upon the number of tons of iron salt given each year which are promptly passed on and out through the bowel. Iron tablets are, however, a relatively innocuous form of psychotherapy if nothing else.

The body iron is freely used in the synthesis of hemoglobin and the ultimate formation of red blood cells in the bone marrow. These blood cells go through a number of preliminary stages before being released into general circulation as erythrocytes.

Certain maturation factors are necessary before the progressive changes from one stage to another take place. In the abscence of the chemicals which promote maturation, the process may be halted or vastly depressed at any given point. The most common example of this is the failure of maturation of red cells in pernicious anemia due to lack of vitamin B_{12} or some of its end products.

If our concepts of living tissue are correct, the red blood cell suffers one of the most lengthy and traumatic dissolutions that it is possible to imagine. Before it leaves the bone marrow the nucleus has degenerated, and by our usual standards the cell is in the process of death. After leaving the bone marrow it continues to exist for three to four weeks and travels, according to some calculations, as much as 700 miles through the vessels. During this course it is juggled and jostled by other cells, repeatedly squeezed through small openings, forced to change shape, and may be attacked by all kinds of noxious influences. The cells literally are "beat to pieces" during their traumatic existence and old cells can frequently be identified by proper microscopic procedures.

The aged erythrocytes are ultimately destroyed by the reticulo-endothelial system and their iron content largely reutilized. Just what impulse is responsible for the destruction of these cells we do not know.

For practical purposes, all circulating hemoglobin is contained in the red blood cells, and for further practical consideration one may look upon the transport of oxygen as the only function of hemoglobin.

When a determination of hemoglobin is made it is, in essentiality, a measurement of the concentration of hemoglobin per unit of blood or a measurement of the oxygen-carrying capacity per unit of blood.

The principal reasons why hemoglobin should be lowered are deficiency of iron intake and utilization, loss of large quantities of iron-containing pigment, and interruption of the maturation process in the bone marrow.

Considering these facts in the light of cases usually seen in the office, there are three conditions of great importance. They are (1) the iron deficiency anemias, (2) the pernicious anemias, and (3) chronic hemorrhage.

Technique

The technique as represented in the colorimeter instruction book is entirely adequate.

Errors

The two most common errors seen in the office are inaccurate filling of the hemoglobin pipette and allowing the blood to clot in the pipette before the chemical diluent is added.

The first has a certain unavoidable error inherent within itself. In attempting to pull blood up through a pipette to a certain mark it is almost impossible to obtain great exactitude. On the other hand, with careful technique this inherent error should be considerably less than 5 per cent.

It is tempting to say that allowing the blood to clot in the pipette is simply a matter of carelessness and should not be tolerated, but when one has actually done the procedure, attempting occasionally to control a crying baby, stop a wound from bleeding, and quiet the fears of a desperately anxious mother, meanwhile carrying out the test, it is easy to have a profound sympathy for the technician.

Should a blood clot form in the pipette, let it stand overnight in a solution of strong hydrochloric acid and rinse out in the morning with the usual cleaning solutions.

Interpretation

In the normal individual who has adequate processes of blood formation and who is otherwise in good health, the hemoglobin concentration is a function of oxygen tension in the blood. Such a person will respond to high altitude (and therefore lowered oxygen tension) by formation of additional erythrocytes and will respond to increased tension by exhibiting a slight lowering of hemoglobin concentration.

The test for hemoglobin is a much more sensitive indicator than the older red blood count. In our own clinic we have practically eliminated the routine erythrocyte count and have resorted almost entirely to hematocrit and hemoglobin determinations.

Lowered hemoglobin readings are most often due to the anemias and occasionally may reflect a physiologic dilution of the blood. An example of such physiologic dilution is that which occurs during the last trimester of pregnancy or immediately after moderate hemorrhage.

There is no precise normal hemoglobin content. Under ordinary circumstances a healthy adult male usually has from 14.5 to 16 grams of hemoglobin and the healthy adult female from 14 to 15 grams. Minor deviations from these levels, either upward or downward, are probably of no significance.

Newborn infants usually have about 20 grams of hemoglobin, but this falls in the first few weeks to normal or below as the peculiar hemoglobin formed in intrauterine life is taken from the blood stream and replaced with the usual hemoglobin of extrauterine life.

There is no difficulty in interpretating extreme deviations of hemoglobin. For example, the woman who shows 6 grams of hemoglobin does not present any problem. But another type of case can often be difficult to diagnose. This is an example:

Mrs. C. L. B. is a 34-year-old housewife, obviously quite intelligent and somewhat modern in outlook and also quite obviously a psychoneurotic. She complains of extreme lassitude and weakness, and although she goes to bed early at night, she sleeps poorly. Her heart pounds and occasionally skips a beat. She feels "nervous and rundown" and blames this on the existence of anemia which she has had for five years.

The hemoglobin is reported as 13.2. A careful physical examination produces nothing but the scars of time, and a careful history points to no organic disease but does show a surprising coincidence between the onset of her neurotic symptoms and the onset of the so-called anemia.

Previously, Mrs. C. L. B. has taken a black capsule containing iron, liver extract, and a half dozen other ingredients to which she responded very well. The druggist in our drug room is asked to empty the contents of 100 such capsules and to substitute milk sugar for the contents. Mrs. C. L. B. is given these capsules and told that "they are the same capsules that she has taken before, but with a special ingredient"—which is truthful in a way.

One month later this woman has a hemoglobin of 14.8 grams and feels fine. Since Mrs. C. L. B. is an intelligent patient she is taken into the clinic study for a cup of coffee and given a frank explanation of what occurred, and is asked to help us figure out her case.

She has been most cooperative and a year later can tell no difference between lactose capsules and the multitherapeutic capsules insofar as result is concerned. Several times when she had "a fall in hemoglobin," capsules were given, and she was told to decide specifically whether they were the placebo or the effective capsule. She could not tell.

This woman's symptoms, of course, were due to psychoneurosis, but what caused the small drop in hemoglobin? I believe that stress with its increased depth and frequency of respiration causes a slight increase in oxygen tension and, therefore, a decrease in hemoglobin.

If such is the mechanism, one would suspect that approximately 40 per cent of the so-called "minor anemias" in the United States are directly related to stress through its influence on the respiratory system.

Increase in hemoglobin is more difficult to interpret. Usually it is due to decreased oxygen tension and this is most often seen in slowing of the general circulation. Cardiac decompensation is the most frequently seen entity in the average office practice in which hemoglobin values might be increased.

Body fluids show more rapid changes in infants than in adults and dehydration is most often a cause of increased hemoglobin readings. Even in minor diseases children may lose enough fluids to cause hemoconcentration and increased hemoglobin readings.

True polycythemia with its inordinately high reading is a rare disease. It has been mentioned under the red blood count on page 22.

In general, the physician should remember that the hemoglobin concentration is a reflection of the oxygen-carrying capacity per unit of blood. If normal blood formation is taking place it also is a reflection of the state of hydration and speed of the circulation. Numerous other inferences can be drawn from changes in the hemoglobin, but they have little significance in office practice.

BLOOD UREA NITROGEN

Determination of the blood urea nitrogen is a much more simple test than the determination of nonprotein nitrogen. Since the information to be gained is essentially the same, in the small office laboratory it will be well to concentrate on the blood urea nitrogen (BUN) determination and seldom, if ever, resort to the more difficult nonprotein nitrogen determination.

So far as we know urea is a waste product. It has no utility whatever in the human body.

Proteins are often used repeatedly in the body, being partially broken down, reused, partially broken down when rebuilt again and going through this cycle many, many times. However, there is some complete breakdown of proteins into carbon dioxide, water, and urea.

This breakdown of proteins and utilization of energy obtained can apparently occur in any cellular tissue of the body, but one of the final steps, deamination with formation of urea, for practical purposes occurs entirely in the liver. The urea thus formed is released into the general circulation and is eliminated by the kidneys.

Since the urea molecule is small it readily diffuses through the glomerular filter. Unfortunately, urea is extremely soluble in water and tends to "go along" when water is resorbed by the tubules. Approximately 40 per cent of the urea that passes through the glomerular filter is passively reabsorbed with water. This, of course, means that for every 100 grams that passes through the filter, only 60 grams are excreted in the urine.

Since it passes the glomerular filter so readily it is only in rare instances that urea can be formed so rapidly that it is not eliminated quickly and efficiently by the kidney.

In the exceptional case, so much protein will be deaminated so fast that the BUN rises in spite of normal kidneys. This is always a temporary process and the rise seldom lasts more than forty-eight hours. This is quite obvious, for the human body cannot undergo such an extensive protein breakdown for more than a temporary period without death intervening.

In trauma, particularly to the extremities, we sometimes see a rise in BUN. Possibly this is due as often to kidney damage as to the release of large quantities of urea. There is, however, one instance where this rise may be used as a diagnostic sign. In the case of massive hemorrhage into the gut there is a rise in BUN which may last for as much as twenty-four hours. Hemorrhage into other body cavities usually does not produce such a rise. Here, again, the reason is obvious. The digestive juices act upon blood protein and large quantities are absorbed in a few hours. Breakdown in deamination occurs in a significant fashion in this resorption of protein, and BUN rises.

The other possible cause of an elevated BUN is glomerular damage. It is this cause that is most often sought out in the office laboratory.

Technique

As with other blood chemistry tests, directions furnished with the photocolorimeter are entirely adequate.

Errors

Occasionally ammonia ions may be present in the reagents and will make a slight difference in the final reading. This can be obviated by running a blank determination and subtracting the results of the blank determination from the test reading. This occasionally is a major source of error and it is probably wise to run blanks each time the test is needed.

Interpretation

The name of the disease with which we are most concerned indicates its relationship to the BUN—uremia. The BUN determination is a sensitive indicator of the accumulation of nitrogenous waste in the blood.

Ordinarily values are accepted as from 12 to 15 mg. for 100 ml. of blood when calculated in the form of urea nitrogen. A gradually rising BUN is evidence of serious kidney damage and insipient uremia. There are no confusing extraneous factors in this determination.

One must, however, keep in mind that the BUN will fluctuate from day to day and that transient, small rises have little or no significance. It is only in the case that shows a sustained rise with gradually increasing amounts of BUN in which the findings point toward uremia and dissolution that it is significant.

A surprisingly large number of cases seen in office practice show that serious kidney damage and elevated blood urea nitrogen are present, but the patients manage to stay in a reasonably well-compensated state for one or two years. It is to follow such a case that the test may be highly recommended.

The BUN is much like the test of kidney function. It does not measure organic damage to the kidneys but is rather an indication of their functional capacity in the secretion of urea. We have found it valuable to keep BUN charts on those patients with serious renal disease.

Here is the chart of a patient who rapidly developed uremia and died. You will notice from the chart that this fact is predictable several months before its occurrence.

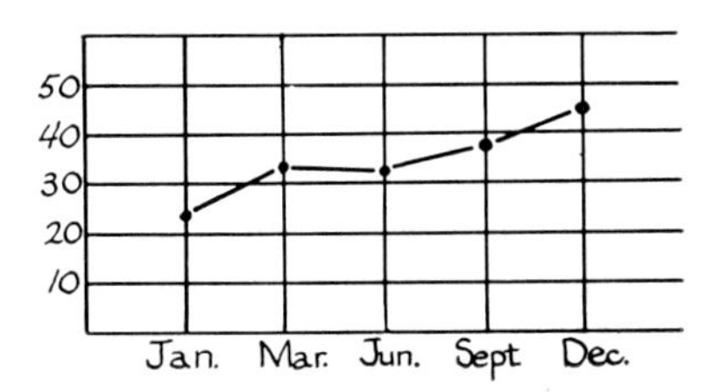

Here is the chart of a patient with a serious kidney lesion who was doing well when last seen but who had an ultimately bad prognosis.

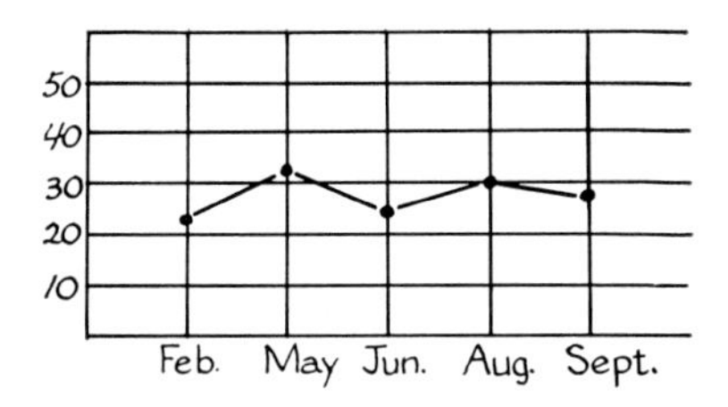

A lowered BUN implies poor protein nutrition or liver disease but clinical signs are so definite in such cases and other tests so much more valuable that the BUN is of little importance.

THYMOL TURBIDITY TEST

As it stands now the thymol turbidity test is a purely empirical procedure and, therefore, we are in no position to explain why it occurs or exactly what it indicates. It is only on the basis of clinical experience that we can make any statement at all.

It has been postulated that thymol turbidity measures in some degree the amount of gamma globulin in the serum, but this has not been proved.

The test came about following the observation that when patients' serums are added to a solution of thymol, varying degrees of turbidity result. This then was applied to clinical patients and it was noted that the degree of turbidity reflected with some accuracy hepatocellular function, particularly in cases of some hepatitis and cirrhosis.

Technique

All the newer photocolorimeters can be calibrated for the thymol turbidity test and the technique suggested in the instruction book is entirely adequate.

Errors

Since we do not know exactly what we are doing or why the test works, it is not possible to chart out probable errors. The only caution would be to follow exactly a standard technique so that the determinations may be comparable one with another.

Interpretation

The test is utilized mainly in cases of suspected cirrhosis and hepatitis. Since it has an inherent accuracy of approximately 80 to 90 per cent, in the event that it is positive, one may assume the existence of hepatocellular damage. Beyond this point interpretation is hazardous in the extreme because of the empirical nature of the procedure.

All of this does not lower the value of the test. It is simple, easily performed, and certainly one of the most valuable devices we have for the exploration of liver disease. It should be a frequent procedure in the office laboratory, and because of its extreme ease of performance it will probably take precedence over the cephalin-cholesterol flocculation.

The physician should remember that we have no proof that the thymol turbidity and cephalin flocculation tests measure the same thing. For practical purposes we assume that they do at least measure closely related entities but at times one may be positive when the other is negative. If after performing a thymol turbidity test you still feel that the patient has a liver disease, it is better to have a cephalin-cholesterol flocculation run than to accept the results of the thymol test as perfect. The cephalin-cholesterol test is a procedure better done in larger laboratories and, while it can be done in the small office, it is not to be highly recommended.

BROMSULPHALEIN LIVER FUNCTION TEST

A number of substances are selectively taken up from the blood stream and excreted by liver cells. Any such substance could conceivably be used as a means of testing the function of the liver cells. The one most commonly used is Bromsulphalein. In alkaline solution this is a reddish purple dye. It is practically without toxic side effects and may be readily measured by simple chemical procedures.

Recently there has been some comment that cells of the reticulo-endothelial system also remove the dye from the general circulation, but it would seem that only insignificant amounts are absorbed.

The test is based on injecting a measured amount of dye according to the patient's weight. Thirty minutes are then allowed to elapse and blood is drawn for testing. Simple alkalinization of the plasma brings forth a degree of color if any of the dye is present. Practically always in the presence of actively functioning liver cells all dye has been removed within the thirty-minute period.

Technique

No special preparation is needed, although we usually ask the patient to report to the clinic in the morning, having taken only a cup of black coffee for breakfast. A standard solution in 5 per cent strength is used for injection. The patient is weighed and his weight divided by 55. The result is the number of milliliters of solution that should be injected. This dose is equivalent to 2 mg. of dye substance per kilogram of body weight. The injection is made with moderate rapidity into one antecubital vein and the exact time taken. Thirty minutes later 5 to 10 ml. of blood are withdrawn and treated as specified in the directions that come with the colorimeter.

In the event that some dye retention is indicated, a second specimen is taken one hour after the original injection and again tested.

Errors

The most frequent error in the test is the administering of an incorrect amount of dye. Trivial discrepancies in amount probably influence the results very little, but 0.25 ml. one way or the other may have some influence. It is best to use a tuberculin syringe in order to give the calculated dosage.

Interpretation

For practical purposes Bromsulphalein is selectively taken up from the blood and quantitatively excreted by liver cells. There are only two common circumstances under which this is not done:

1. Damage to hepatic cells
2. Occlusion of the bile duct system between the lobule and the duodenum

In occlusive biliary disease the test is of little value, for other methods of examination are more specific. One must, however, be sure that occlusive biliary disease does not exist before attempting to test for hepatocellular damage. An accurate history is usually sufficient, but rarely gross examination of the stools may be necessary to determine whether or not obstructive disease is present.

If there is no obstructive disease, one may then assume that any failure to pick up the dye from the blood is due to changes in the hepatic cells. Normally at the end of thirty minutes no dye at all is found in the blood serum. In the presence of disease of the liver cells from 5 to 100 per cent may be found still circulating. The amount is a rough measure of the extent of liver damage.

This test as well as those discussed in the preceding chapter must be envisioned as a test of function, not necessarily as a test for organic damage.

Severe functional damage may exist in the liver with few permanent organic changes and the Bromsulphalein test is very sensitive to such functional changes. A rough grading of functional impairment may be listed as follows:

1. Five to 15 per cent retention: minor liver damage
2. Fifteen to 40 per cent retention: moderate liver damage
3. More than 40 per cent retention: serious liver damage
4. Retention greater than 80 per cent: dangerous liver damage

In the event of retention, a second determination should be made one hour after injection of the original test substance. In the presence of minor or even moderate damage, uptake should be sufficient so that less than 10 per cent of the dye is retained at the end of one hour.

Most workers feel that the Bromsulphalein test should not be resorted to in cases of jaundice and this is certainly true in office practice. The test, however, in conjunction with the thymol turbidity test just described is probably the best indicator of hepatocellular damage available for the small laboratory.

ICTERUS INDEX

Jaundice is simply defined as staining of the tissues by bile pigments. It is commonly seen in office practice and the great majority of patients may be adequately diagnosed and treated in the office.

Many classifications have been proposed but the simplest and most useful is that of Ducci. For purposes of office practice, even this may be somewhat simplified. Jaundice may be classified into three basic types, the prehepatic, hepatic, and posthepatic.

Prehepatic jaundice presupposes hemolysis of red blood cells and a production of a breakdown product—a bilirubin-protein complex—more readily than liver cells can dispose of it. Few of these patients are followed in the office.

Hepatic jaundice presupposes one of two conditions. The first, which comprises at least 90 per cent of all cases, is damage to the hepatic cells. When injured these hepatic cells do not break down the bilirubin protein complex and excrete the bilirubin in the bile as do normal liver cells. For that reason the bilirubin is literally piled up in the circulation, awaiting the action of these cells.

The more rare type consists of some malfunction of the tiny bile canaliculi which dam up the bilirubin acted on by its cells and will not allow its entrance into the bile duct. It is probable, though by no means proved, that inflammatory reaction along the walls of these canaliculi effectively stops deposition of bile in them by the liver cells.

The third type of jaundice, or the posthepatic jaundice, presupposes obstruction to the bile flow at some point between the collecting ducts in the liver and the duodenum. The most frequent cause of such an obstruction is a stone; perhaps the next most frequent, inflammatory stricture, usually following an operation; and the least frequent, carcinoma.

Any of these three mechanisms (undue hemolysis, hepatocellular, and damage or outflow obstruction) will cause clinically appreciable jaundice. The icterus index gives no information as to which type of jaundice is present. The test is simply a measurement of the yellow coloration in plasma. As such, it is a rough guide to the amount of bile or bilirubin in the general circulation.

Normal results are approximately 4 to 6 units, and clinically appreciable jaundice occurs when the icterus index reaches 10 to 16 units. As one can see from this, there is a period during which jaundice is clinically nonappreciable but readily suggested from the results of the icterus index.

For this reason it is a valuable test and may often give information in suspected cases of liver disease. In addition to its use for detecting jaundice before the discoloration becomes clinically apparent, it also furnishes a guide to the amount of pigment in the plasma, a consistently increasing icterus index being decidedly unfavorable.

Various investigators have shown beyond doubt that keratin in the blood may interfere with the icterus reading, but such interference is so rare and of such slight amount that it is insignificant from the standpoint of office practice.

Technique

Blood is withdrawn and treated as specified in the colorimeter manual.

Errors

The test as done by colorimetric technique is so simple and straightforward that an error is practically unheard of even with the most inexperienced technician.

Interpretation

Since the icterus index is only a rough measurement of the color of plasma, it is not subject to detailed ultrascientific interpretation. In general, the following table encompasses just about as much as can be said of the results of the test.

ICTERUS INDEX	INTERPRETATION
0 to 6 units	Normal
7 to 9 units	Probable incipient jaundice
9 to 14 units	Almost certain incipient jaundice
14 units or over	Jaundice clinically appreciable

In some cases of hepatocellular or posthepatic jaundice, repeated determinations of the icterus index give an excellent picture of the progress of the disease. Hepatocellular disease with a steadily increasing index will, of course, indicate increasing functional impairment of liver cells, while a steadily decreasing index will indicate restoration of normal function.

In posthepatic disease a slowly increasing but unremittent icterus index usually indicates complete obstruction and one should certainly be suspicious of cancer. A fluctuating index, on the other hand, is more often found with stones in the common duct. Here is why:

When complete obstruction occurs from stones, the hepatic secretory pressure gradually builds up and the duct is gradually dilated proximally to the stone, like this:

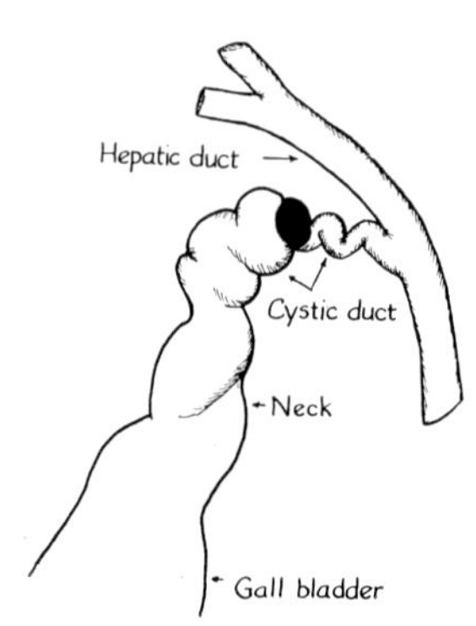

The icterus index rises. As the pressure builds still higher, some of the bile escapes around the stone and the icterus index falls. This may be repeated during relatively short intervals for months at a time. Finally, however, back pressure will cause irreversible damage in the liver and real difficulties will begin.

TOTAL SERUM PROTEIN

The process of protein metabolism is so intensely complicated by the extreme size and complexity of the molecules involved that a clear exposition has never been made. For practical working purposes, the cycle goes something like this:

Proteins are absorbed from the intestinal tract largely in the form of amino acids. Some of these amino acids may be taken directly from the blood stream by the general tissues and used for cellular metabolism, but the great majority are first acted upon by the liver.

After having been taken from the circulation by the liver cells, proteins have several possible fates. They may be used to replenish the blood protein or may be resynthesized into compounds utilizable by the general tissues. If protein intake is adequate, a number of amino acids may go through the process of deamination and be resynthesized into carbohydrates or fat breakdown products, such as the ketone bodies. In the usual person seen in the office probably the larger part of ingested protein is altered into carbohydrates or fat before being utilized.

Waste protein metabolites from the general body cells are often returned to the blood stream and picked up by the liver for resynthesis or deamination and complete breakdown. The end products of protein metabolism are carbon dioxide, water, and urea, but few protein molecules are likely to reach this stage without having gone through several episodes of use and resynthesis. The exception to this statement would be those proteins immediately deaminated to the liver and used as suppliers of energy.

Of the serum proteins only the albumin fraction is principally formed in the liver. It has been proved beyond question that while a significant portion of the globulins may be formed by hepatic tissues, other cells of the body are also capable of their synthesis.

The plasma proteins are, in a sense, a reserve protein pool and are in a state of constant flux. Sometimes a graphic example is of service in understanding this function: Picture a long freight train and draw an analogy between it and a plasma protein molecule. Let each car of the freight train be an amino acid. In circulating around the system of tracks or blood vessels, these proteins approach contact with most of the body cells. These cells are capable of side-tracking the freight train and removing certain cars containing foodstuff while replacing them with empties or cars of waste material. When the train gets back to the freight yard (in this case the liver) empty cars or waste cars are taken away and replaced with filled freight cars. From this analogy one can see that there is a constant interchange between the liver, the general cellular tissue, and plasma proteins.

Let me repeat: I know full well that this is an inexact chemical analogy. Nonetheless, it is a good working illustration.

A point to remember is that the plasma proteins are not constant bodies immutably kept in position but are, in actuality, in a state of continual interchange with the cellular tissues and the liver.

Much of the dynamics of the actual circulation is based upon proper levels of plasma proteins. The capillaries are walls with semipermeable membranes through which solutes freely diffuse but which hold back most molecules of plasma protein. This, of course, creates an osmotic pressure tending to suck fluids through capillary walls into the vessels. Opposed to this pressure is the pressure within the vessels as generated by the heart. In the average capillary the relations may be presented like this:

In the arterial end the head of pressure generated by the heart is greater than the osmotic pressure tending to bring fluids back into the vessels. For that reason solutes freely diffuse through the capillary membranes and into the tissue spaces.

In the venous end of the capillary the blood pressure has fallen somewhat and the diffusion of solutes into tissues has slightly concentrated the remaining proteins so that osmotic pressure is somewhat increased. Fluid is then returned from the tissue spaces into the capillaries. It is upon this constant process of fluid extrusion and return that cellular life depends.

If the capillary membranes are damaged they may lose their semipermeable quality and freely permit the egress of proteins. Once these proteins have escaped the vessels, their osmotic pressure is exerted to bring additional fluids from within the lumen out into the tissue spaces. In such case, the existing head of blood pressure and the osmotic pressure of the proteins abet one another to remove fluids from the vessels.

Such a process represents the syndrome we call shock and is not compatible with life unless overcome and reversed by compensatory mechanisms or by active treatment.

By no means are the plasma proteins the only arbiters of edema formation. It is true, however, that edema is seen relatively often when total protein is lowered below 4½ grams per 100 ml.

In summary, one may say that the basic functions of the proteins are (1) osmotic, (2) nutritive, and (3) immunologic.

There are three mechanisms which may cause change in the protein level. All three are seen with some frequency:

1. Deficient uptake. This is often nutritive and is rarely due to changes in intestinal absorption.

2. Liver disease. This is more rarely seen in the office, for it is a manifestation principally of severe and often terminal changes. In the average office patient, we may see an occasional ambulatory cirrhotic with vastly altered proteins. Toxic damage to liver cells may render them incapable of proper protein processing, but this is most often of a transitory nature and is seldom tested for in office practice.

3. Excessive loss. Large quantities of proteins may be lost in the urine, particularly in the nephroses. It is a tribute to the remarkable ability of the hepatic cells that this excessive protein loss does not immediately progress to the extent that death is inevitable. Even so, in most cases wherein the disease is severe, protein is usually lost beyond the ability of the liver to replace it.

Technique

This is fully explained in the manual accompanying the photocolorimeter. One point is worthy of emphasis. The test is done on serum—not plasma. The withdrawn sample of blood is allowed to clot, which removes the fibrinogen, and then the serum is removed by pipette.

Errors

The most frequent error is not allowing the blood sufficient time in which to clot. One may thereby get a number of red cells into the serum and greatly increase the reading. There is no exact time that can be given during which the blood should be allowed to stand and clot, but it is probably wise to let it stay in place for at least one hour before removing serum from the test tube.

This test, of course, depends upon the old salting-out process which is an inefficient means of separating the plasma proteins. It is the only means available to the average office laboratory and most of the textbooks are written utilizing the findings of this test rather than the much more accurate electrophoretic determinations. For that reason it maintains its position as the most utilizable of the tests.

Interpretation

Serum proteins are extremely variable. The normal finding is usually given as 6 to 8 grams per 100 ml. of blood, but it is possible that even greater variations still remain in the range of normal.

Changes in the fluid concentration of the blood, which go on constantly, may change the relative level of plasma proteins per 100 ml. without changing the total amount of circulating protein, and unquestionably some of our findings are related to this rather than to an actual change in quantity of circulating protein in the blood.

There are three possible mechanisms which may account for lowered plasma proteins:

1. The first is deficiency of intake which is most often seen in the moderately severe infections, when patients do not eat. The fall in such instances is usually not great, seldom exceeding 1 or 2 grams per 100 ml., so that the total protein determination reads from 4½ to 6 grams. It was formally thought that the lack of nutrition was solely responsible for this, but now there is good evidence that the dilution of blood in response to an infection may be the true factor. Be that as it may, it is possible to starve a human body until plasma proteins begin to fall. On the other hand, mechanisms of formation are such that other than this slight fall, which may be seen relatively early, there is practically no alteration in the protein until immediately before death.

It has been said quite accurately that the plasma protein level is one of the most protected systems in the human body.

For entirely practical purposes, one may say that while the debilitated patient may show a slight fall in total serum protein, this is overshadowed in significance by other elements of the disease and the test is of little or no help.

2. Deficiencies in manufacture of proteins may cause a lowering in the level. Slight depressions may unuestionably be due to minor toxic effect upon liver cells. This is an interesting but not very practical finding in such cases. When severe liver damage occurs, the proteins may become depleted.

As has been said previously, the protein system is maintained almost as long as any vital metabolic function, and it is only in severe liver disease that there is a significant drop in total liver protein. For that reason this test is more interesting academically than in practice. In fact, one might say that it is almost an admission of incompetency to see a patient with proved liver disease, monstrous ascites, edema formation, and then request a serum protein determination to see whether or not the proteins are depleted. They are.

The mechanisms of ascites and the collection of fluids in other serious cavities in advanced liver disease are not completely understood. When the plasma proteins are definitely lowered, some of these patients respond reasonably well (but not excellently well) to the administration of albumin concentrate. Occasionally such a patient may be treated in the home and a total protein determination may be of some value.

3. The third method of depletion is loss of the proteins. The obvious loss in nephrosis is so apparent and so well understood that little need be written about it. When the pathologic excretion of albumin is great enough to cause plasma protein levels to fall markedly, even as much as 2 or 3 grams a day, therapy may be urgently indicated and the test for total serum proteins of value. These patients are more often seen in the hospital than in the office laboratory.

A major loss of plasma proteins, which is often unsuspected, may occur from draining wounds. Enough proteins may be lost in the drainage from a large abscess to impair seriously the plasma protein level. When this occurs some of the amino acid needed for repair of tissues is not readily available, and healing may be so slow that the physician is alarmed. In office practice, this is an excellent point to keep in mind. Particularly is it true in chronic cases of osteomyelitis or large perirectal abscesses that drain repeatedly and in profusion.

I have seen many cases in which patients who did not heal readily were given large quantities of vitamins when steaks would have been more beneficial. Occasionally office determination of total serum protein will serve to clarify the reason for delay in healing in such a patient.

We know little about the reasons for heightened serum protein levels. Such do occur in many diseases. The most commonly seen in the office is the collagen group, including rheumatic fever, rheumatoid arthritis, periarthritis nodosa, and other similar entities. It has never been fully explained just why the increase in plasma proteins should occur, and since this increase is inconstant and may occur in a number of diseases, it has no present diagnostic significance.

Based upon what we know now one should certainly not try to draw any inference from the finding of increased plasma protein.

In office use the total serum protein determination is not often a test of great value but occasionally it is greatly needed. We have applied it most often to suspected cases of chronic malnutrition (with questionable results) and to cases of profusely draining wounds (with excellent diagnostic results). In the rarely seen cases of nephrosis and early cirrhosis the test is of value but such cases are not common in the office.

It has been our experience that the determination of albumin and globulin and the resultant A/G ratio are seldom of much utility in office practice. We feel that the salting-out error involved is often so great that little dependability can be placed on the test.

URIC ACID

Findings during the past three years have almost completely changed our outlook on purine metabolism and the pathogenesis of gout. Before this time it had been believed that abnormalities in the metabolism of ingested purine were reflected in the blood uric acid level and that this was always related to gout or a tendency toward gout.

Now it appears that various uric acid producers can be and are synthesized in the human body from nonpurine precursors. The blood uric acid level is inconstant and fluctuates markedly in either the presence or absence of gout. This does not mean that the uric acid test is valueless, but it does mean that interpretation is, of necessity, more restricted than we have formerly thought.

Picture, if you will, a lake fed by several streams and kept at a certain level by a dam with floodgates. The water in the lake may be taken to represent what we might call the uric acid pool of the human body. The inflow streams represent the intake of uric acid into the body and the outflow stream the release of uric acid into the blood.

This pool of urate is greatly increased in those persons who have a tendency toward gout and this increase seems to bear some almost direct relationship to the intensity and frequency of symptoms.

As an example, one might say that in a person with a tendency toward gout, the lake would be twice or three times the size of normal, while in the person undergoing severe gouty changes, the lake might be ten times the size of normal. We do not know the mechanisms that regulate the inflow to the urate pool, nor do we know what regulates release of urates from the pool into circulation.

We do know that sooner or later if the lake keeps enlarging there is going to be an increased outflow. In other words, there is going to be enough release of urates into the blood stream so that the test for uric acids will become positive. From this example, however, you can see that the increase in blood uric acid might fluctuate from moment to moment, even though the urate pool is constantly and slowly enlarging.

Technique

The technique as elaborated in the colorimeter handbook is entirely adequate.

Errors

Errors of the test are most often those of interpretation rather than mistakes in chemical technique.

Interpretation

Since the uric acid content of blood fluctuates a great deal, there is some active question as to what constitutes an entirely normal finding. In my colorimeter book, normal is given as 2 to 4 mg. per cent, but in line with others who have made many of these determinations I believe that these figures are too low. Probably 4 to 6 mg. per cent may be taken as normal for women and 5 to 7 mg. per cent for men.

There are not many diseases other than gout in which there is likely to be a rise in blood uric acid. Occasionally, in a renal disease there may be a hyperuricemia, and this conceivably could be (though it seldom is) confused with gout. Determination of the blood urea nitrogen which is not elevated in gout is a laboratory means of verifying the picture.

Now suppose we are given a male who has had acute arthritic symptoms and we suspect gout. A blood serum uric acid level is done and reported as 9 mg. per cent. What are the possible interpretations?

In the first place there seems to be an inherited familial tendency toward hyperuricemia in gout. On the basis of a single uric acid test we can assume that the patient *probably* has this inherited hyperuricemia. On the other hand, beyond this assumption we cannot proceed. At this stage of the game a history of an acute attack is a much more reliable diagnostic criterion than is the blood uric acid test.

Determination of blood uric acid at monthly intervals for three to six months is the next logical step. If it remains elevated in five out of six of the determinations, one may be reasonably certain that the familial hyperuricemia is present. Now the problems of age and sex come into play.

For some reason which we do not understand this abnormality in the uric acid pool usually does not become manifest in males until puberty and in females until the menopausal stage. If the patient is a 12-year-old boy or a 30-year-old woman, it is probably wise to take a long time before believing the results of the test.

But, let us assume that we have established that hyperuricemia exists. Still the best criterion of the existence of gout is historic and the test has only assumptive value. This does not mean that the test should not be done, but it does mean that the physician should not proceed to unfounded assumption. Most important, it does mean that the patient should not be allowed to formulate an opinion because of the results of the test.

I hope you will permit a digression from the matter at hand to let me consider with you this problem of test interpretation by a patient. We are practicing medicine in an era where wild and foolish ideas regarding tests are rampant. Through our own shortcomings patients have come to believe that the laboratory test is the final arbiter in their disease. If the test, for example, shows gout, they have gout and there is no possible other outlook.

I cannot advise you too strongly, in talking with patients about laboratory tests, to make the point constantly and firmly that the clinical judgment of the physician outweighs the value of tests approximately 100 to 1. Your laboratory and your x-ray are useful and valuable tools, just like the carpenter's square and level. When used in the light of your clinical judgment, they can build a remarkable diagnostic structure. When used without clinical judgment, the structure is likely to look much like a house built by an 8-year-old boy with the level and square. No test is the final arbiter in any situation and, again, I cannot advise you too strongly to make this point well known to the patient.

After that little outburst, let us return to the problem of uric acid levels. Assume that the case seen seems unquestionably one of gout and that uric acid determinations have supported the diagnosis of a gouty tendency. Now the uric acid determination in and of itself becomes essentially worthless. It does not always rise before an attack nor does it always fall when an attack is over. It should be used occasionally to follow the case and to demonstrate that serum uric acid remains elevated. Beyond this point of "reassurance" it has no value whatever.

BLOOD CHOLESTEROL

Cholesterol is manufactured in the liver and is also ingested with foodstuffs and absorbed. Since the capacity of the liver to synthesize it is far greater than the daily need for the compound, it seems unlikely that a question of deficient intake could ever exist in the person eating a diet even partially normal.

Apparently not only the liver but also most of the other cellular tissues of the body have some ability at cholesterol synthesis. It is excreted principally in the bile.

The compound is so protean in distribution and the intermediary steps in its metabolism so poorly known that testing for cholesterol level has little value except in one specific instance.

The level of thyroid hormone seems to control, to some degree, both liver synthesis of cholesterol and its removal from the body by way of the bile. In hyperthyroidism both liver synthesis and excretion are increased, but the excretion is increased to a far greater degree, resulting in a lowering of cholesterol level. In hypothyroidism, on the other hand, both formation and excretion are decreased, but the excretion is decreased to a much greater extent and blood levels rise.

Unfortunately the basic normal blood level of cholesterol seems to be an individual matter, like the size of the nose or configuration of the hand. Normals fluctuate very widely. Some studies have indicated that normal may range between 100 and 300 mg. per cent. You must remember that *no individual* range is this great. The cholesterol level for any one person seems relatively constant, but one disease-free individual may have a normal level set at 150 mg. per cent and another equally disease-free individual establish his normal at 250 mg. per cent. Why this is so, we have no idea.

Since it is so, the interpretation of the test must be limited by this factor.

Technique

Have the patient report to the laboratory in the morning without breakfast and follow the colorimeter manual technique.

Errors

The technique requires some chemical extractions which must be precisely done, but further than this it is relatively simple. Most errors lie in the field of interpretation. The test solution sometimes degenerates, and for this reason a blank determination is best run with each test. Should the blank exceed more than 50 mg. of cholesterol, the solution had best be discarded and a new one made.

Interpretation

In actuality there is only one condition observed in office practice in which blood cholesterol determinations are of great value. This is hypothyroidism.

In hyperthyroidism the lowering of the blood cholesterol is so inconstant and results are so uncertain that in general it is best not to use the test. Clinical diagnostic means are far more accurate and far superior to anything that can be offered by the small office laboratory.

The rise in cholesterol seen in hypothyroidism is limited in diagnostic value by the fact that only in an occasional patient do we know the individual normal cholesterol level. However, as the hypothyroidism progresses, blood cholesterol often reaches 300 or 400 mg. per cent and sometimes as much as 500 mg. per cent, at which time it is distinctly diagnostic.

Given a suspected case of hypothyroidism the inference to be drawn from a rise in blood cholesterol remains of extensive value. For example, a woman evincing some of the symptoms and signs of hypothyroidism reports to the office. The first question is whether the signs are of psychoneurotic or hypothyroid origin.

A painstaking history and physical examination will usually give clear indication, *but not positive indication,* as to this differentiation. If, then, a blood cholesterol is reported as 310 mg. per cent, one has a confirming test although by no means a diagnostic test.

Since it seems almost a standard error in the medical profession to diagnose psychoneurotics as hypothyroids, the test can be of great value. As an example the other way, take this one:

A 35-year-old woman has reported to the office complaining of weakness, general fatigue, and other symptoms which might be taken as a borderline hypothyroid or as an absolute psychoneurosis. She had, of course, been told many times that her thyroid gland was the root of all evil and that thyroid medication was necessary.

The only difference she noticed after taking a grain of thyroid daily for one month was a tremendous increase in nervousness. A careful history and examination disclosed no signs or symptoms entirely typical of hypothyroidism and there was ample reason to believe that tension was at the root of symptomatology.

The case was quite clear at this point, but for the sake of confirmation the patient was taken off thyroid for one month and a blood cholesterol was run at the end of this thirty-day period. It was reported as 190 mg. per cent. In such a case one may certainly infer that thyroid function is relatively normal and that tension is at the root of the symptoms.

Let me emphasize again that the blood cholesterol is an excellent test, but the results are only indicative. To use it as a means of positive differentiation is simply asking for trouble.

GENERAL DISCUSSION

There are many other tests which have been or might be applied in the office laboratory. For example, the van den Bergh test for bilirubin in the blood, including the direct and indirect reaction, perhaps should be included.

On the other hand, the blood cholesterol test has been largely discredited in the past few years and many fine authorities in the field believe that it does not show what it was originally claimed to show. Until the problem is clarified the practitioner should not rely on it.

Tests for such things as calcium level in the blood, creatinine, amylase, alkaline phosphatase, etc., may all be performed in the office laboratory, but, in general, they are more applicable to patients who are far too ill to be carried as outpatients and, therefore, these tests have been omitted.

There is a great temptation to perform many of these procedures in the office before hospitalizing a patient. Experience has taught us, however, that the tests are likely to be repeated in the hospital during the first few days of the patient's stay and that good hospitals are understandably chary about having the results of office tests entered upon their records.

As an economic measure it is probably wise to use the office laboratory only to make determinations on the patients who will be followed in the office or upon those patients who must be followed until it is decided whether or not hospitalization will be necessary. This would seem to restrict the office laboratory unnecessarily, but, as a matter of fact, it actually works out better when this policy is followed.

CHAPTER SIX

Physical Observations Upon Blood

There are six simple procedures which may be done in any laboratory and which will offer much information. Many other tests are available but these six form a basic group which will supply most of the diagnostic information needed.

SEDIMENTATION RATE

The erythrocyte sedimentation rate is a measure of the rapidity with which the red blood cells settle out of a citrated solution of blood. We do not know all the many various factors that control the process, but certain empirical facts are demonstrable.

Probably due to complex electrochemical reaction, red blood cells tend to remain individualistic under certain circumstances and under other circumstances form stacks or piles called rouleaux. When these rouleaux are formed, each clump presents less surface area per unit of weight than do the cells when individually suspended. Because of this obvious physical change, blood cells formed into rouleaux will settle out of solution with much greater rapidity than cells which remain isolated individuals. This, apparently, is the basis for changing rates of sedimentation.

Processes in which tissue destruction occurs seem to release into the blood stream certain elements that promote rouleaux formation. When this occurs the final sedimentation rate roughly parallels the rate of tissue destruction and it is a useful indicator that some such process is in progress.

Other factors besides tissue destruction may influence the sedimentation rate. For example, it has never been explained why the rate should be increased during the middle trimester and perhaps the first part of the last trimester of pregnancy.

In diseases that cause hemoconcentration, such as congestive failure, the rate is slowed by the simple factor of crowding, and in marked anemias the rate may be speeded by the relative isolation of each red blood cell. These factors must be taken into consideration in attempting to interpret.

The sedimentation rate is somewhat more rapid in women than in men, though why this is so has not been clearly elucidated.

It is essential to keep in mind that the rate parallels tissue destruction and not the speed with which a process advances. Here are some examples: In the earlier hours of acute appendicitis, during the stages of invasion and before there is necrosis or gangrene of the appendix or even minor cellular destruction involved in the inflammatory reaction, the sedimentation rate is essentially normal. After approximately twenty-four hours it may become greatly increased. The same is true of acute myocardial infarction, the rate remaining normal until tissue destruction becomes pronounced. Usually this means a twenty-four-hour period of relative normalcy before the rate changes.

It has been postulated that changes in plasma protein, particularly the fibrinogen factor and to a less pronounced extent the globulin fraction, are responsible for the changes in sedimentation. Perhaps they may be. At present, the process is too complex for ready explanation.

Technique

We have always used the Westergren method, although the Wintrobe method is unquestionably just as good. Our reason is this: In the Wintrobe method one has to fill a narrow bore test tube with blood, whereas in the Westergren method blood may be sucked up into a calibrated pipette which is much easier.

In the Westergren method, proceed as follows:

1. Use a pipette to transfer 0.5 ml. of 3.8 per cent sodium citrate solution to a test tube.

2. Using a 5 ml. syringe, withdraw from the antecubital vein a little more than 4.5 ml. of blood. Squirt out the excess so that there remains exactly 4.5 ml. of blood in the syringe and then put this blood into the tube containing citrate. Invert the tube several times to mix the blood-citrate solution.

3. Using the Westergren sedimentation pipette and mouth suction, fill the Westergren pipette until the column of blood comes just above the 0 mark.

4. Wipe the Westergren pipette tip and allow enough blood to escape so that the meniscus is almost exactly on 0.

5. Place the Westergren pipette in the rack especially designed for it and clamp it in as near vertical position as possible.

6. In exactly sixty minutes read the test and report the amount of sedimentation.

Errors

There are several common errors. Going through the technique a step at a time, probably the first and one of the most common is to squirt the freshly obtained blood into the citrate solution with so much force that cells are hemolyzed. This becomes apparent from the reddish color of the plasma in the sedimentation tube at the time of reading. Such a test is not accurate and should be discarded.

Another common error is to place the tube at a slight slant, which increases the speed of sedimentation and makes accurate interpretation difficult.

Still another common error occurs when two or three sedimentation rate tests are being made at the same time and are mixed up so that the reports are not attached to the records of the right individuals. This can be avoided by labeling each tube with a piece of adhesive tape bearing the patient's name at the time the sedimentation rate is started.

Interpretation

There are only a few prime facts which must be kept in mind in accurately interpreting the results of the sedimentation rate. In the first place, remember that it is a measure of tissue destruction and has absolutely no specific significance whatsoever. This point may be emphasized by the following case.

One morning an otherwise healthy 8-year-old boy fell out of a hayloft and lit, buttocks foremost, on a sawhorse. Extensive examination showed no major damage but severe contusion to both buttocks, with extensive hemorrhage under the skin. He was sent home and told to rest. Three days later his mother brought him in with the terrified complaint that he had "been exposed to 'romantic' fever"* and had fever and aching in his joints. The boy did have a temperature of 101° F. and did complain of mild joint symptoms. His heart was normal and there were absolutely no other findings. I completely forgot about the bruised buttocks.

The sedimentation rate was taken and reported as 38. The boy was put to bed, and I made daily calls to examine his heart, looking for evidence of terrific damage. In three days we found nothing and the boy seemed quite chipper and happy. About that time I realized that the hemorrhage in the tissues from the blow on the buttocks had caused both the fever and increased sedimentation rate.

In retrospect the story sounds a little foolish, but such misinterpretations are extremely common in office practice, even with doctors far wiser than I. You *must* keep in mind that the sedimentation rate is totally nonspecific and that it will become positive in the presence of any tissue destruction.

There are certain specific office uses in which the sedimentation rate may be of value. Among them are the following:

1. A normal sedimentation rate means nothing in the distinction between functional and organic disease, but a patient suspected of functional disease who has an increased sedimentation rate should require explanation of the increase before definite pronouncement is made as to the functional aspect of the case. Often it is wise to do a single test of the sedimentation on what seems to be a purely functional case, and if the sedimentation rate is increased make a further diligent search for organic pathology.

2. In rheumatic fever the sedimentation rate is the best single index of activity that we have. In general, the degree of sedimentation parallels with some exactitude the degree of rheumatic activity. There are two areas in which the sedimentation rate may be grossly misleading.

Under the influence of cortisone or ACTH the sedimentation rate may approach normal even though rheumatic activity continues unabated. In the patient taking such medication, the sedimentation rate should be interpreted with exceeding care.

In rheumatic carditis the onset of congestive failure, even in its earliest stages, may produce enough hemoconcentration to bring the sedimentation rate back to normal. In any case of rheumatic heart disease the sedimentation rate should never be taken as the final arbiter, unless one is sure that no congestive failure exists.

3. Most dangerous neoplasms have enough malignant activity to result in some destruction of tissue. In such cases the sedimentation rate will be increased. Occasionally this is useful in differentiating benign gastric ulcer from gastric malignancy. The ulcer, unless extremely large or virulent in attacking the tissue, will not cause enough degeneration to change the sedimentation rate greatly, while the carcinoma probably will do so.

4. In rheumatoid arthritis the sedimentation rate is an excellent way of deciding when there is activity. The treatment of the disease, of course, differs markedly in active and nonactive periods, and changes in sedimentation rate are an excellent reflection as to the degree of activity.

5. Measurement of the degree of tissue destruction in any infectious process may have some importance to the clinician and the sedimentation rate will provide this. For example, an apical tooth abscess, which is a strictly localized process without major tissue destruction, will seldom show an increased sedimentation rate but an active osteomyelitis of the jaw will. Another example: Ordinary infectious sinusitis shows no change in sedimentation rate but virulent sinus infection with necrosis of the mem-

*At his age it seemed improbable.

branes shows a marked increase. Similar criteria of tissue destruction may be applied to almost any infection any place in the body and this is certainly one of the most important uses of the sedimentation rate.

MEAN CORPUSCULAR HEMOGLOBIN CONCENTRATION

The mean corpuscular hemoglobin concentration (MCHC) test is a rough calculation and expression of the amount of hemoglobin per red blood cell. It is an excellent and simple method of dividing the anemias into two great classes, the microcytic hypochromic anemias, which will respond to iron, and the macrocytic hyperchromic anemias, which will usually respond to vitamin B_{12} or liver.

Technique

The index is obtained by mathematical calculation of two previously obtained findings. The two findings necessary are hemoglobin, expressed in grams, and the hematocrit. Methods for determining hemoglobin will be found on page 82 and discussion of the hematocrit on this page.

This is the formula for the calculation:

$$\frac{\text{Hb} \times 100}{\text{Hematocrit}} = \text{MCHC}$$

For example, let the hemoglobin equal 14.5 and the hematocrit equal 41. The figures would then read $\frac{14.5 \times 100}{41} = 35.3$.

Normal readings may be considered from 31 to 35.

Errors

If the index seems a rather odd figure, check the multiplication and division involved. Surprisingly, most errors happen in the process of the simple calculations involved.

Interpretation

If the index is less than 30, the chances are that one is dealing with a microcytic hypochromic anemia which will respond to iron. If the index is above 36, a macrocytic anemia is probably present and will respond to vitamin B_{12} or liver. If the index is between 30 and 36, chances are greatest that there is some error in either the hemoglobin or the hematocrit, but there is a secondary possibility that a normocytic normochromic anemia might be present. This second possibility is very, very remote.

THE HEMATOCRIT

The hematocrit test consists of centrifuging a known quantity of blood containing anticoagulants until a near-maximum packing of cellular elements occurs. Then by means of calibration on the tube one can read off the percentage of red blood cells, of white blood cells, and of plasma per unit of whole blood. This simple test, in conjunction with a hemoglobin determination and blood smears as indicated, will give near-maximum information about the cellular elements of the blood.

Technique

Special tubes in which blood from the veins is to be received must be prepared. Make up a solution as follows:

Ammonium oxalate	1.2 Gm.
Potassium oxalate	0.8 Gm.
Distilled water	100.0 ml.

Pipette exactly 0.5 ml. of this mixture into each of a series of test tubes and remove the water by evaporation. Cork the tubes which are now ready for use.

Withdraw 5 ml. of venous blood from the patient, placing it in one of these tubes. The quantity should be measured as accurately as possible using an ordinary syringe for the purpose. Recork the tube and invert it several times to mix the anticoagulant thoroughly with the blood. The blood in this tube may then be used for sedimentation or hemoglobin determination and for the hematocrit. It should not be used to make blood smears.

A special hematocrit tube which looks like this:

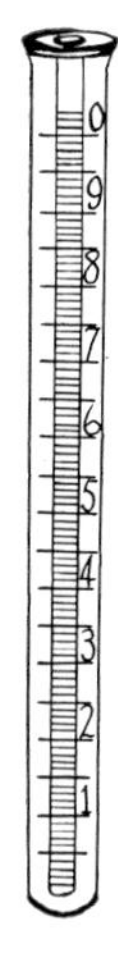

should be used to make this determination. Using a micropipette, fill the hematocrit tube exactly to the 0 or 10 mark with the blood and anticoagulant mixture. Then cap the tube and centrifuge it at a speed of at least 3,000 r.p.m. (most modern office laboratory centrifuges have a maximum speed of 3,600 r.p.m.) for fully fifteen minutes and longer if possible.

When packing is nearly complete there are actually five discernible layers in many bloods. For our purposes we need consider only two:

A red blood cell layer in adults should reach from the bottom of the tube at 0 to between the 40 and 50 marks. Anywhere between 40 and 51 or 52 may be considered within the range of normal.

A second layer, the buffy coat, should extend from the top of the red blood cell layer toward the top of the tube from 0.4 to 1.0 mg.

Errors

The most frequent error is insufficient spinning of the sample to pack the cells. Actually, fifteen minutes' centrifugation is not enough to gain maximum packing but it is usually enough to allow a good estimate. It is better to spin for a half hour, or longer if time permits. Other than this, errors are practically nonexistent.

Interpretation

Only inferences may be drawn from the results of the hematocrit test but these inferences are so specific and so generally reliable that the test is one of the most valuable procedures performed in the office laboratory. We use it and the hemoglobin determination almost to the exclusion of the red blood count.

If the volume of packed red blood cells is slightly less than 40, say, 34 to 40, it is possible that one is dealing with a minor anemia or with a physiologic or pathologic hemodilution. Minor anemia would be clarified when the hemoglobin estimation is run and the MCHC calculated. Pathologic blood dilutions are seldom seen in the office and the most common physiologic dilution is that seen in the latter trimester of pregnancy.

The volume of packed red blood cells when decreased to less than 34 or 35 ordinarily are indicative of moderate to severe anemia. Changes this great can be, but scarcely need be, confirmed by determination of hemoglobin.

Increased volume of packed red blood cells indicates either polycythemia or hemoconcentration. Since true polycythemias are exceedingly rare and usually present a clearly indicated symptomatology, the test is seldom necessary for such cases and when needed is only confirmatory. Much more important is the hemoconcentration which may be elucidated by the test.

Perhaps the most frequent cause of hemoconcentration in adults is cardiac decompensation and in children, the diarrheal and vomiting diseases. In the cardiac patient, hemoconcentration gradually increasing in spite of treatment is an extremely bad prognostic sign.

Since children normally show a somewhat lower hematocrit reading than adults (usually in the 35 to 40 range normally), a reading of 55 or more usually indicates serious disease and points up the desirability of hospitalization.

The normal buffy layer of 1 mg. represents a white blood count of approximately 10,000 per cubic millimeter of blood. The count can usually be estimated, using this as a criterion. Probably up to 1.5 mg. of buffy layer is not too significant, but should the buffy layer be greater than 1.5 on the tube scale one is unquestionably dealing with a leukocytosis which is best clarified by means of a smear. In our own practice the measurement of this buffy coat has been just as satisfactory as the white blood count in determining whether or not an infectious process exists.

I have never seen a buffy coat pathologically decreased, but logic would lead one to believe that in cases of leukopenia the thickness of the buffy coat would decrease down to the point where it is perceptible but not measurable. If this should happen, certainly a stained smear and an immediate white blood count would be in order.

There are two discolorations of the supernatant plasma which may be of some interpretive significance. The first is the yellow staining in icterus and the second is the red staining of laked erythrocytes. If the yellow staining is present, an icterus index should be done, but if red staining is present, one should suspect laking of the blood cells at some point of the test procedure after having withdrawn the blood from the patient's vein. Few people with intravascular hemolysis of sufficient degree to be apparent in this test are seen in the office.

All in all, the hematocrit is one of our best office tests.

CLOTTING AND BLEEDING TIME

The mechanics of blood coagulation are still a hotly disputed physiologic problem. For that reason it is not readily possible to discuss the processes leading up to alterations in the clotting and bleeding time. These are empirical tests which, while useful, are not applied on a foundation of known physiology.

Technique

If the technician is careful, both tests may be done at one time. After cleansing the patient's finger, make a stab wound sufficiently deep to produce a free flow of blood. Timing is begun when the first drop of blood appears. Fill a capillary tube from this first drop and then at thirty-second intervals touch the wound with a sheet of filter paper. Break a short piece off the capillary tube after scarifying the glass with an ampule file.

The end point of the bleeding time test is reached when the filter paper after touching the wound does not have a deep red blood stain but only a faintly pinkish stain of extruded plasma. The end point of the clotting time test is taken to be the point at which a string of fibrin is seen between the two ends of the capillary tube when they are pulled apart like this:

Normal clotting time is usually considered to be from three to five minutes by this method, and bleeding time is usually one to three minutes, although normals may extend up as far as five to seven minutes.

Errors

It is difficult to buy new capillary tubes with the same diameter, but those obtained from any reliable surgical supply house are usually accurate enough to make the tests comparable. One should remember that results of these tests cannot be freely compared with the results of other types of coagulation and bleeding time tests. Each type has its normal.

Interpretation

Any bleeding time of more than ten minutes may be considered abnormal. There are two classes of condition which cause such a prolongation. The first is liver disease of destructive nature, such as acute yellow atrophy or terminal cirrhosis. The second is any condition resulting in extreme lowering of the blood platelets, such as purpura hemorrhagica, aplastic anemia, and occasional cases of leukemia.

The test is of principal value as a preoperative measure before performing even simple office surgery. A number of physicians still do office tonsillectomies (and there is certainly no criticism of this if the office is properly equipped) and this test should be applied before such a surgical procedure.

Coagulation time is prolonged in many of the major and minor infectious diseases, but prolongation is for relatively short periods of time, perhaps up to ten minutes. On the other hand, in patients with hemophilia and in certain cases of jaundice, prolongation is most pronounced. This test has some diagnostic value in hemophilia because often the coagulation time is prolonged as much as an hour or more in such disease. In other conditions it is more a preoperative measure than an actual test with diagnostic value. As a safety factor it should always be performed preoperatively.

CLOT RETRACTION

Clot retraction is apparently due to the presence of blood platelets. Exactly how they act has never been completely elucidated, but since retraction parallels almost exactly the number of platelets, their action in clot retraction has been assumed. In the absence or severe diminution of the number of platelets there is no clot retraction.

Technique

Place 1 or 2 ml. of blood in a test tube and observe from time to time. Normally the clot begins to retract within twenty to 120 minutes after it is formed and gradually withdraws from the side of the vessel and becomes increasingly smaller.

No particular measurements are needed, for visual observation of the retraction will give the information required from the office laboratory.

Errors

None.

Interpretation

Failure of the clot to retract indicates diminution of the number of platelets. While this occurs in several pathologic processes such as aplastic anemias, leukemias, etc., its principal significance in the office laboratory is in the diagnosis of thrombocytopenic purpura. In such cases no clot retraction may occur from twelve to twenty-four hours, and the duration of time before clot retraction bears an inverse relation to the number of platelets. Other than this, the test has no particular significance, but it is often just as accurate as a platelet count in the diagnosis of thrombocytopenic disease.

CHAPTER SEVEN

Microscopic Observations Upon Blood

The hematopoietic system of the human body may be looked upon as a complex factory with all the problems inherent to such an enterprise. A supply of raw materials must be kept constantly available for every step of the process if it is to succeed. Every step of manufacturing must be carefully controlled—in the case of the body, by a complex chemical system. Production must be coordinated so that there are the right number of finished products available at the right time, for storage space is limited and an overplus of products will inevitably block other manufacturing elements in the factory. Orders for delivery must be received and coordinated and the product released at the proper time.

The parallel is exact.

The hematopoietic system must receive raw materials in the proper amount and kind or it cannot take the first steps in manufacturing blood elements. The steps in production must be coordinated by complex chemical mechanisms or abnormal forms will result. An overproduction of one product, such as granulocytes in certain forms of leukemia, will result in literally crowding out the production of other elements and finally, unless enough of the complex chemicals necessary to mature and develop the cells are available, the finished product cannot be delivered in an adequate amount.

Such a process represents a complexity far beyond the scope of this book and equally far beyond the scope of the average office laboratory. In this chapter we will consider the most commonly sought for pathologic indications and discuss briefly their interpretations.

STAINS AND ROUTINE STAINING

At least two hundred stains are currently available for the staining of blood and marrow smears. In spite of this plethora of material with which to work, four or five simple techniques will suffice for all procedures in the office laboratory. Rarely can the practicing physician be so expert in interpreting blood films that he needs special stains to bring out the finer details of cells.

Taking and Fixing the Smear

Methods of drawing blood and the cautions to be observed are discussed on page 19. For routine leukocyte counts a thick smear is most valuable, and for delineating cellular characteristics the thin smear is preferred. A simple little technique is available to regulate this thickness of the smear.

Begin by placing a drop of blood near one end of a microscopic slide, like this:

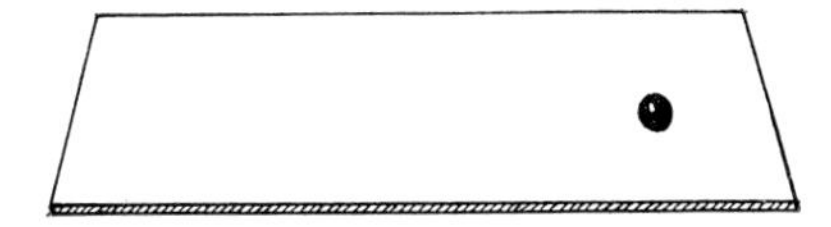

Try to use a drop of nearly uniform size each time you make a smear.

Now apply the edge of a second slide to the first and allow the drop of blood to spread along the edge of the second slide. Move the second slide along the surface of the first, like this:

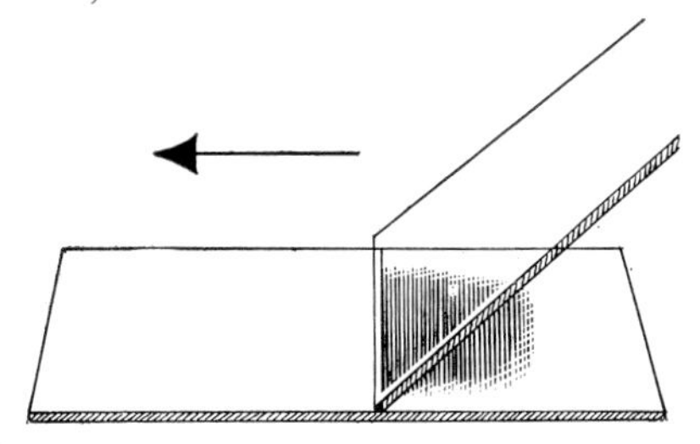

Try to maintain a uniform speed of movement so that each smear is made exactly as its predecessors. If one does this, the thickness of the smear can be regulated by changing the angle between the slides.

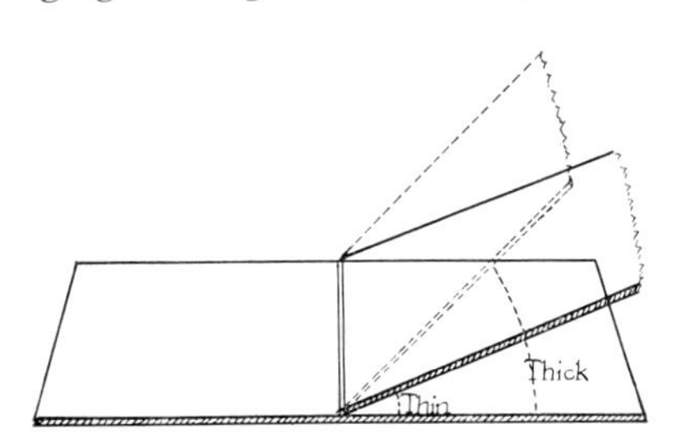

The most frequent error in spreading blood films is to use dirty or scratched slides. Scratched slides should be put aside to be used for more gross purposes, such as examination of feces.

Slides for diagnostic blood work should be washed thoroughly after use and then immersed in a staining dish of glacial acetic acid for ten minutes. Following this they should be washed in water and then stored, pending use, in a solution of alcohol. When the slide is removed from the alcohol it should be polished dry with a bit of lens paper.

Wright's stain does not require fixation before staining, nor, of course, do the supravital stains. On the other hand, films to be stained with Giemsa's preparation should be fixed by immersion for two minutes in absolute methyl alcohol.

For a Wright's stain the smear is allowed to air dry and then the commercial stain solution is applied. Actual staining time varies from batch to batch and should be determined experimentally for each bottle purchased. In general, it is about one minute.

After expiration of the primary staining time, distilled water is added to the stain on the slide. It is best to add a volume of water approximately equal to the volume of stain previously applied. This mixture should remain in place for about three minutes. The slide is then washed in tap water and dried.

Errors in staining with Wright's stain are legion. The solution is temperamental and does not lend itself well to the extreme conditions often found in the office laboratory. For that reason we use the Giemsa stain almost exclusively.

The most frequent mistake is pouring the stain and water solution off the slide and then washing it. When the stain is poured off first and then the slide is washed, a fine film of stain particles clings to the slide and may cause difficulty in visualizing finer structures seen through the microscope. Avoid this by holding the slide, with the stain solution still on it, under the water tap and washing copiously.

The next most frequent mistake is allowing the stain-water mixture to stay on the slide too long. This will produce a precipitate which cannot easily be washed away.

Wright's stain consists of dyes dissolved in pure methyl alcohol. At first the solution is usually too alkaline, and the resultant slide shows red blood cells colored a dirty blue instead of their normal yellowish red.

As time goes on there is gradual oxidation of some of the methyl alcohol to formic acid. First the solution becomes "just right" with near-perfect results and then, finally, it becomes too acid. At this point erythrocytes stain reddish pink or even distinctly red and the nuclear structures in leukocytes are pale blue or not visable at all.

Individual batches of stain do not correct easily, but one may mix old and new solutions to gain a proper stain. A little practice usually makes it possible to keep the stain just right for consistent good results.

The Giemsa stain takes longer to accomplish than the Wright's but has many advantages. Using dilute solutions one does not have to be concerned with precipitates. In case staining seems inadequate one merely immerses the slide in solution again. This can be done as many times as may seem necessary.

For this procedure the blood film should be fixed in absolute methyl alcohol for at least one minute. More time may be necessary. Place 5 ml. of stain solution in a covered staining dish and fill to near the top with distilled water. Mix gently.

When the slides have been fixed, simply put them in the staining dish like this:

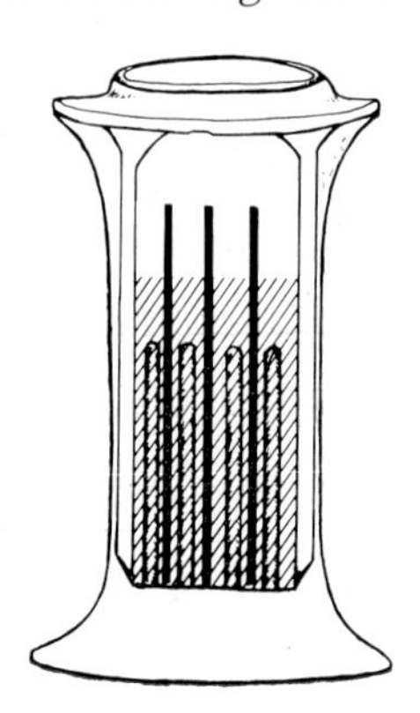

Staining time is extremely variable, extending from a few minutes to as much as thirty minutes. The quantity of stain in the solution may be adjusted to shorten the time. We generally get the best results with a sufficient concentration to allow adequate staining in ten to fifteen minutes.

Reticulocyte Stains

The following special solution is used:

Brilliant cresyl blue	0.5 Gm.
Sodium citrate	0.4 Gm.
Physiologic saline solution	100.0 ml.

A small drop of this solution is placed on a microscopic slide and one drop of blood from the patient's finger is mixed with it. The mixture of blood and stain is smeared, using the standard technique, and the smear is allowed to air dry. It is then stained, using either the Wright or Giemsa technique.

All the cells in two fields are counted and the relative number of reticulocytes noted. At least 200 cells are counted, utilizing more than two fields when necessary. The percentage of reticulocytes is calculated. Incidentally, for this and other mathematical procedures, a $2.00 slide rule will save many times its value in minutes preserved for other tasks.

Supravital Staining

The reading of supravital smears is one of the most difficult tasks in hematology and detailed interpretation is not within the province of the average physician with an office laboratory. Nevertheless, it is easy to learn to differentiate mature from primitive cells by this technique and such a differentiation may be of the utmost diagnostic value. The principal interpretative error to avoid is attempting to read too much from the preparation. With great skill and constant study much is to be learned. We beginners must be content to identify primitive cells.

Slides and cover slips for the preparation must be scrupulously clean. Wash them in soap and water, rinse in acetone, and polish with lens paper. Be particularly cautious about bits of dust or fibrils from the paper, which will invalidate the preparation.

The stains used are a 0.25 per cent solution of neutral red chloride and a 0.33 per cent solution of Janus green B. The latter stain is toxic to cells and must be used in the smallest quantity possible to obtain adequate staining.

For each preparation a mixture of the two stains should be made as follows: Using an 80-unit insulin syringe, draw the Janus green B to the 1 unit mark. Then add neutral red to the 80-unit mark. This will result in about a 20 to 1 mixture,* which is proper for ordinary purposes.

Gently mix the two stains for several minutes. Place one drop of the mixture on a *clean microscopic slide and smear exactly as one does in making a blood smear.* Allow this to air dry. Discard the slide if the stain does not seem to be evenly spread.

Secure a drop of blood on a clean cover slip and place it gently on the prepared slide, making no effort to spread the blood. Use sealing wax or paraffin to seal the edges of the cover glass to the slide. *Be sure* the seal is airtight.

Put the preparation in an incubator at body temperature (see Bacteriology section, page 154) and wait twenty minutes. When the preparation is withdrawn for examination a penny should be warmed in the Bunsen flame and placed on one end of the glass slide. This will serve to keep the slide warm. If the examination continues for more than a minute or two the penny should, of course, be reheated.

Some common errors that may be made:

1. Unclean glassware. White blood cells will clump around particulate matter and make accurate diagnosis impossible. Maximum cleanliness is imperative.

2. Too much Janus green. This will kill the white blood cells. Particularly notice the granulocytes. They are usually the most active of the commonly seen cells in such a preparation. They normally move by smooth, flowing motion in one direction only. As death approaches they become "undecided" and may put out pseudopodia in several directions at once or may repeatedly alter direction. Instead of smooth, flowing motion the cytoplasm shows a jerky, vibratory, or trembling motion.

Words offer a poor description. Make such a preparation of your own blood and watch the cells die. Once this process has been seen it will never be forgotten. Preparations that exhibit this phenomenon of decease should not be used for interpretative purposes.

3. Allowing the preparation to cool. This causes the same phenomenon of decease mentioned above. Such preparations are completely useless.

*The "extra" Janus green is in the syringe tip.

Eosinophil Counts

Eosinophils are enumerated exactly as one does a white blood cell count (see page 24) except that a different diluting fluid is used. The one we prefer is made up as follows:

Eosin Y	0.05	Gm.
Acetone	5.0	ml.
Distilled water q.s.ad.	100.0	ml.

After the counting chamber is loaded—again exactly as for a white count—one then sets the condenser of the microscope to furnish the maximum amount of light easily tolerated by the eye. With this procedure white blood cells other than the eosinophils will not be seen and the eosinophils will look like red dots. Calculation for the count is in no way different than for the standard white blood count.

ERYTHROCYTES

While we certainly can pin point the various reasons for failure in hematopoiesis, it still remains true that we know next to nothing about the synthesis of the hemoglobin molecules. We are not even certain how much of this is done in the bone marrow and how much may be done in other portions of the body.

Required Factors

Any list of those factors required for synthesis for hemoglobin could be dragged out interminably by adding the name of every known chemical compound which is required in human nutrition. Actually, there are only a few positively known factors which absolutely must be present if red blood cells are to be manufactured. They are as follows:

1. Adequate foodstuff. The intake of proteins and possibly carbohydrates is necessary for the formation of the hemoglobin molecule. However, we practically never see an anemia that could be based on inadequate intake of these basic compounds. It has been demonstrated experimentally that proteins forming hemoglobin will be taken by the bone marrow, even at the expense of a plasma protein if necessary. Except in cases of extreme starvation there is little possibility that we will ever see in the office a patient with anemia due to inadequate protein intake.

2. Iron. There is a difference between gross iron intake and the amount of utilizable or absorbable iron. On the average American diet it is practically unheard of not to get a sufficient total amount of iron for routine hematopoietic need. On the other hand, this does not mean that the diet provides enough absorable iron. Particularly in those people with poor dietary habits—the person who snatches a bite and runs—can there be a question about the adequacy of absorbable iron intake.

The human body does not store large quantities of iron, but it does reutilize the iron in hemoglobin, time and time again, so that it is only in cases of excessive blood loss or extremely low intake that iron-deficiency anemia occurs.

Cells seem to be made adequately in the absence of iron but they are deficient in hemoglobin. It is simply as if an empty package were sent through the mail. Under such circumstances one may expect lowered hemoglobin concentration and probably smaller cells than the "full" cells. This is exactly what happens.

3. There seems to be a maturation factor which has to do with controlling the proper development of the erythrocyte. This factor is probably vitamin B_{12} combined with another compound, but for the sake of simplicity we shall refer to it as B_{12}. In the absence of the factor the bone marrow functions well but does not release normal cells. The final products are "overstuffed" with hemoglobin.

4. An adequately functioning bone marrow is, of course, a primary requirement for erythrocyte formation.

These four factors, adequate protein foodstuffs, iron, B_{12}, and a properly functioning bone marrow, are positive essentials for the formation of red blood cells. In considering them from the standpoint of pathology, one may eliminate the first and thereby arrive at three basic factors in consideration of the anemias.

There must be (1) adequate utilizable iron, (2) adequate maturation factor, and (3) adequate bone marrow. Carrying this simple idea still further, one might actually classify the anemias due to deficient formation as those resulting from iron lack, maturation factor lack, and bone marrow damage. This is not a good scientific classification but it is an excellent working device.

Control of Hematopoiesis

Assuming adequacy of the necessary building factors, we next have to answer the question of just what controls the formation of erythrocytes. How does the bone marrow know when to stop or when extra cells are needed?

At least a hundred factors are known that have something to do with the rate of cell formation, but basically the most important factor seems to be that of oxygen tension. If erythrocytes are normal the degree of oxygenation of any tissue is related proportionately to the number of circulating red blood cells in approximation to it. For example, take the heart muscle. Each red cell has a certain capacity to supply oxygen. Each red cell that passes the heart muscle can supply oxygen to that muscle in proportion to its hemoglobin content. If a number of red cells containing adequate hemoglobin pass by, the muscle will be adequately oxygenated. If only a few red cells pass by it will not be adequately oxygenated.

It is possible to have an anemia so pronounced that the heart muscle cannot be adequately oxygenated after minor exertion. In such a case anginal pain occurs in the absence of damage to the coronary arteries.

It has been proved time and time again that the bone marrow is exquisitely sensitive to oxygen tension. A slight reduction in oxygen supply will stimulate it to produce more red blood cells and an increase in oxygen supply will cause a slight but measurable depression in the production of erythrocytes. For working purposes we can assume that the production of erythrocytes is an inverse function of oxygen tension, provided the factors discussed in the preceding section are normal.

Microscopic Appearance

Since the early stem cells are seldom seen in the office laboratory and are most difficult to identify they will not be discussed here. The first cell in the chain—which is rarely seen in the circulation—is the early normoblast. It is approximately three times the diameter of a red blood cell and looks like this:

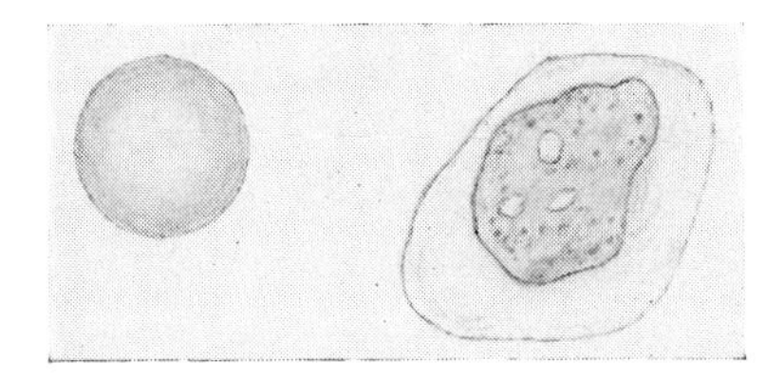

A typical red blood cell is shown for comparison.

Notice the knobby-appearing nucleus and the lack of nucleoli. The cytoplasm of this cell, since it contains little hemoglobin, usually stains a moderately dense blue.

Next in line is the intermediate normoblast which looks like this:

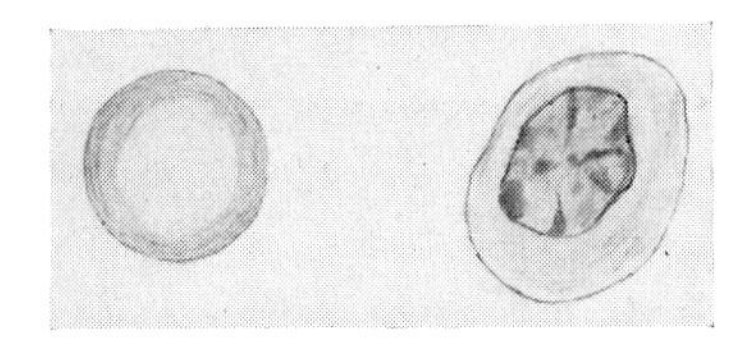

The nucleus is increasingly smaller and the cytoplasm has begun to lose its blue-staining properties. This cell is sometimes found in the circulating blood when the bone marrow is extremely hyperactive.

The late normoblast, which is simply a further progression, is a still smaller cell that by now contains much hemoglobin and therefore shows pinkish staining of the cytoplasm. It looks like this:

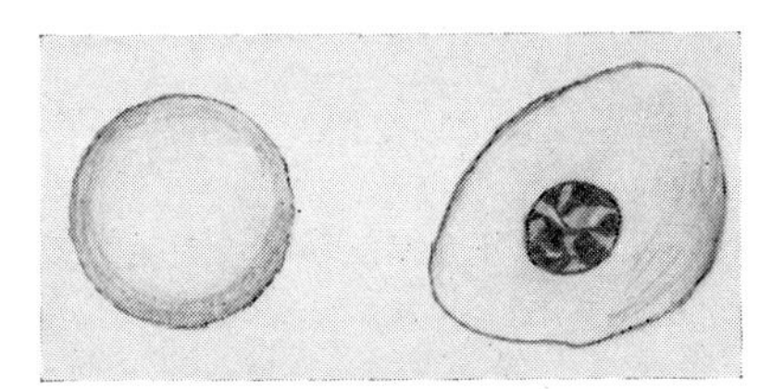

The nucleus is small and gives the impression of being densely packed. Such a cell may be seen in the process of extrusion of the nucleus or with obvious fragmentation of the nucleus. They are often found in the circulating blood when hematopoiesis is active.

The next cell in the series is the reticulocyte which is simply a red blood cell still showing some fragments of nuclear material and looks like this:

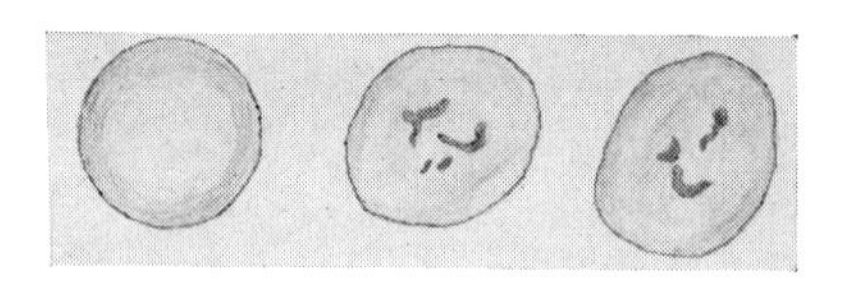

These fragments of material usually leave within a short time after the cell is extruded into the circulation.

Normal peripheral blood usually contains from 1 to 2 per cent of reticulocytes. When there is a deficiency in blood formation, the number of reticulocytes may be so small as not to be calculable, and when there is extreme active hematopoiesis the per cent may rise as high as 20 per cent or more.

The final result, the normal erythrocyte, is so well known that it needs no comment here.

Abnormal Cells

In the absence of proper maturation factors, a completely different chain of development takes place. This is characterized by two particular findings. The first is the large size of the cells in the developmental chain and the second is that hemoglobinization of the cytoplasm takes place quicker than the nuclear development. This means that the nucleus does not become compact as quickly as it does in normal maturation processes and that throughout the process it is relatively immature. These cells are called megaloblasts.

This is a normal early normoblast with an early megaloblast drawn to the right of it for comparison:

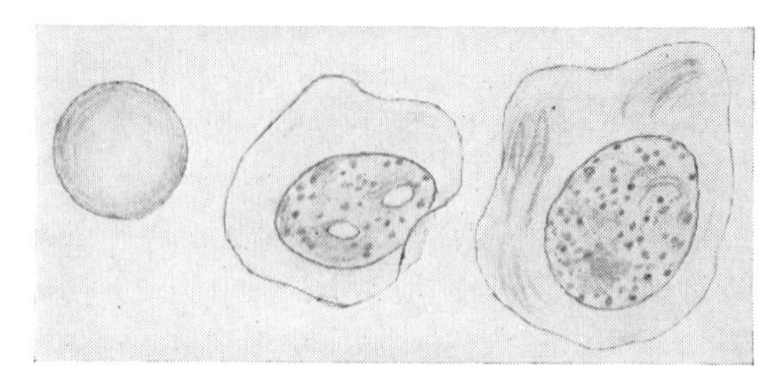

The practitioner will practically never see such an early megaloblast in the blood stream.

This is a late normoblast compared with a late megaloblast:

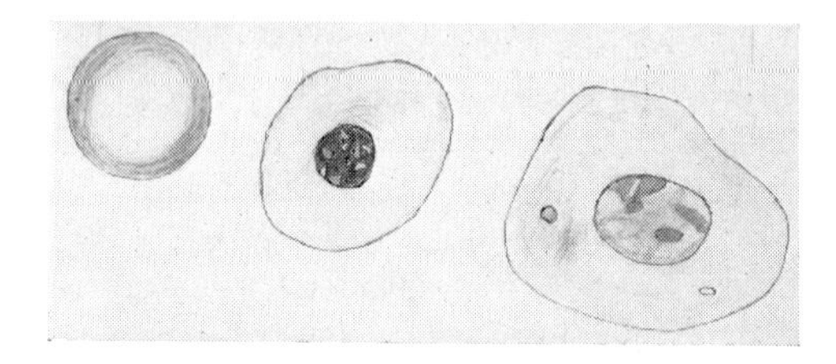

Notice particularly the megaloblastic nucleus. Both cells have pink-staining cytoplasm and a normal complement of hemoglobin, but the nuclear changes in the megaloblast are lagging behind.

The final result is a megalocyte, a macrocytic, often hyperchromic, cell.

In actual practice it seems difficult for the average physician to interpret the finer changes in red cell structure. Actually, if one can appreciate gross changes one can do much toward proper hematologic diagnosis and treatment. Summarized in pictorial form, here is a good standard to follow:

These are erythrocytes in normal size and coloration. Ordinarily no treatment is needed in the presence of such erythrocytes.

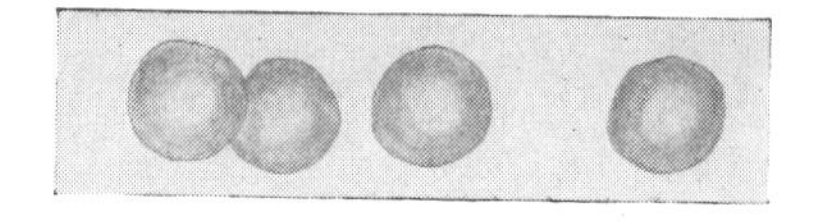

Next are macrocytic hyperchromic cells. Actually the hyperchromia may be relative due to the size and thickness of the cells, but at least they are macrocytes, and factors containing vitamin B_{12} are the proper treatment.

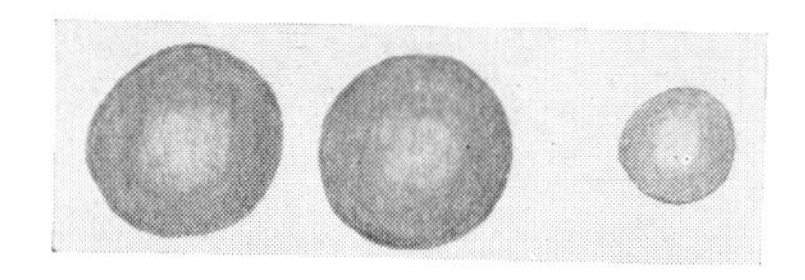

These cells are normal in size but hypochromic. Iron is the indicated treatment.

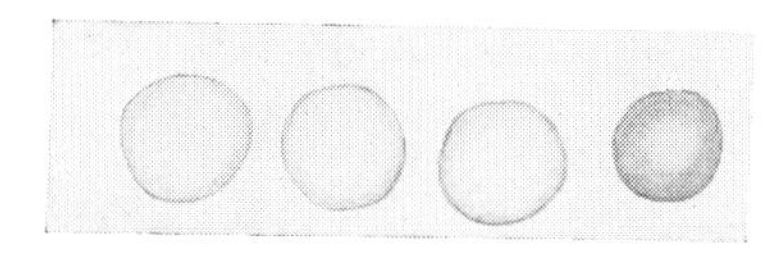

These cells are microcytic and hypochromic. Iron is usually the desired treatment.

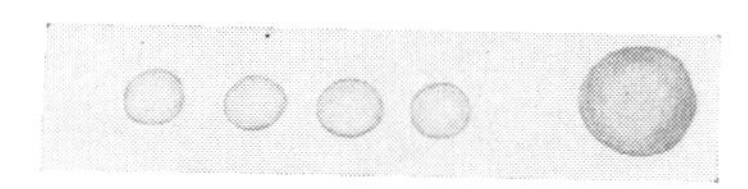

These cells are macrocytic but hypochromic. When such a rare combination is seen, usually both liver and iron are indicated.

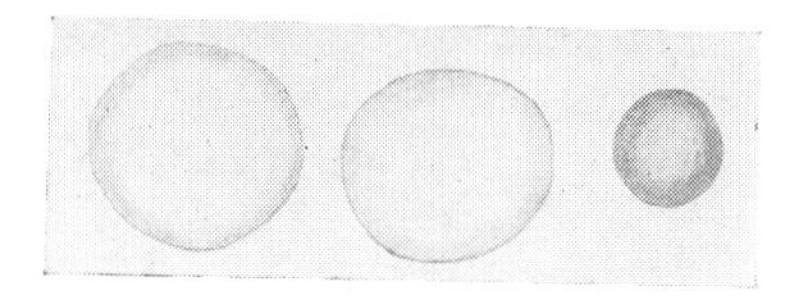

Reticulocytes

The presence of reticulocytes simply indicates that the bone marrow is in the process of manufacturing red blood cells. In the normal person there will be 2 per cent or less of such reticulated cells in the general circulation. If there should be more than 2 per cent, one may assume an abnormally intense reaction of the bone marrow, of which there are several possible causes.

The most frequent consideration, of course, is the response to treatment for anemia. The drugs which usually engender a reticulocyte response do not often do so in a patient with adequate circulating hemoglobin. The anemic patient, on the other hand, will show a reticulocyte response within one week if the treatment is adequate. If such a response does not occur, one may assume that the treatment is inadequate or, possibly, the diagnosis is improper. In the small office this is perhaps the greatest use of the reticulocyte count. If anemia is severe this procedure is very much indicated.

In the otherwise normal person, when one suspects but cannot prove the presence of hemorrhage, a reticulocyte response in the peripheral blood is an excellent indication that such hemorrhage has occurred. A good example would be the girl who states that she had a prolonged menstrual period, and actually looks tired and weak, but who violently denies that she had a uterine hemorrhage. A reticulocyte response is definite evidence of bleeding over and above normal.

Another typical example would be the suspected but unproved gastrointestinal hemorrhage. In actual practice this is seldom of much moment, but in an occasional case it is a valuable point to remember.

Also in the occasional case in which the bone marrow is severely encroached upon by some invasive process an increase in reticulocytes indicates that the remaining normal marrow is at least making an attempt to keep up with the demand for erythrocytes.

In general, the only real value of the reticulocyte count in the office laboratory is to assess the treatment of anemia.

Interpretation of Findings

Detailed hematologic interpretation is not within the competence of the average office laboratory. There are certain basic facts, however, that any practitioner should be able to elicit from the study of stained smears.

These are best studied from the standpoint of etiology.

Iron deficiency. Blood findings reveal that the process of iron deficiency, no matter what the cause, passes through three stages:

First, the cells are manufactured in a normal number and contain a normal amount of hemoglobin, but they are smaller than usual. The red cells look like this:

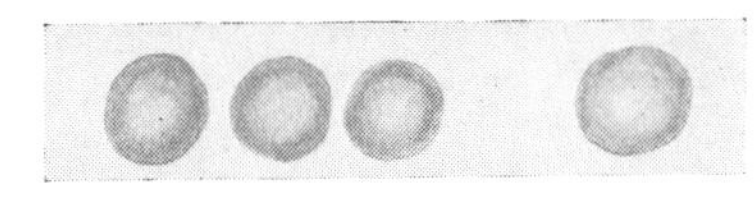

Only a person skilled in hematologic interpretation will detect an iron deficiency at this stage. It cannot often be done in the office laboratory.

Second, as hemoglobin synthesis becomes more and more impaired, not enough of the compound is manufactured to "fill up" the microcytic cells and a hypochromia results. Even at this point enough erythrocytes are being made so that the count remains relatively high, usually in the 4.2 to 4.5 million area. The blood cells look like this:

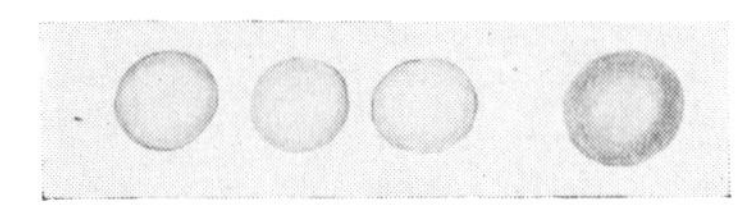

Hemoglobin, determined in grams per 100 ml., drops while the number of cells remains high. This results in a lowering of the mean corpuscular hemoglobin concentration (page 102) and gives a tip-off to the type of anemia with which one is dealing.

It also reveals a pernicious error in the red blood count, for the count at this stage remains relatively normal. Incidentally, most patients are seen by physicians at about this point.

The third stage is that in which microcytic and hypochromic cells are the rule and in which there begins a drop in the number of total red blood cells. Few patients progress to this stage before being seen. Those patients who usually do progress the furthest before medical advice is sought are the ones with "milk anemias" from childhood. There is an unfortunate impression among a segment of people that milk represents the perfect food for the infant and growing child. In some ways this is true, but it does not supply sufficient iron. Some of the most vicious anemias we have ever seen are in this category.

In examining the blood smear from such a case, one should not be confused by the presence of occasional macrocytes or abnormal forms. Microcytic, hypochromic cells predominate and can scarcely be mistaken.

Reticulocytes are normal or reduced in number. In the earlier cases they usually range from 1 to 2 per cent, but in later cases they become progressively more rare.

Treatment of such a patient may be followed with great accuracy by periodic reticulocyte counts. After the administration of adequate quantities of iron the reticulocytes usually begin to increase within three days. Within a week or ten days the response reaches its height.

The extent of the reticulocyte response should be related in inverse ratio to the hemoglobin level. The lower the original hemoglobin level, the higher the response may be expected to be. A typical response is this one:

	Hb	R (%)
Original determination	8.2	1
3 days of treatment	8.1	3
6 days of treatment	8.4	11
11 days of treatment	9.1	8
15 days of treatment	9.8	6
22 days of treatment	10.2	3

During such a response to treatment an occasional normoblast may be seen in the peripheral blood. It has no particular significance other than to show that the marrow is exhibiting a marked response.

Megaloblastic anemias. Interference with normal cell maturation is the principal characteristic of these anemias, the best example of which is typical pernicious anemia. Clinically, they are characterized by the extreme grades of anemia which may develop before symptoms cause the patient to seek medical advice.

Seldom is such a case seen before the red count has dropped below 2.5 million and patients may not seek advice until the count is lower than 1.0 million. For this reason we will describe the blood findings as seen in such an advanced case.

Early in the disease only an occasional macrocyte is seen, but usually by the time the office laboratory is called into use the majority of cells are macrocytic. As the anemia gets progressively worse, poikilocytosis becomes more and more pronounced. Cells assume fantastic and "lopsided" shapes, but all are well filled with hemoglobin.

A typical blood smear looks like this:

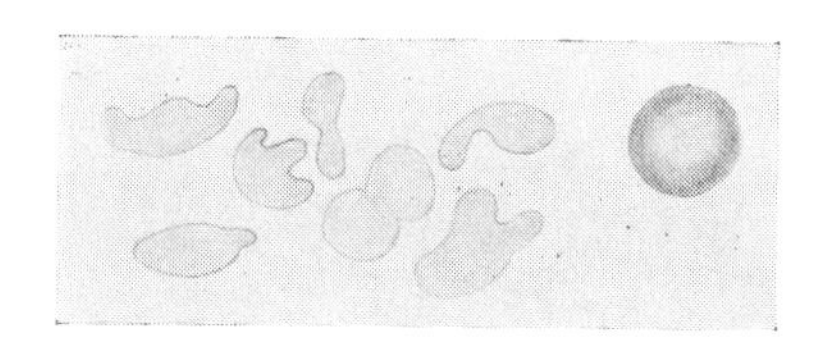

Careful search of the peripheral blood usually will reveal a few megaloblasts which look like this:

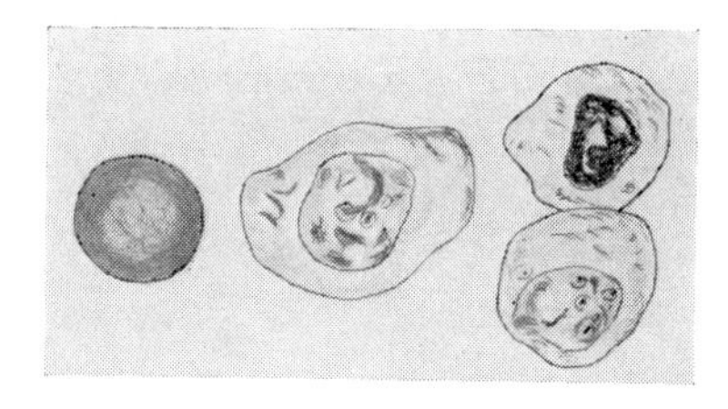

Since the cells carry much hemoglobin the MCHC is increased to above 35 or 36.

If there are many nucleated forms before treatment is started, a bad prognosis may be assumed, and immediate transfusion is the procedure of choice. Such a picture usually indicates a final gallant effort on the part of the marrow to keep up with demand.

The same phenomenon in the presence of adequate treatment may be taken to mean an adequate response and nothing else. When liver or vitamin B_{12} is given, the result may be followed with great accuracy by means of the reticulocyte count.

Reticulocyte response is actually somewhat slower in the megaloblastic anemias but tends to persevere longer. This is a typical chart:

DAYS OF TREATMENT	Hb	R (%)
0	7.4	1.1
3	7.5	1.4
6	7.5	3.2
10	8.0	6.4
15	8.4	11.0
22	9.1	10.6
30	10.2	5.7
40	12.6	3.0

In following a typical case one should remember that the first sign of relapse is the appearance of a few macrocytes in the blood. Even before there is anemia sufficient to allow diagnosis, circulating macrocytes increase in number. Treatment should be aimed at relief of all clinical signs *and* establishment of a blood picture in which macrocytes are excessively rare.

Infections. Anemia is almost a characteristic finding in any severe and long-continued infection. Investigations have indicated but have not proved that there is a fundamental interference with hemoglobin synthesis.

Most such anemias are normocytic and normochromic. The blood picture is in no way abnormal except for the scarcity of erythrocytes and the relative or absolute increase of leukocytes. In cases of long-standing, a hypochromic, microcytic anemia may develop, but this usually takes from thirty to one hundred twenty days and there will be no doubt as to the cause of the anemia.

It is noteworthy that the usual therapeutic agents give little or no reticulocyte response in such a case.

Other normocytic, normochromic anemias involving hemolytic disease, etc., are scarcely within the province of the office laboratory.

Aplastic anemias show uniform reduction of both erythrocytes and leukocytes. Usually they are normocytic and normochromic. There is, of course, a relative lymphocytosis. The only problem in diagnosis is differentiation of aleukemic, chronic, lymphoid leukemia. In this disease there are signs of attempted red cell regeneration, while in aplastic anemia such signs are absent.

Comment

From the amount written (and from the material presented here) one would think that the anemias are a major problem in clinical practice. Actually the average practitioner sees perhaps one puzzling anemia case per year.

An accurate history will make the diagnosis in the great majority of cases, though it certainly must be confirmed by other means. The simple MCHC (page 102) will separate the anemias into three great classes:

Below 30, iron deficiency

30 to 36, normochromic, normocytic; probably chronic infection

Above 36, macrocytic, hyperchromic; to be treated with liver or vitamin B_{12}

A therapeutic trial should be made with the indicated medication and followed by reticulocyte counts. If a reticulocytic reaction fails to occur within the specified time, a further careful search should be made for etiologic factors.

It is just that simple.

LYMPHOCYTES

If there is one theoretically known fact about the lymphocytes that has not been seriously questioned, I do not know what it is. Our information about these cells is woefully inadequate. While it is possible to draw some inferences from their microscopic appearance and number, one should remember that our lack of knowledge makes detailed interpretation difficult.

Maturation

The lymphocytes are formed principally in lymph glands throughout the body. Some hematologists contend that there are foci of lymphoblastic tissue of the bone marrow, which may or may not be true.

We are not even positive of the exact precursor of the lymphocytes, but the later steps in their development are fairly well known. The cell which should be known to the practitioner is the lymphoblast and looks like this:

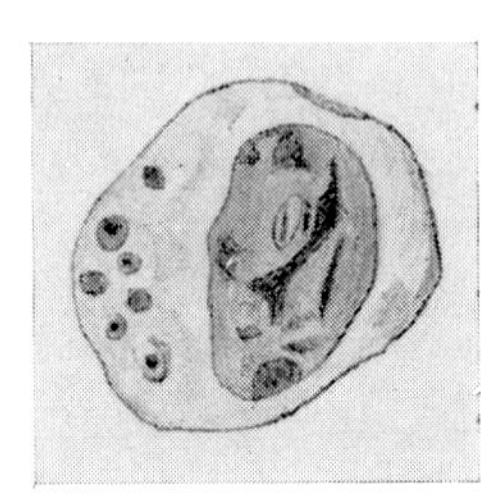

The lymphoblast and myeloblast, which are precursors of the granulocytes, are astonishingly similar. Here is a drawing of a lymphoblast and a myeloblast side by side:

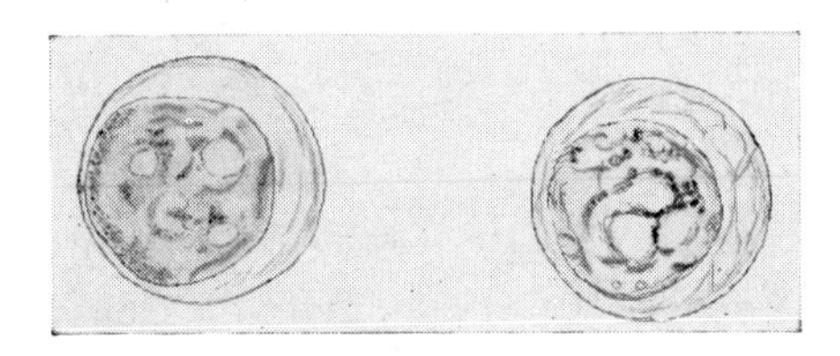

Notice that the nuclear structure of the lymphoblast is coarser than that of the myeloblast. Now notice the clear-cut nuclear

membrane in the lymphoblast and the feathery irregular edge of the nucleus of the myeloblast. Notice, too, that the nucleoli of the myeloblast are indistinct, with feathery edges and a rather mottled look to the cytoplasm, whereas the nucleoli in the lymphoblast are clear-cut and stain a faint sky-blue.

Even with these points of differentiation it often becomes a matter for the expert hematologist rather than the practitioner to tell the difference between these cells. The important point of differentiation is in aleukemic leukemias, and clinical symptoms usually serve to differentiate the lymphocytic from the myelocytic type.

In the chain of development the next cell after the lymphoblast is a large lymphocyte which is found in small numbers in the general circulation. It shows an abundance of pale blue cytoplasm in which an occasional small granule may be seen and a dense dark-staining nucleus like this:

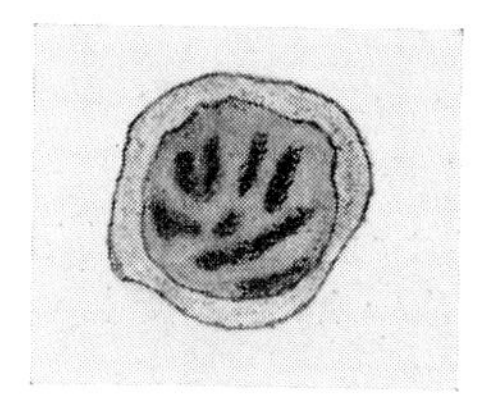

It is assumed that when these cells age they form the typical small lymphocytes with which we are all familiar.

If this represents a true picture of the development and aging of the lymphocyte, then the large lymphocyte has somewhat the same connotation as do reticulocytes in the ordinary circulation. The number indicates the relative activity of the lymph glands in providing young cells.

We do not know the exact fate of the lymphocyte. Large numbers are lost by migration into the intestinal tract, but it has been proved that destruction must take place in other sites. Recent studies would indicate that the life of a typical lymphocyte ranges from twelve to twenty-four hours, so that there is almost a complete daily turnover in the circulation.

Known Physiology

Here we come upon a stumbling block of importance, for little is known about the function of these cells. Probably they are active in tissue repair.

During the reconstructive stage of any pathologic process, including inflammation, wounds, and infection, there is invasion of the damaged tissue by lymphocytes. Some authorities feel that their role in tissue repair is essential; others label it more as incidental.

Apparently the lymphocytes are concerned in the manufacture of antibodies. Cytochemical methods have demonstrated this, but it would seem that in view of their short life and the relatively long time it takes to form the circulating antibody this is an unusual function, if true. Nonetheless, we have the immutable fact that cytochemical processes indicate antibody formation by lymphocytes.

The cells do contain globin which is concerned in immune reaction. Other than this we can say little about their function.

Abnormal Cells

Only one real abnormality of interest in the laboratory occurs so far as the lymphocytes are concerned. That is the presence of blast cells in the general circulation. Here is a blood smear showing several normal mature lymphocytes and a blast form:

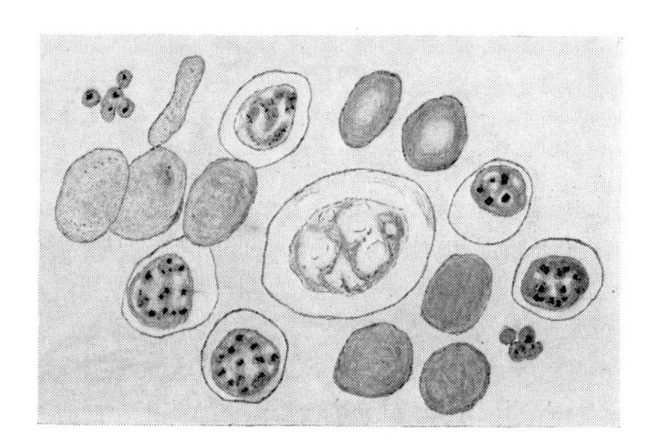

Lymphatic Leukemia

Acute lymphatic leukemia is considered to be the most common form of acute leukemia which we see. It has an age incidence almost altogether in children under 5 years of age and, incidentally, an interesting point is the fact that nearly one third of the cases are aleukemic leukemia.

The blood changes in the leukemic phase are so obvious that diagnosis in excessively easy. The count usually ranges around 60 to 80 thousand per cubic millimeter and lymphocytes make up more than 95 per cent of the white blood cells. A great many of these cells are of the blast series.

Occasionally, but not often, a supravital stain with Janus green and neutral red as described on page 108 will be of service.

The supravitally stained lymphoblast has mitochondria at least twice as big (and often larger) as those of the myeloblast and approximately half the number. This one point in the mitochondrial differences in supravital staining will serve to differentiate clearly these two types of cells.

As the cell matures, neutral red bodies may begin to appear. This is a typical supravitally stained lymphoblast and myeloblast:

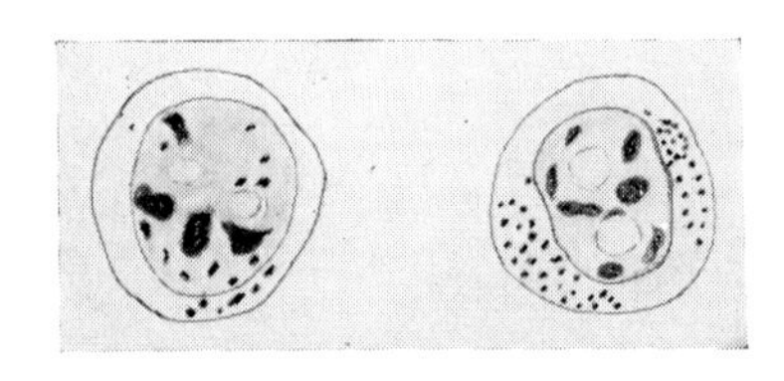

In examining peripheral blood of children one should never forget that whooping cough and occasionally infectious mononucleosis will cause an extremely high lymphocyte count, with rare blast forms in the circulating blood. Clinical differentiation is usually easy and one should not be stampeded into making a diagnosis on the basis of a high white blood count.

Chronic lymphatic leukemia is a disease often found in older people. The commonest incidence is in the 60's and patients are seldom seen before the age of 35.

The white blood count is strikingly variable but usually ranges from 50,000 to 150,000 per cubic millimeter. There are few blast forms.

In all cases the predominant cell is the small lymphocyte and these often appear to be more fragile than normal, sometimes bursting when a smear is made and giving an appearance like this:

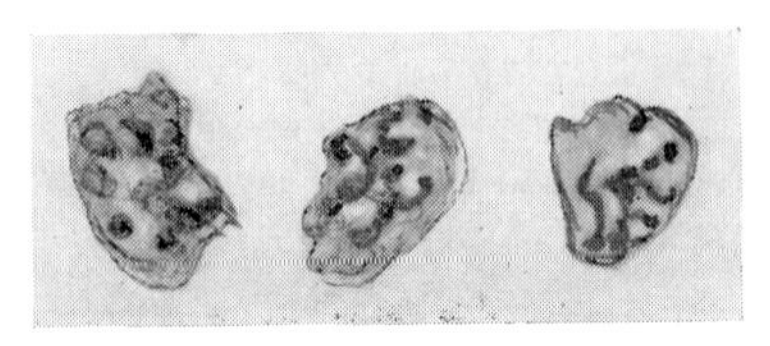

The diagnosis of this disease is actually more of a clinical problem than a hematologic problem. Given an extremely high white blood count with at least 90 per cent small lymphocytes, one may assume chronic lymphatic leukemia and begin clinical search for the well-known signs.

When blast cells are found in the circulating blood, they have a bad prognostic significance.

Either the acute or chronic form may go through an aleukemic stage. In acute aleukemic leukemia careful search of the peripheral blood will still usually show an occasional blast form and furnish a tip-off to the diagnosis. In the aleukemic stages of the chronic form, on the other hand, blast forms may be extremely rare and bone marrow biopsy may be necessary to make the diagnosis.

Ordinarily the reading of bone marrow smears is not in the province of the office laboratory, but the slides may be taken, fixed, and stained with Geimsa before being sent to the nearest hematologist.

It is well to make several slides, sending two to the hematologist and retaining two for office use. Take his report and carefully work out his findings while examining the slides yourself. In a period of a year or so you will be doing excellent, though amateur, hematology.

EOSINOPHILS

Eosinophils are produced from myeloid tissue exactly as the neutrophils. This is mentioned in brief detail in the next section. Certain characteristics of these cells are important.

The granules are big. Ordinary polymorphonuclear leukocytes contain granules, some of which will stain red, and it is not rare for physicians to mistake eosinophils for such cells. As a comparative device, if the average polymorphonuclear granule were the size of a baseball, then the eosinophil granule would be at least the size of a basketball. There is actually that much difference in granular size.

Eosinophils often have the typical spectacle nucleus like this:

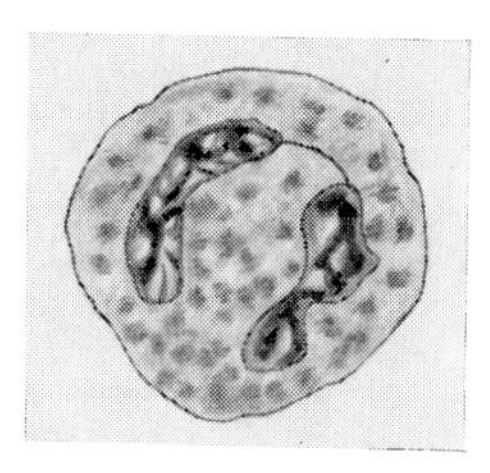

Occasionally one will see a single-lobed or a trilobed nucleus in the eosinophil, but most of them are of the typical spectacle arrangement.

The cells are in some way related to allergic reactions and contain histamine. They are usually increased in various allergies. This point is of some diagnostic value. An increase in circulating eosinophils should suggest (1) direct allergic disease such as bronchial asthma or hay fever, and (2) parasitic infections, particularly with intestinal helminths.

In acute infections it is customary for the eosinophils to be greatly diminished or even to disappear from the circulating blood. Why, we do not know. As convalescence begins, the eosinophils return. Perhaps a personal example of this might be of interest:

I attended medical school before penicillin and the other antibiotics were in use. One of my professors was capable of making absolutely astounding prognoses in cases of acute lobar pneumonia. As the crisis approached he would take a drop of the patient's blood and study it intensely for several minutes. Then he would say decisively, "This patient will live" or "This patient will die." He was right so much of the time that we suspected him of some form of necromancy. After puzzling us for some time, he let us in on the secret. He was simply looking for the eosinophils. When these cells return, the prognosis is good. If there are no eosinophils present when the crisis approaches, the prognosis is bad.

If the pituitary gland is functioning adequately the number of circulating eosinophils is depressed by the administration of epinephrine. This can be the basis for the test for pituitary function, but in actual practice the clinical differentiation is just as easy as interpreting the results of this test.

POLYMORPHONUCLEAR NEUTROPHIL

In other portions of this chapter we have covered briefly the developmental cycle of some typical blood cells. The neutrophils, of course, follow the same cycle as all myeloid tissue and are derived from the primitive myeloblasts, going through these phases:

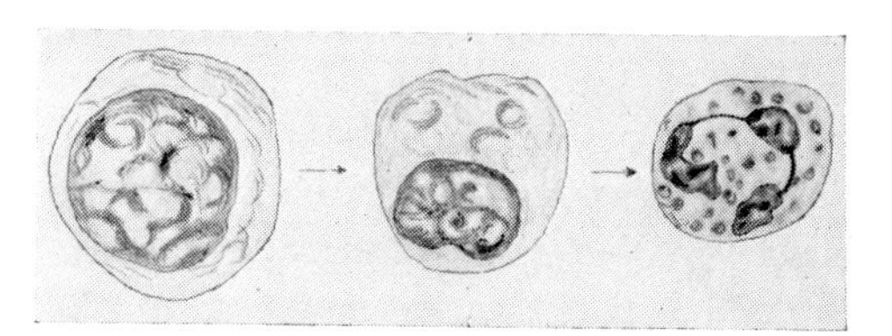

Polymorphonuclear neutrophils are actively motile, phagocytic cells which apparently put up an active defense against invasion by bacteria. Not only do they attack bacteria cells enzymatically but they also actually ingest and seemingly digest bacteria. Many other important functions have been attributed to these cells, but from the standpoint of the average practice they are the principal internal defense of the body against invasion by pathogens.

The relationship of the white blood count to infection will be mentioned in the next section. Here, we are concerned with abnormal forms that occur in the circulating blood in the leukemias.

Myeloid Leukemia

The acute myeloid leukemias are about one third aleukemic and are seen most frequently in children and young adults. They may, however, be seen throughout life. For some reason which we do not understand this disease seems to be becoming more frequent. Practitioners of a generation or two ago lived an entire medical life without seeing more than one or two cases. Now you may expect, with confidence, several cases each year. Why, no one knows.

The total leukocyte count is usually about 40,000 per cubic millimeter but varies greatly from day to day.

The disease is simple to diagnose because myeloblasts make up from 60 to 80 per cent of the circulating white cells and the majority of adult white cells in the circulation are polymorphonuclears. With careful examination one can usually find myeloid cells undergoing division in the peripheral blood.

Even in the aleukemic form a careful search will usually reveal an occasional blast cell. One does see cases in which diagnosis is not possible without bone marrow studies. In general, even a cursory examination of a well-prepared blood smear will allow accurate diagnosis. A typical picture is this one:

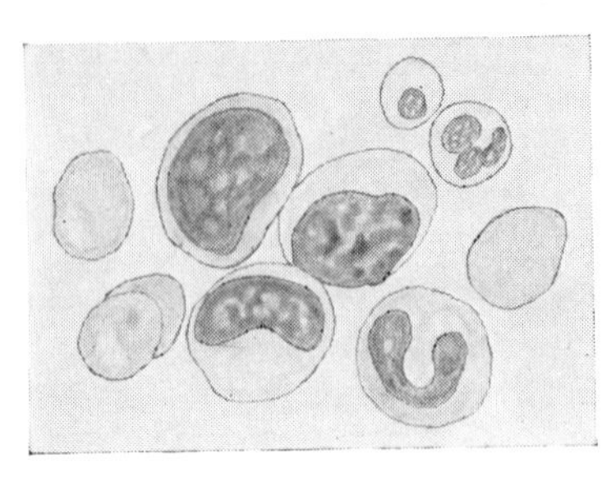

Chronic myeloid leukemia occurs more frequently in persons between 55 and 80 years.

The disease has the highest average white blood cell count of any of the leukemias and it is not unusual to find more than a quarter of a million white cells per cubic millimeter in the general circulation. Of the myeloid cells, usually at least 20 per cent will be immature forms which, again, makes the diagnosis easy. A typical field looks like this:

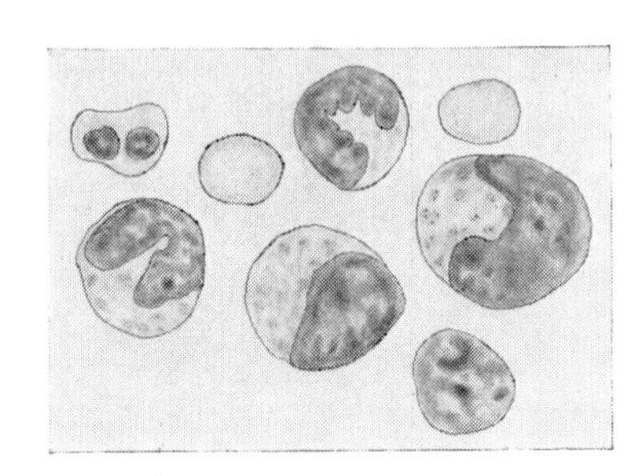

An increasing number of myeloblastic forms indicates a poor prognosis and a significant number of cases terminate with a myeloblastic crisis.

WHITE BLOOD CELL COUNT

Many times our crude attempts at precise mathematical delineation of medical findings merely obscure the picture we seek to see. The differential count is sometimes a good example of this.

Almost limitless information is available from examination of the stained smear and sometimes the general expressions of an experienced hematologist are of more value than any precise numerical determination. It is as if one were to try analysis of a Goya painting by mathematics. Of course, it could be done, but the over-all effect of the picture might be more marred than helped by the mathematical analysis.

Let me give you an example. How would you express in mathematical terms this meaningful but slightly silly phrase: "These poor old beat-up polys look like they had gone through the Battle of Bull Run?" I know only too well that many qualified hematologists would shudder at such an asinine statement, but it means more to me than a count of nuclear lobes and a bare statement that toxic granulations are present.

The point is this: The blood smear is a natural picture reflecting momentary changes in body economy and stating with the sublime artistry of nature a concise picture of bodily conditions. As such, it is not fully subject to mathematical pronouncements.

This does not mean that mathematical readings should not be taken. Let your technician make them all, but learn to look at the cells yourself.

Maturation

For purposes of discussion and without naming the various forms, the white blood cells go through the following stages in aging:

This is the youngest normal cell:

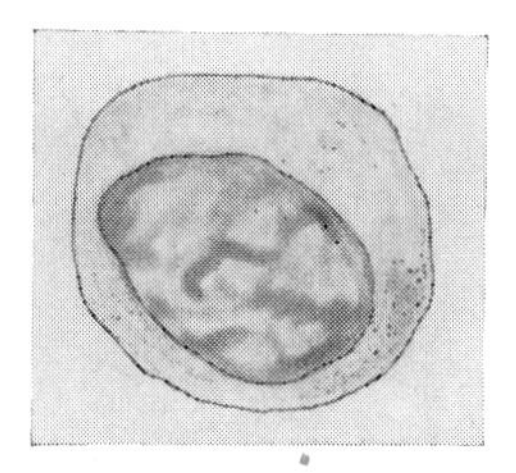

Then the nucleus begins to segment.

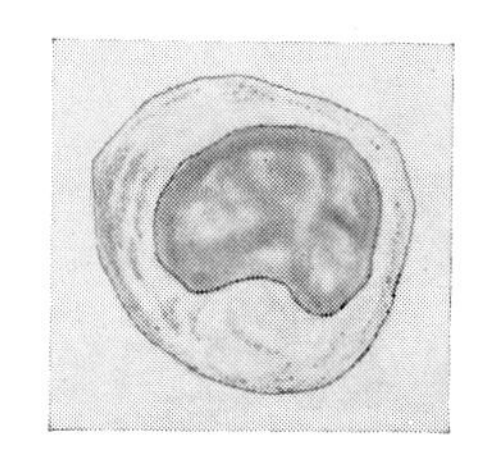

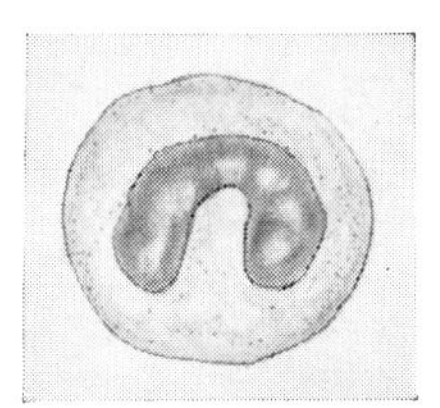

Segmentation increases.

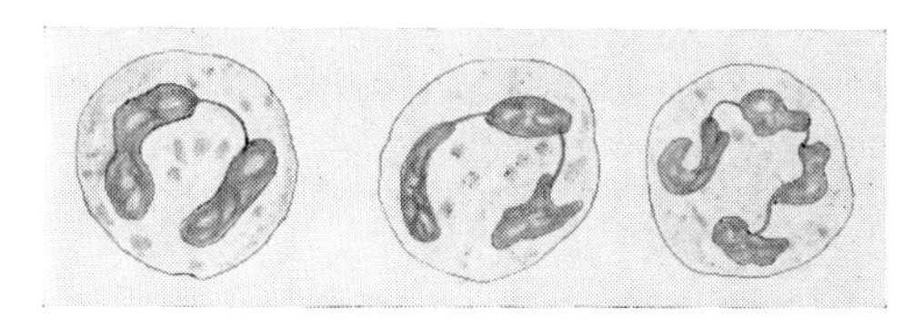

At this stage the cells usually disappear from the circulation. During infectious processes the cells may be injured. The first sign is toxic granulation like this:

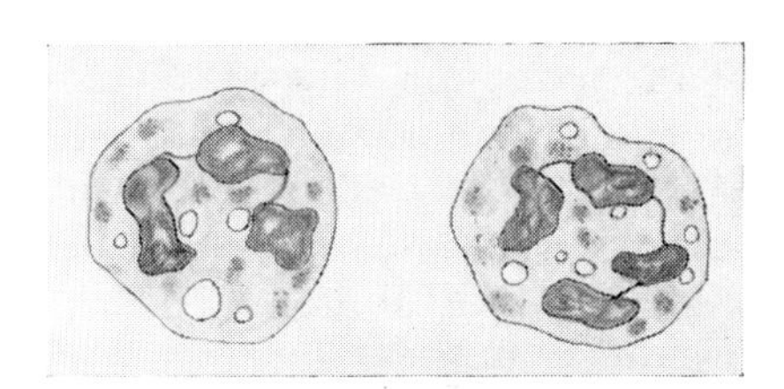

Then the cells actually disintegrate like this:

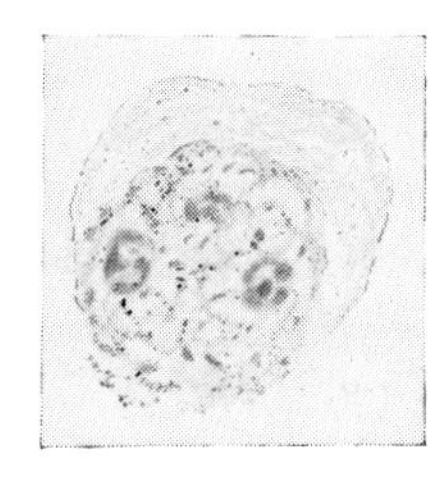

Technique

The technique of white blood cell counting has been specified on page 25 and the technique of making blood smears on page 107.

Errors

Actually the principal error in interpreting the differential count and the smear is an attempt to mathematize, which excludes common sense interpretation.

Interpretation

Although the physiologic background is sketchy, to say the least, one may separate blood count reactions into three specific categories.

1. Mobilization. Any potentially stressful situation produces a general mobilization of white blood cells. This, of course, includes cells of the lymphocytic series as well as granulocytes. An example would be a cold bath which may run the white blood count up to as much as 20,000. Careful analysis of the smears will show that these cells are mostly mature forms and that the proportion betwen lymphocytes and polymorphonuclear leukocytes remains the same. A heavy meal will do the same thing. So will pain.

When one sees an increased number of white blood cells, most of the cells being fully mature and the differential count remaining in approximately the 70-30 range, one should be chary of diagnosing anything except a stressful situation.

It is certainly true that in the early stages of some infections traumatic episodes and other entities may begin as essentially stressful situations, *but one cannot make any other interpretation* in the presence of an increased mobilization of relatively mature cells.

Here is a clinical example:

A 15-year-old girl was seen with pain in the right lower quadrant. There was no rigidity and only tenderness on deep palpation. The white blood count was 14,000, with a 70-30 differential, and upon examining the cells they were found to be largely mature with only a few young forms and no "old beat-up cells."

The diagnosis is probably Mittelschmerz with trivial chemical peritonitis. A stressful situation, this time a chemical insult, has been inaugurated and the body has met it by mobilization of existing white blood cells without calling forth any additional manufacture of new cells.

2. Manufacture of new cells. In the case of infectious disease these cells are, of course, usually polymorphonuclear leukocytes. When this second type of reaction occurs one may assume the presence of inflammatory, *not necessarily infectious,* disease. The differential count rises in favor of the polymorphonuclears, a moderate process usually evoking a response of approximately 80-20 and a severe process of 90-10 or greater. Such a response indicates a serious enough insult that not only are cells mobilized but also new cells are released from the bone marrow to meet the threat. Careful examination of the blood smear usually shows a number of young cells much greater than normally found, often as many as 20 per cent or more.

The body is actually meeting the insult for the present, at least, but such a count should indicate to the physician that he must soon know what the pathology is and take care to meet it with therapeutic effort if needed.

3. The third type of reaction is when the cells literally become "beat-up." Toxic granulation appears in a variable percentage of the cells and, at times, older cells are seen to begin fragmentation.

The number of cells exhibiting toxic granulation is a fairly good prognostic device. In ordinary moderately severe infections this number seldom exceeds 25 to 35 per cent. In definitely dangerous infections as many as 50 per cent of the cells may look weather-worn. Should about 75 per cent of the cells begin to show damage, then a dangerous stage has been reached. Unless treatment is immediate, vigorous, and successful the patient will probably die.

Here, again, I have committed the error of trying to classify in the old one-two-three order. Actually the blood picture is one of shading rather than one of positive numerical quality. If you learn to examine your own smears and examine them carefully, you will see, first, this mobilization of available white blood cells, the manufacture of new cells with increasing numbers of "youngsters"; then there will be degenerative changes and, finally, signs of bone marrow exhaustion when the youngsters no longer appear and old cells are damaged past the point of adequate function.

At the risk of being boresomely repetitious, I cannot emphasize too strongly that the picture is more important in diagnosis and treatment than is any mathematical analysis.

Lymphocytes are concerned with reparative processes and with immunologic reaction. From the standpoint of the differential smear, we are mainly interested in lymphocyte increases, as they indicate the existence of these reparative processes.

Actually a true increase in lymphocytes is a rarity during the acute phase of any disease. Perhaps the principal exception is whooping cough.

During the active stage of repair, however, an absolute lymphocytosis is common.

CHAPTER EIGHT

The Sputum

Few tests done on sputum in the office laboratory are of much value. Gross examination, determination of the relative eosinophil count, examination for heart failure cells, and the examination for tubercle bacilli are the important procedures.

GROSS EXAMINATION

Many of the gross observations upon the sputum as it appears in any transparent in the past actually have little value. A few signs, however, will give worth-while information.

Technique

Actually all that is needed is to observe the sputum as it appears in any transparent container. If there is any doubt, pour a little into a Petri dish and hold the dish over a black background.

Errors

The most frequent mistake is perhaps to read too much into the findings.

Interpretation

Copious production of foamy sputum seen to be tinged with a pink color is almost pathognomonic of cardiac decompensation. It occurs when fluid is present in the alveoli and there is diapedesis of blood due to back pressure. This finding is so specific that it can often be elicited historically without recourse to the laboratory. In an occasional case gross examination of the sputum will clarify an otherwise obscure diagnosis.

In the pneumonic process, blood in the alveoli is first of a normal color, and then an autodigestive process gradually changes the color to a russet brown about the color of a rusty nail. Sputum in early cases shows streaking with bright red blood, and as the condition progresses an admixture of rust-colored fluid. This finding is so characteristic as to be considered diagnostic of the pneumonic process and probably rightly so.

Exceptionally foul-smelling sputum containing white homogenous flecks of caseous material is characteristic of disease involving tissue destruction in the lung or bronchial tubes. It is not often seen in examinations conducted by the office laboratory.

EOSINOPHILS

Eosinophils are extruded to the surface of the mucous membranes in large numbers in the presence of various allergic conditions. Why, we do not know. Their presence in profusion is essentially diagnostic of allergy.

Technique

Make a smear of the sputum and, preferably, fix by immersion in absolute methyl alcohol. Then stain it by either Wright's or Geimsa's method and count 100 leukocytes under the microscope. From this calculate the percentage of eosinophils.

Errors

This procedure must be done on sputum while it is relatively fresh. Degenerative processes in the cells take place after an hour or so and make the examination worth progressively less and less as time passes. Other than this time factor, errors are most rare. It is important that you count only cells that show no degeneration. If there is any sign of loss of clear-cut nuclear borders of cell outline, do not count. Almost without exception there will be enough normal cells.

Interpretation

The eosonophil is a relatively rare cell in the bronchial secretions. Ordinary smears seldom show more than 1 or 2 per cent at most. In the infectious diseases the percentage is greatly lessened. Actually, in such disease, it is rare to even find an eosinophil. In allergy, on the other hand, the percentage is usually at least 10 and in some cases may run up to as much as 90 per cent.

This technique is little used in the office laboratory but it is valuable in some cases and should not be neglected. Particularly is it valuable in the case of an obscure cough which is difficult to diagnose.

HEART FAILURE CELLS

There are normally large, phagocytic cells on and about the mucous membrane of the lung and in the sputum. In any case where blood pigment is available for some time, these cells phagocytize particles of the pigment and become laden with reddish brown granules. They look like this:

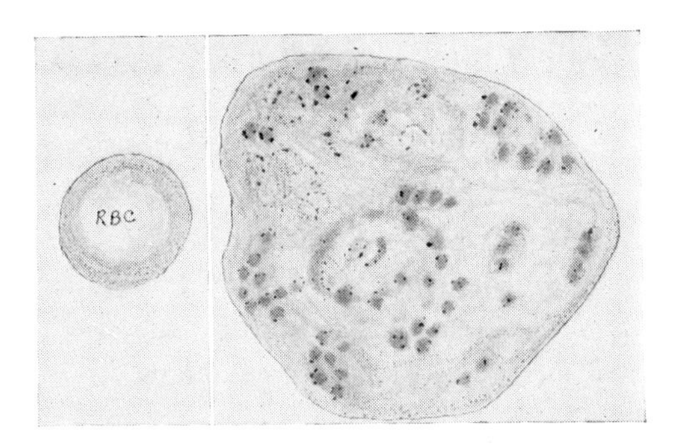

Notice that the nucleus is almost obscured by the granules and that the cells are quite large, often four to five times the diameter of a red blood cell.

Technique

Examine the sputum unstained in greatly reduced light. Cells containing particulate matter of a brown color are almost certainly heart failure cells.

Errors

Persons who work in the carboniferous industries, mines, carbon black plants, etc., often show phagocytized particles of carbon which greatly resemble the hemoglobin pigments except for their darker color.

If there is any confusion, fix the sputum with absolute alcohol. Then flood the slide with a few drops of 10 per cent potassium ferrocyanide solution for three or four minutes. Wash in tap water and put a few drops of 0.1 N hydrochloric acid on the slide for one minute. Wash again and examine. If the pigment in the cells is iron-containing (and, therefore, probably derived from hemoglobin), some of the spots will turn a bright blue.

With the crude technique used in this test, seldom do all the pigment granules turn blue. If as many as 10 per cent of them show a bluish discoloration you may assume that hemoglobin is the principal contained pigment in the cells.

Interpretation

Two relatively unimportant conditions from the standpoint of laboratory diagnosis will show deposition of pigment. They are pulmonary infarction and pulmonary hemorrhage for as long as two weeks after hemorrhage. The laboratory, of course, is of little use in diagnosing these conditions and their diagnosis by this means is, as mentioned, unimportant.

The third condition is of the utmost importance. The application of this test may result in clearing up an obscure situation that has been troublesome from a diagnostic standpoint. In even slight grades of left heart failure, there is some pulmonary congestion. Back pressure causes at least a few red blood cells to escape from normal channels and to lie free in the alveoli.

As these cells are broken up the pigment escapes and begins the process of degeneration. It is taken up by the phagocytes and the presence of such pigments is an excellent indication of mild chronic left heart failure.

TUBERCLE BACILLI

With modern methods of chemotherapy constantly being improved, we have a better understanding of how to treat tuberculosis. This disease is becoming progressively more rare. By no means should this lull the practitioner into a false sense of security. Early cases are still seen relatively often in a busy practice, particularly in some sections of the country. The office laboratory is far too seldom used in the diagnosis of tuberculosis.

Search for the tubercle bacilli is an exacting task which is useless unless carefully done. The significance of finding acid-fast rods is too well known to be discussed here.

Technique

Using an applicator stick, dish out a bit of caseous material from the sputum and smear it well on a clean slide. For several years we have used a different staining technique than the one generally accepted. It has been so reliable that we have come to depend upon it. Perhaps you may like it, too. This is it:

1. Air dry the smear for a minute or so and fix by immersion in 1 per cent aqueous bichloride of mercury. The slide should be actually submerged in a staining dish full of this solution and left for four or five minutes.

2. Wash in tap water.

3. Immerse in a staining dish full of carbofuchsin solution for approximately fifteen minutes. Heating is not necessary with this method, but the staining time will vary from batch to batch of the dye. A known positive specimen should be stained with each new batch of dye and proper time for staining determined.

4. Wash in tap water.

5. Put a few drops of acid alcohol on the slide and shake it gently and then discard the acid alcohol. Repeat this until no more stain flows from the slide when the acid alcohol is agitated gently on the surface.

Standard acid alcohol solution is made up of 3 ml. of concentrated hydrochloric acid and 97 ml. of ordinary 70 per cent alcohol.

6. Wash in tap water.

7. Counterstain for one minute with picric acid stain. This is made up of equal parts of 70 per cent alcohol and saturated aqueous solution of picric acid.

The picric acid stain will make a faint yellow background but will not selectively stain either bacteria or cells. Acid-fast bacilli appear as bright red rods against this faint yellow background. They are more prominent when stained by this procedure than when stained by the conventional carbofuchsin–methylene blue technique.

Errors

The most common error is to mistake a fleck of degenerating food from between the teeth for caseous material. Warn the patient during the time he is collecting the sputum to brush his teeth thoroughly and often and not to expectorate material from the mouth into the sputum cup. He is to place in the cup only material coughed up.

Occasionally the edge of a cell will take the acid-fast stain and will be most stubborn about decolorization. When this happens the technician sometimes mistakes such a cell edge for a tubercle bacilli. In our own clinic we make it a standard procedure for the physician to check all slides reported as positive.

Interpretation

All acid-fast bacilli, of course, are not *Mycobacterium tuberculosis.* Nonetheless, in the average practice the physician will probably not see one case in a lifetime where a sputum is consistently positive for acid-fast organisms and where the patient does not have tuberculosis. For all practical purposes, the *repeated* presence of acid-fast rods in sputum smears is positive evidence of tuberculosis.

Concentration Procedures

Actually, in our experience concentration procedures have offered little advantage. If tubercle bacilli are not found in a carefully done sputum smear and x-ray evidence is equivocal, we believe that the patient should be sent to a diagnostic center for final determination.

There is a method for quick sputum culture which will be mentioned in the section on office bacteriology.

CHAPTER NINE

The Gastric Content

One never ceases to wonder at the remarkable resiliency of the human stomach. Throughout life it is insulted with impunity by alcohol, various vile foods, and swallowed tobacco smoke and tarry residues. Almost every conceivable type of chemical insult is rendered. Beginning in youth and continuing to the dietary excesses of middle age, we literally shatter the stomach with a barrage of potentially toxic material.

Not only does the stomach bear chemical and thermal insult but emotional insult as well. The human stomach seems to be one of the organs most readily affected by emotional tension. When a business man refers to a particularly harrowing occupation as an "ulcer factory," he is talking exactly and concisely. In spite of all this, the stomach usually continues to function adequately.

VOMITUS

In any patient who is vomiting one should make an attempt, if possible, to examine the vomitus, for much information can be gained. The stomach itself responds to a sufficiently noxious stimulus by engendering relaxation of the esophagus and contraction of the abdominal musculature, resulting in the regurgitation of the stomach contents. It is probable that a distended bowel may undergo reverse peristalsis which will ultimately place the offending material and the other bowel content back in the stomach and allow vomiting to take place.

Technique

Examine vomitus carefully for particulate matter, for blood or blood pigment, and for other colored material. If at all possible, smell it, and, finally, dip a strip of nitrazine paper in it to determine the pH.

Errors

The most frequent error concerns the problem of blood. The intensive pressure changes involved in the act of vomiting may rupture a small vessel and allow a few streaks of blood to be present. This in itself does not indicate pathology. It simply shows that the vomiting was intense enough to cause rupture of a vessel.

Interpretation

If there are undigested particles of food in the vomitus, several reasonable assumptions can be made. The first, of course, is that the patient has not been vomiting for a long period of time. If he had been he would be too sick to eat and, therefore, not likely to have taken anything in the way of aliments. The one exception to this statement is the regurgitation found in a diverticulum of the esophagus. Vomitus in such a case will show a conspicuous absence of action by the digestive juices and will usually show a pH in the 6.5-to-8 range, which is not consistent with that expected from food that has been in a secreting stomach.

If blood is present, one should note carefully the degree of digestion. Fresh blood, of course, is of normal color and usually indicates intensive bleeding. Older blood gradually becomes dark brown and then black and is usually coagulated into flecks by action of the stomach acids.

Streaks of bright red blood mean nothing as mentioned above. Small quantities of partially digested blood (i.e., spots of blood in the vomitus) are probably relatively insignificant also.

The most common conditions one thinks of in the presence of large quantities of fresh blood are ruptured esophageal varices and extensive bleeding from carcinoma. The latter condition will probably not be seen in the office, for this seldom occurs except as a more or less terminal event.

Quantities of digested blood, the "coffee-ground" vomitus, are significant mainly of bleeding peptic ulcer, although varices that are leaking steadily but not bleeding actively may show digested blood in the vomitus.

Green-colored vomitus simply indicates that duodenal material is being regurgitated along with stomach content. This has no great significance since it can be caused by intense vomiting which results from a noxious gastric stimulus as well as from vomiting induced by the small intestine.

Ordinary stomach content has a pungent, acidulous odor, and a physician with a normal sense of smell can usually detect the acidic tinge. For comparison, smell an open bottle of hydrochloric acid.

If gastric content is vomited and this smell is absent, one thinks immediately of lowered acid secretion which occurs most frequently in the gastritic type of disease and the next most frequent disease, carcinoma of the stomach.

A foul, fecal smell usually indicates regurgitation of partially digested material from the small intestine and should remind one of the possibility of intestinal obstruction, although when this vomiting occurs it is a little late to be reminded. Remember, too, that a large necrotic gastric carcinoma can impart the same odor to the vomitus. As a matter of fact, if anything, it smells worse.

A strip of nitrazine paper will indicate quickly whether the material is from a normally secreting stomach. Such material will be distinctly acid, whereas material that has been in the small intestine for some time is alkaline and material that has not reached the stomach is alkaline.

TEST MEALS

Many physicians have designed meals to be administered as a test for gastric function. In actuality, all of them are good and work reasonably well, but none is perfect. The one described here is simply the one we have used and probably has no advantage over the others.

In using these tests there are certain basic points that might be kept in mind. The first, of course, is that the test is simply a spot check. Gastric function is probably relatively constant for any person under basal conditions, but there is no such thing as a basal condition seen in office practice.

The secretory functions change somewhat as the type and degree of emotional pressure upon a person change. There is change according to diet which is varied from time to time, and the test itself has certain fundamental inaccuracies that are difficult to overcome.

For example, we theoretically aspirate the complete stomach content. Chances are probably better than a thousand to one that we never actually get anything like the total content. Also, the adsorption of acid is a variable factor, depending upon many, many conditions not controlled in the test meal. In addition, the neutralization of acids by saliva depends upon both the pH of the saliva and the amount secreted and may vary from meal to meal.

By no means is it implied that the test is not a valuable one. Many times we modern physicians forget the fine old tests and simply order an x-ray. There are occasions when such a test will give information of value far above that obtainable by roentgen examination.

Another factor which many physicians forget in doing the test-meal examination is that far more people show a diminution in acidity than ever show hyperacidity. The proportion is perhaps four to one. This hypoacidity can be just as important from the clinical standpoint as the hyperacidity and, in fact, is often more so.

Apparently there is a gradual atrophy or a gradual functional failure of the gastric mucosa, beginning at about the age of 20 years and progressing throughout life. In some 10 per cent of the people this failure becomes fixed early in life, and by the age of 60, 20 to 30 per cent show definite, if partial, failure of the gastric mucosa. Whether or not this partial failure has clinical significance, I do not know.

There are many controls of gastric secretion, including nervous, humoral, and mechanical. From the standpoint of disease seen in the office, the most important of these is the nervous control.

It has been amply proved that various tension states will produce profound changes in both gastric secretion and motility. In all probability these changes have some basic etiologic relationship to gastric dysfunction and peptic ulcer.

It is well known, also, that pepsin and hydrochloric acid will digest any tissue of the human body. Therefore, it is entirely possible to assume that some protective mechanism must exist in the mucous membrane lining the stomach and the upper duodenum that prevents this digestive activity.

Probably the most important mechanism is the adsorption of acids by gastric mucin. It is known that profound alterations in both type and quantity of mucous secretion may be influenced by the nervous mechanism.

There is a gradual diminution in the amount of acid and pepsin secretion by the stomach, beginning at approximately the age of 20 years and continuing until death. This is found in such a great percentage of the population that it has been conjectured to be an involutional phenomena.

Technique

Instruct the patient to dine early, immediately upon finishing work (usually best at 4:30 or 5:00 in the afternoon), after which he is not to sup. Further instruct him to take, just before retiring, a tablespoonful of uncooked finely chopped spinach with a little water.

When he reports to the office the next morning, give him a test meal. A good one is a shredded wheat biscuit and a glass of water. One hour later pass the stomach tube and aspirate the contents. There is an exacting technique for passing the tube which greatly aids in securing the confidence of the patient and should be followed at all times. First chill the tube in a pan of ice water and then lubricate it with olive oil. Usually the small stomach tube is best passed through the nose and the patient will be grateful if the nose and pharyngeal membranes are sprayed with 2 per cent Pontocaine before this is done. Now have the patient flex his neck slightly and thrust his chin forward in a position like this:

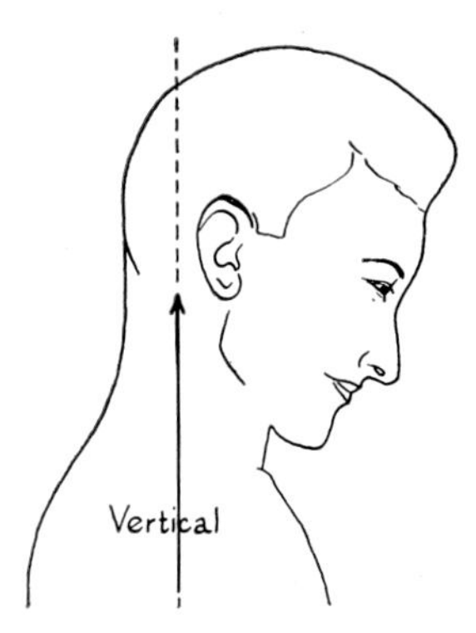

Give the patient a small glass of water and have him take a mouthful and *hold* it in his mouth. When the tube has reached the pharynx ask him to swallow, and when he does so push the tube gently forward. Several repetitions of this maneuver will usually pass the tube well into the esophagus.

Caution the patient after swallowing to open his mouth and breathe deeply for several breaths. Then have him repeat the swallowing process.

Be sure not to attempt to force the tube along faster than it is carried by normal swallowing, for this induces extreme discomfort and will often make the patient retch and gag. If there is a question about the tube entering the trachea instead of the esophagus, ask the patient to hum. It is impossible to make an adequate humming sound with a tube between the vocal cords.

When the tube is in the stomach, have the patient lie down and turn on his right side for five or ten minutes; then aspirate the total stomach content. Have the patient change position slightly once or twice during this aspiration to make certain that the tube enters all parts of the stomach.

Begin the analysis by looking for fragments of the spinach ingested the night before. They may be slightly discolored by the action of the stomach ferment but will usually be appreciable if present. They indicate gastric retention.

Next, test the acidity of the stomach content with nitrazine paper. Neutral or alkaline fluid would suggest, first, contamination of the content with large quantities of saliva in an apprehensive or neurotic patient. Gastric neuritis or cancer often shows alkaline fluid.

Next filter the stomach contents and preserve the filtrate.

Continue by putting 5 ml. of fresh milk in a test tube and add five drops of gastric juice. Cork the test tube tightly and put it in your shirt pocket where your body warmth will act as an incubator. If normal rennin is present, coagulation will occur in fifteen to twenty minutes.

Next place 10 ml. of filtered gastric juice in each of two beakers. To the first beaker add four drops of 1 per cent alcoholic solution of phenolphthalein. Use a 10 ml. graduated pipette or burette to add 0.1 N sodium hydroxide solution, a drop or two at a time until the solution turns a faint purple and remains so after gentle agitation. Note the number of milliliters of 0.1 N sodium hydroxide required to achieve this end point and multiply by ten. This expresses degrees of total acidity. The normal is considered between 50 and 100.

To a second beaker containing 10 ml. of filtered stomach content add five drops of Topfer's reagent. If free hydrochloric acid is present the solution will immediately turn a reddish pink color. Titrate as mentioned above with 0.1 sodium hydroxide until the last trace of red disappears and the solution is a canary yellow color. During the titration the fluid should be gently agitated constantly. The number of milliliters of 0.1 N sodium hydroxide used to reach the end point multiplied by ten is an expression of the total free acid. Normal range is usually considered as 30 to 60 units.

Next place a drop of the stomach fluid on a microscopic slide and cover with a cover glass. Examine immediately before drying occurs. Leukocytes are normally extruded into the stomach in numbers sufficient to be detected in this unstained preparation.

If a normal amount of hydrochloric acid is present in the stomach, however, these cells are almost immediately digested and only a few unidentifiable nuclear remnants remain in the fluid. If you find leukocytes in a good state of preservation you may assume practical absence of hydrochloric acid from the secretion.

Errors

The excessively nervous patient will frequently swallow a large quantity of saliva, which completely nullifies the value of the test. In insertion of the tube, if one causes a great deal of retching and gagging, duodenal contents will almost certainly be regurgitated into the stomach and will also interfere with the test. Unless you are certain that neither of these happenings has occurred, it is better to discard the results of the test and try again another day.

The chemical manipulations involved are so simple that errors practically never occur. Occasionally one will accidentally titrate past the end point, but there is usually sufficient gastric residual that the procedure may be done again and proper precaution used as the end point is approached.

Interpretation

Diminution in gastric secretion may occur in various cachetic diseases, but in such cases it has little meaning. Simply, it is one among many manifestations of disintegration. It may occur as a manifestation of time and regarding this there is a great argument.

Some experts maintain that the dissolutional process itself is represented in the stomach, with a gradual lessening of the potency of the gastric solution. Others maintain that this lessening of gastric activity is always a result of chronic gastritis. We practicing physicians are scarcely in a position to take part in this argument.

For practical purposes we are usually inclined to look upon those cases of diminished function in patients under the age of 50 as indications of at least functional disease of the stomach (i.e., psychoneurosis or extended chronic gastritis). This is true, of course, only after other diseases such as carcinoma are ruled out.

In patients over 50 years of age, on the other hand, we are inclined to look upon the condition, at least in part, as an involutional process and not altogether manifestations of a disease called chronic gastritis.

Since a discussion of gastritis is completely out of line in this volume, I suggest that you read the chapter on it in Meakins' *The Practice of Medicine.**

Regardless of what exactly the pathology may be, one usually notices that this diminution in stomach function is a gradual process, the patient showing first a loss of free acids, then a hypochlorhydria, and finally a relative anacidity. Ultimately there also will be a diminution in enzymatic content as shown by the milk test.

When one finds an excess of acids, the old problem of the chicken or the egg comes immediately to the forefront. Which was first, an irritative phenomenon that caused excessive secretion or an excessive secretion that caused the irritative phenomenon? We do not know the answer to this question. All current evidence points to the fact that in most cases an excessive secretion of acids is of neurogenic origin.

We can say with absolute certainty that all psychoneurotics do not show excessive gas-

*Meakins, J. C.: The Practice of Medicine, St. Louis, 1956, The C. V. Mosby Co.

tric acidity, but we can say with equal certainty that it is a rare case of gastric hyperacidity in which we cannot find sufficient psychic trauma to account for the findings. *This does not mean that all gastric hyperacidity is a result of emotional disease.* It is perfectly possible for a person to be tense and under pressure without showing any further manifestations of a psychoneurosis.

Without begging the question further, exactly what do we mean when one finds evidence of gastric hyperacidity? First of all, it can mean that the patient was frightened of the test and, being tense and nervous before the test was undertaken, may have excreted more acid than usual. A repetition of the test in several weeks, if both the original and the repeat test are done gently, will usually clarify this point.

Second, a positive test for hyperacidity does not mean peptic ulcer. It means that the stage is set for an ulcer but not that the pathology has occurred. Incidentally, high free and total acids are almost always found in duodenal ulcers and may be said to be a characteristic of the disease. This is not so in gastric ulcer. Ulceration of the stomach itself may occur in the absence of gross hyperacidity. In older persons with arteriosclerosis, vascular insults may cause gastric ulceration in the presence of entirely normal acidity.

Comment

The test meal is much more valuable than we usually realize and should not be totally discarded in favor of x-ray. Here is why: An obvious ulcer crater will be demonstrated almost invariably upon repeated x-ray. The irritable, hyperacidic stomach is not nearly as easily discovered roentgenographically as many would have us believe, but a simple gastric test meal will often clarify the picture when x-rays fail to do so.

There are some who claim that most cases of pernicious anemia actually start with a malfunctioning mucosa which does not secrete a sufficient quantity of acid and intrinsic factor. This seems within the realm of possibility but it is by no means proved. Certainly a gastric analysis should be made in all cases of anemia that are the slightest bit puzzling.

In young people, particularly in young women, with what appears to be obvious functional disease, a gastric analysis will sometimes clarify a microcytic hypochromic anemia. Such patients often exhibit gross lowering in gastric function.

CHAPTER TEN

The Feces

Examination of the stool is a valuable procedure in the office laboratory. Often much more information can be gained from careful stool examination than we realize. A significant percentage of the complaints seen in the office pertain to the gastrointestinal system, and precise stool examination will often elicit positive information regarding these complaints.

GROSS EXAMINATION

In all cases of gastrointestinal disease, at least one examination should be made of the stool and this should include a careful gross inspection. A normal or constipated stool may be secured at home by the patient and simply brought to the office immediately in a cardboard container. We have found entirely satisfactory the cardboard ice-cream containers stocked by all drugstores. The examination should not be delayed more than an hour or two. Diarrheal stools should be collected at the office and examined while fresh.

For easier understanding we shall list the abnormalities found upon gross inspection according to age groups rather than following the usual format of this book.

Newborn Infant

Meconium stools are usually a greenish-black color and of sticky, pasty consistency. The stools of every newborn infant should be inspected carefully to see that this meconium passes from the intestinal tract. If it does not do so it will become inspissated and may give rise to intestinal obstruction.

If there is a question about the patency of the intestinal tract, take a small bit of meconium and dilute it with normal saline in about equal amounts. Smear the resultant solution on a slide, air dry, stain it with gentian violet and decolorize with acid alcohol. Such a specimen will normally show a number of cornified epithelial cells which look like this:

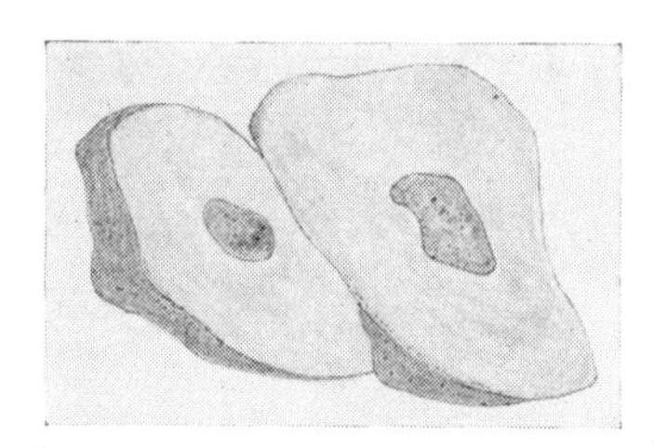

When they are present they are proof of the patency of the gut, and when absent bespeak some congenital abnormality resulting in the gut closure. This test should be run two or three times before assuming that the cells are absent.

Within a week or less bacterial flora have invaded the intestinal tract and normal digestive processes are being set up. The stools assume what is called the transitional character. During this period there may be mucus and occasionally tiny streaks of blood admixed with the stools. This is apparently due to irritation in the intestinal tract caused by the invasion of bacteria. It is not abnormal.

At this time stools may be relatively frequent, numbering from five to ten daily, and will ordinarily gradually assume a brown or greenish color. They may contain incompletely digested milk curds. This, too, is of no significance during the transitional period. After a week or ten days, digestive processes should have become relatively normal, the stools being of a pasty consistency and from golden yellow to pale brown in color. An occasional bit of green at this time is not abnormal.

Children

The digestive tract in children is somewhat more sensitive than it is in adults and responds to minor irritation with copious outpouring of mucus. An example of this would be the response to an irritant laxative. A large dose of castor oil or phenolphthalein may cause excessive production of mucus and much mucus in the stools. Occasionally such mucus will be lightly blood-tinged.

When stools have such an appearance it does not necessarily indicate pathology but indicates an irritative phenomenon of the gastrointestinal tract. A careful history should be taken before any pronouncements can be made about the presence of disease. The most extreme example of this mucoid stool is the typical stool seen after intussusception. It consists principally of mucus deeply stained with blood pigments. During starvation the same kind of stool may be seen, but it is not nearly so copious nor is the blood staining present. Usually a brown tint of bile pigments predominates.

Inadequate digestive processes or poor feeding, particularly in the smaller child, will produce fatty stools which have a greasy, wet soap appearance. To test for this put a bit of stool on a small square of filter paper and leave it for three minutes; then shake it off. A grease spot will remain on the paper in the presence of fatty stools.

During poor carbohydrate digestion the stools appear frothy and green or light yellow in color. At times they are watery. Such a stool has a pungent, acidic odor and a marked acidic reaction when tested with nitrazine paper.

Adults

Much information can be gained about the colonic function by gross study of the adult stool. The normal diameter is one to one and a half inches and segments of two to six inches are passed at one time. Small hard stools and stools in the form of balls or small segments usually indicate excessive spasticity of the descending colon, and consistent passage of such stools should make one suspicious of a psychogenic disorder of the colon.

The presence of mucus in any quantity is indicative of colonic irritation, and consistent presence of large quantities of mucus indicates the ill-defined entity known as "mucous colitis," which is assumed to be another psychogenic disorder.

Streaks of bright red blood clinging to the outside of the stool indicate anal disease, usually a fissure or a small hemorrhoid. Large quantities of bright red blood are most often due to active bleeding from a large hemorrhoid but may be associated with a lesion, such as carcinoma of the rectum.

Blood from higher in the intestinal tract is usually of black color and tarry consistency. This is by no means a certain test, for blood in the gut is an irritant and occasionally may cause a mild diarrhea and, therefore, be passed through the tract before the digestive ferments have time to complete their action. Such blood will usually be dark red in color and show the earliest changes in consistency and color toward the typical tarry stools.

When the entrance of bile into the duodenum is prevented, the stools show characteristic change. They are about the color of gray window putty and obviously contain large amounts of fat. Again, this may be tested for by placing a small bit of stool on filter paper, allowing it to remain for a minute or two, and then shaking it free. A spot of grease is a typical finding.

With two exceptions undigested food is seldom seen in the stools of adults except in pathologic states. The two exceptions are corn and beets, and particularly is corn an offender. Apparently the digestive ferments do not act upon the intact kernel of corn and, unless thoroughly masticated, the kernel covering will be passed in the stool much as it entered the intestinal tract.

Gross pus is not often seen in stool specimens. When it is present one may assume that he is dealing with either an ulcerative colitis or a chronic bacillary dysentery. Since chronic bacillary dysentery is a rare disease in most parts of this country, diagnosis is almost certain to be ulcerative colitis.

The detection of parasites in gross stool samples will be mentioned in the section beginning on page 139.

MICROSCOPIC EXAMINATION

Microscopic examination of the stool is an important part of the total stool examination and it has great value in addition to that usually assigned to it, which is diagnosis of parasitism. Many diseases show somewhat characteristic microscopic findings and one should always search for these.

To take a bit of material from the outside of the stool and smear it for microscopic examination is not good technique. Ordinarily the best way to do it is as follows:

In the event the patient does not have loose stools, give a small dosage of saline cathartic the night before the stool sample is to be collected for examination. Do not give enough to cause a copious watery diarrhea but just enough to be sure that loose movements will be evacuated. Be sure not to use the oily laxatives, such as mineral oil or castor oil, but use the mild salines such as a half teaspoonful of Epsom salts.

Proper stools should be mushy in consistency and should be gently stirred up and emulsified before a sample is taken. When this has been done a wire loop is used to transfer a bit of the stool, about half the size of a lead pencil eraser, to each of four test tubes.

In the first test tube, 1 ml. of Lugol's solution is added and the stool thoroughly mixed with this. In each of the remaining test tubes 1 ml. of normal saline is added. Tube 1 then contains Lugol's solution; tube 2, normal saline. To tube 3, in addition to the normal saline, add one small drop of methylene blue stain, and to tube 4, which also contains normal saline, add one small drop of Sudan III. Emulsify a small bit of the stool in each of the test tubes.

Cells

Use a drop of the methylene-blue-stained feces specimen to examine for cellular content. If cells appear to be degenerating to the extent that adequate readings cannot be taken, discard the slide and use a drop of the plain saline and feces combination. Put a drop of this on a slide, add a cover glass, and put one drop of 30 per cent acetic acid solution at one side of the cover glass. This will clear the cytoplasm of the cells and allow the nucleus to be seen plainly. After this a drop of methylene blue may be added at the side of the cover glass and the nuclei will promptly take the stain.

If there are a large number of leukocytes which appear to have bilobed nuclei and look as if they contain coarse granules, use a bit of the saline-feces solution to make a smear. Air dry it, fix in methyl alcohol, and stain with Giemsa's stain for eosinophils.

Ordinarily neutrophilic leukocytes are not common in the exudate of the normal colon. Their presence is pathognomonic of some inflammatory process. The most common is a minor inflammation in the anal canal, such as an anal fissure or ulcer. However, cells from this are usually not grossly admixed with the stool and, therefore, are relatively few in number. The presence of large numbers of these cells is almost certain indication of gross inflammatory change in the colon itself. The most common chronic cause is ulcerative colitis and, next, chronic bacillary infections.

In amebiasis the enzymes secreted by the ameba usually destroy or partially destroy these cells so that they are not present in exceptionally large numbers.

Erythrocytes are usually present in any disease of the colon, even the relatively minor ones. The presence of large numbers of erythrocytes along with relatively large numbers of polymorphonuclear cells indicates an acute ulcerative process and it is quite frequently associated with carcinoma. The frequency is such that detailed x-ray studies are most assuredly indicated.

Eosinophils are rarely found in bowel exudate and are practically never seen in the bowel exudate containing pus. When they are present in large numbers they probably indicate some allergic manifestation in the bowel. This test may be used as an accurate means of differentiating inflammatory from allergic disease.

Food Residue

First, place a drop of the emulsion with Sudan III on the slide and add a cover glass. Examine several high-power fields for fat globules which will stain a pink or light orange color in the presence of the Sudan III. There should not be more than one or two globules per high-power field. If there are more than eight to ten per high-power field, one thinks of the disease in which fat is improperly digested, such as regional enteritis, intestinal tuberculosis, celiac disease, idiopathic steatorrhea, or pancreatic insufficiency.

Often small globules of soap may be seen. They look like this:

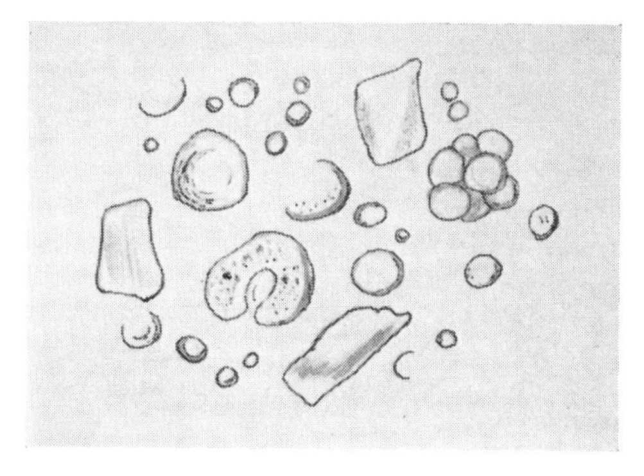

They do not take Sudan III stain. If there is any question add three drops of 30 per cent acetic acid to the test tube containing the Sudan III and heat gently to boiling. This will break down the soap and after cooling will allow accurate assessment of fat by repeating the microscopic examination.

In the normal person a few muscle fibers from ingested meat escape complete digestion but they are usually so changed as to make detailed identification impossible. If there are muscle fibers present which contain staining nuclei in the methylene blue preparation, you may assume some inadequacy of pancreatic digestion. Usually the fibers that escape digestion are a structureless homogenous mass. Occasionally one sees both striation and nuclei clearly apparent. This might happen once in one high-power field by accident, but if a number of such fibers are found again, one may assume pancreatic insufficiency.

In the Lugol's solution, starch granules stain red if partially digested or blue if digestive ferments have acted very little. Actually this does not mean much so far as the presence or absence of the ferments is concerned because there are practically no demonstrated cases of live patients who cannot digest starches. It does, however, usually indicate intestinal hypermotility and that the material has passed through the gut so rapidly that the ferments have not been allowed time to complete their digestive action. The latter is a valuable point in suspected cases of hyperirritability of the gastrointestinal system, and the examination should not be neglected. Vegetable fibers of all kinds normally appear in the stool and their identification is unimportant from a practical standpoint.

CHEMICAL EXAMINATION

There are only two chemical examinations of great importance and one of these is seldom used. The common one is examination for occult blood and the rarely used one is the examination for pancreatic enzyme activity.

Occult Blood

In the office laboratory the examination for occult blood is ordinarily done with the common Hematest tablet which is quite accurate for all practical purposes. Before making the examination, however, one must realize that blood from the mouth, nose, and throat or from the anal canal will provide a contaminate and invalidate the test.

Ask specifically whether the patient has had bleeding gums, a nose bleed, or "coughed up" any blood in the five days preceding the test. If he is not positive regarding these points, it is best to delay the test for several days while he makes careful observations. Perhaps one of the most common sources of contaminants is bleeding from the gums when the teeth are brushed. The blood is often swallowed and may be sufficient in quantity to interfere with the test.

One must ask careful historic questions about the existence of rectal bleeding also. A rectal fissure or bleeding hemorrhoid, anal ulcer, or other minor complaints about the rectum will completely invalidate the test.

The *technique* is simple and is printed on the side of each bottle of Hematest tablets. The technique should be followed exactly and interpretation done as suggested.

The errors to which the test is subjected are mostly those of contaminants, which have already been suggested.

Interpretation is a matter requiring some careful thought. The presence of occult blood simply means that blood is escaping into the gastrointestinal tract at some point along its course.

Since there are many trivial lesions that allow such escape of blood, one should not base any diagnostic pronouncements upon the finding until it has been demonstrated to be present with some consistency. For example, a trivial gastrointestinal upset will frequently provide enough local irritation at some place along the tract to allow the escape of a few blood cells and the test for occult blood will be positive. I have even found it positive in the typical green persimmon stomach-ache of young boys. Such a thing makes cautious interpretation an absolute must.

I must tell you about one case, if for nothing else than its humorous value. A rancher friend of mine brought to the office his 10-year-old son who was complaining of achy, colicky pain in the right lower quadrant. There were absolutely no findings on physical examination except that the cecum and entire right colon felt somewhat distended. This, of course, is not altogether an unusual finding. A careful examination, going over the boy entirely from head to foot, and a detailed history revealed nothing. He had not vomited, nor had he felt particularly nauseated, although he certainly did not feel as if his gastrointestinal tract were normal. The white blood count was 16,000, but there was a normal differential.

The boy was placed in a hospital. An occult blood test was positive. The white blood count stayed elevated but did not change significantly and the boy complained bitterly of his distress. Both his father and I noticed that when our questions became rather pointed, he was a bit shifty eyed. Finally we both insisted that he tell us exactly what happened. With much hemming and hawing the boy admitted that he had opened a box of rolled oats and eaten several handfuls dry. They had, of course, absorbed water as they passed through the intestinal tract and swelled. The only operative procedure carried out was a good spanking for not telling us what had happened before a $100 hospital bill had accumulated.

The interesting part of the case was this: How did the occult blood test become positive? I questioned the boy carefully (and he was an intelligent lad) about nasal bleeding and bleeding upon brushing his teeth. I examined his rectum thoroughly. There was no source of blood readily demonstrable. The only answer seemed to be that the gut was stretched enough to cause rupture of a small vessel or two and leakage of a few drops of blood into the intestine.

This case illustrates the point only too well. A trivial insult to the gut can cause leakage of a few drops of blood with resultant positive tests. For this reason I am inclined not to put too much stress on the test for occult blood unless it is repeated at weekly intervals and found positive with relative consistency. The repeated positive results indicate a lesion of the tract and should warrant detailed investigation.

Pancreatic Enzymes

Rarely a child suspected of cystic fibrosis of the pancreas will be seen in the practitioner's office. When seen, however, a test for the presence of trypsin in the stool should be performed as follows:

Dilute portions of the stool with distilled water in the ratios of 1:5, 1:10, and 1:100. Use a dental x-ray film and place a large drop of each of these specimens on the surface of one film. Use paper clips to fasten the edge of the film to a cardboard to prevent curling.

Let the preparation set at room temperature for two hours, adding to the drops on the film as necessary to counteract evaporation. At the end of this time gently wash the material off the film with cold water. If trypsin is present the film emulsion should have been digested off in all three specimens. If only the bacteria which liquefy the emulsion are present it is usually digested off in the 1:5 and 1:10 solution specimens but not in the 1:100.

If the test indicates the relative absence of trypsin then a further detailed diagnostic work-up is in order.

The bacteria which digest film emulsion are not sensitive to penicillin and the administration of penicillin for several days preceding the test will allow overgrowth of these organisms and consequently cloud the results. Therefore, the test should not be done during or immediately after penicillin administration.

This test is not absolutely accurate diagnostically, for certain other conditions also may cause the absence of trypsin. In connection with clinical symptoms, however, it is almost specifically diagnostic.

PARASITES

Parasitism is much more common in the United States than the average physician suspects. Possibly because of the large numbers of our people who have been overseas in the past decade or two, amebiasis has become much more widespread than was the case in the early part of this century. In the South, roundworm infestations are quite common and pinworm infestations in children throughout the United States are often found. The laboratory diagnosis of these parasites is extremely important and should be within the province of every small office laboratory.

In this section we will consider only the most common parasites and those which most certainly should be diagnosed in the practitioner's laboratory.

Entamoeba Histolytica

There is no doubt in the minds of most parasitologists that *Entamoeba histolytica* causes severe intestinal disease in man and that its "ally," *Entamoeba coli*, has little, if any, adverse effect. Other amebae found in the bowel, namely, *Endolimax nana, Iodamoeba buetschlii,* and *Dientamoeba fragilis,* are also parasitic to man but are not thought to cause severe symptoms. Identification of the various forms is difficult in the office laboratory but well within the realm of possibility.

For practical purposes, however, most parasitologists agree that any amebae found consistently in the intestinal tract of man should be eradicated. Therefore, whether or not to treat does not become a problem. The practical problem as seen in the office laboratory is differentiating symptoms caused by *Entamoeba histolytica* from other gastrointestinal insults.

Historically, much can be done, for amebiasis has a rather characteristic acute or chronic course and at least the majority of the details of this course are present in nearly every case. The cellular exudate as described previously on page 136 is considerably different in amebiasis than it is in bacterial or ulcerated infections of the colon, and this serves as a point of differentiation.

Technique

In the acute case, one should attempt to find the living trophozoite in the feces. Examine a freshly passed stool. Place a small bit of the blood-stained mucus from the edge of the stool on a warmed slide. If necessary, dilute with a drop of normal saline solution and *be sure* to keep the slide warm. This may best be done by placing a heated penny on one end of the slide.

The trophozoite of *E. histolytica* is actively motile, pushing out knife-blade-shaped pseudopods with relative rapidity for an ameba and seemingly following a purposeful direction. The nucleus is not usually apparent.

In the blood-stained mucus areas, usually a few red cells will have been ingested, and in the unstained preparation they will appear to be disintegrating. In color they will range from a pale yellow to a yellowish green. A typical trophozoite is from four to six times the diameter of a red blood cell and looks like this:

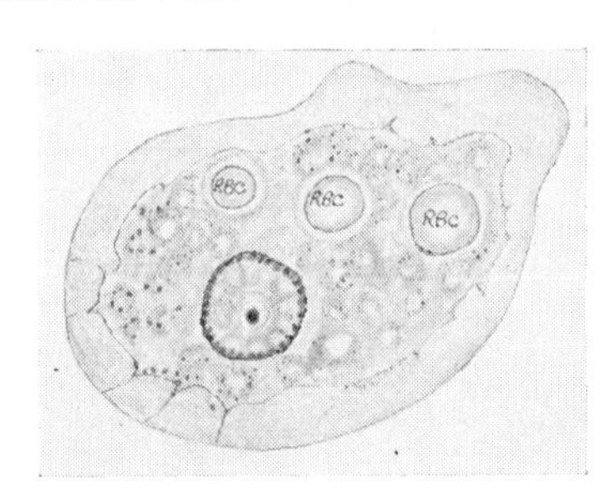

One should never make a diagnosis on the basis of a single ameba. At least eight or ten should be visualized and fully examined before one ventures a positive diagnosis.

In the more chronic case, examination of a routine stool specimen may be made for cystic forms. The typical cyst is one and one half to two times the size of a red blood cell.

When the cyst is stained with Lugol's solution there are usually four small nuclei and upon careful observation a densely staining nucleolus can be seen placed centrally within the nucleus. A typical specimen looks like this:

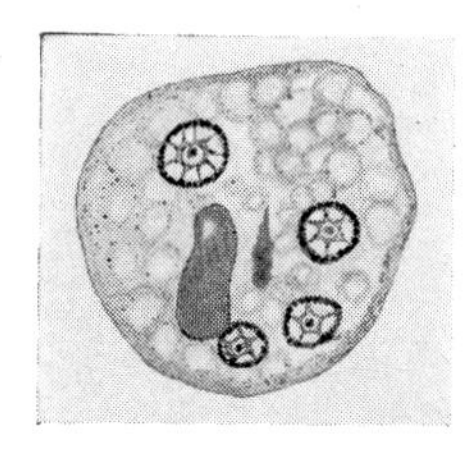

Again, diagnosis should not be based on the finding of a single cyst. At least a dozen cysts should be seen under the oil immersion lens before one offers anything like a positive diagnosis.

Errors

The most frequent point of confusion is *E. coli.* The trophozoite is approximately the same size as *E. histolytica,* but usually the nucleus is seen fairly readily. The nucleolus, if it is seen, is eccentrically placed in the nucleus. Movements are sluggish and *E. coli* will phagocytize debris of all kinds, including bacteria, but seldom phagocytize red blood cells.

A typical trophozoite looks like this:

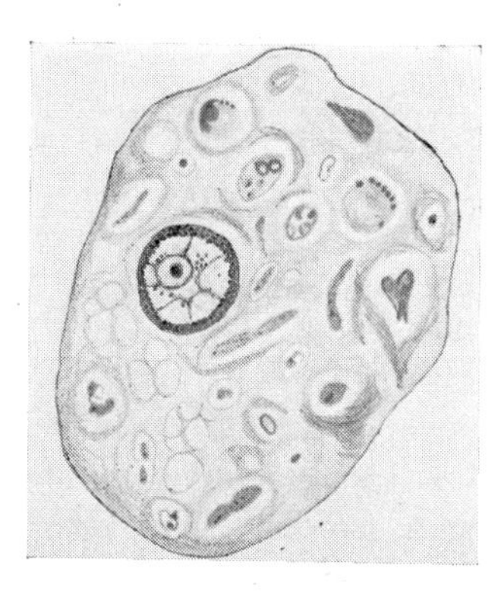

The cystic form is half again as large as the cystic form of *E. histolytica* and has eight nuclei with the nucleoli clearly visible in the stained preparation. These nucleoli are eccentrically placed. A typical cystic form looks like this:

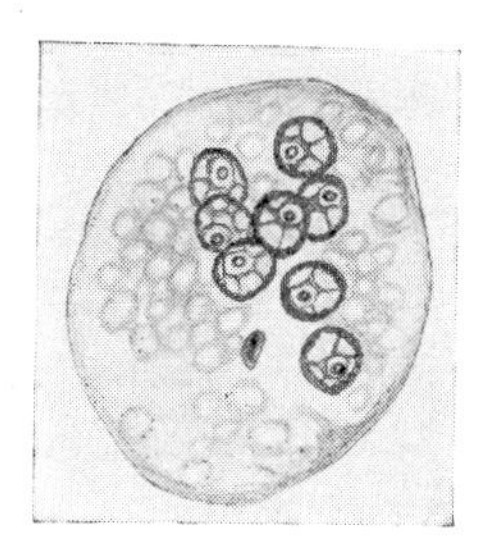

Careful examination will easily serve to differentiate the coli and histolytica forms of Entamoeba, but one should remember that many fine parasitologists make the statement that treatment is indicated if only *E. coli* is found, for there is occasionally an association between histolytica and coli.

Interpretation

In most cases it will be possible for the laboratory to specify the presence or absence of *E. histolytica.* One should remember that the presence of the organism does not mean that it is the cause of the pathology present. Particularly in the so-called chronic, symptomless cases is this important.

A certain number of people are asymptomatic carriers, and intestinal symptomatology may readily be caused by psychoneurosis rather than by the activities of the few entamoebae present.

On the other hand, there is no reason to suppose that entamebae should not be eradicated mercilessly when found. This applies equally well even if the laboratory reports *E. coli,* which is relatively innocuous.

When the laboratory does report *E. histolytica* it is probably wise for the doctor to do two things: (1) examine the slide himself and (2), do repeated examinations if there is any doubt, until one is certain that the structure identified actually is the parasite *E. histolytica.*

Pinworms

Pinworms are among the commonest parasites of man and are found throughout the civilized world. Infestation is seen most acutely in children of school age. In some areas of the United States as many as 25 per cent of children harbor the parasite.

Infestation occurs by ingestion of gravid eggs or larval worms. These multiply and mate in the duodenum and migrate to the colon. They are often visible upon sigmoidoscopic examination. The average worm is approximately 1 cm. in length and about the width of fine sewing thread.

Adult females often migrate out through the anus to deposit their eggs in anal folds. This migration may be the cause of extreme itching. Often the worms may be seen on the perianal skin. Look for them with a reading glass.

Technique

The worms may be seen in great profusion in the stool after a mild saline laxative. They are white and actively motile and may usually be diagnosed by the patient or another member of the family.

Surprisingly enough, this gross examination is probably the most accurate means of diagnosis. The eggs do not ordinarily appear in great quantity in the feces and may be exceedingly difficult to identify even with special concentration techniques.

The next best means of diagnosis is to pick the eggs from the perianal skin, using the sticky side of a cellophane tape such as the Scotch tape purchasable at any drugstore. Simply press the sticky side of the tape firmly into the perianal skin, covering both normal skin surface and the pigmented membrane of the anus itself. Then place the tape, sticky side down, on a microscopic slide and look for typical eggs. These eggs may be seen in all stages of development from the single-celled stage to the eggs containing the moderately well-developed worm. Typical stages look like this:

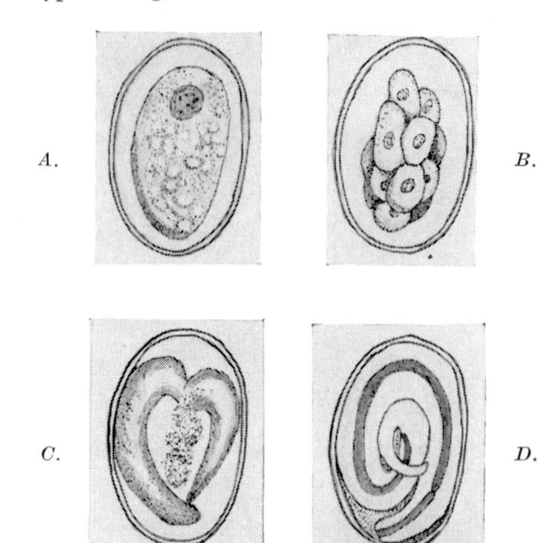

Errors

The most frequent error is not searching diligently enough for the worm. When symptoms and history indicate its presence, at least three or four tape specimens should be taken and at least two mild laxatives administered and the stools carefully examined before one decides that the pinworm is not present.

Ascarides

The adult *Ascaris lumbricoides* looks like a common earthworm or fishworm which has slightly outgrown itself. Normal adults average from 20 to 25 cm. in length and are the most common roundworm parasite of man.

When fertile eggs of the worm are ingested they hatch in the duodenum, releasing minute but active larvi which make their way through the walls of the intestine. Then they migrate by way of the portal circulation, and sometimes by way of the peritoneal cavity, into the liver and lungs, up the trachea into the pharynx where they are swallowed, and again entering into the intestines, this time growing into adult parasites.

Frequently an adult worm will wander into the stomach, be vomited, and brought in indignantly by the patient.

The worms are also often passed from the bowel and may be noticed by the patient in his stool. If identification cannot be made positively either historically or visually, the physician should attempt to find the eggs in a stool sample. Even though the worm is a prolific producer of eggs (several worms in the intestinal tract often produce a million or more eggs daily), they still are not too readily found.

Technique

If a cursory glance at a bit of stool specimen does not show typical eggs which look like this:

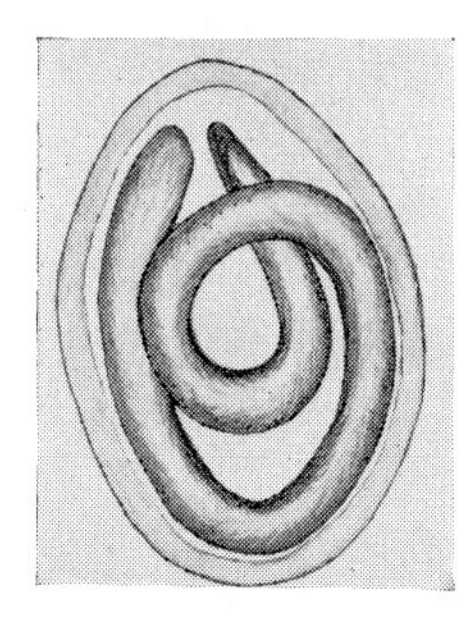

it is probably best to initiate some concentration technique. The one we use is as follows:

Measure approximately 10 ml. of water into a large test tube and saturate it with ordinary table salt. Take a piece of feces about the size of a lead pencil eraser and dilute it with 1 ml. of normal saline. Mix this dilution thoroughly and filter through a surgical sponge to eliminate gross particles. Approximately ten drops of the feces-saline mixture should result from this filtration. If it does not, filter another few particles. Put the filtrate in the brine solution and let it stand fo twenty to thirty minutes.

The eggs and various other fecal particles will float to the top of the brine solution and may be picked up by means of the platinum loop and placed on a slide. When a large drop of this fluid from the top of the brine is present on a microscopic slide (several transfers may be necessary), place a cover drop on this and a drop of Lugol's solution at the side of the cover drop. If eggs are present they will probably be seen in profusion.

Errors

The most common error is failure to be sufficiently persistent in looking for the worm eggs. A quick, casual examination of unconcentrated stool specimen may be negative repeatedly in spite of the presence of several worms in the intestinal tract. It is better to do one or two careful examinations, using the flotation technique, before making any final decision as to whether worms are present or not. Explain to the patient at the outset that several examinations may be needed to be sure whether or not worms exist.

In actuality, few patients come in with complaints leading up to the diagnosis of worms unless they are reasonably certain themselves that they have intestinal parasites. There are few "surprise" cases involving Ascaris.

Necator Americanus

The hookworm is particularly common in the southern United States. It is a small, sluggishly motile worm, 1 or 1½ cm. long and about the diameter of a thread.

The larval hookworm gains entrance through the skin, usually the patient's feet, migrates via the lymphatics or veins to the lungs, and thence up the trachea where they are swallowed and begin their normal intestinal cycle.

These are the real blood-sucking worms which may literally sap the vitality of the patient.

Technique

The feces is put through the flotation technique described in the last section on page 143 and is examined for the typical eggs which look like this:

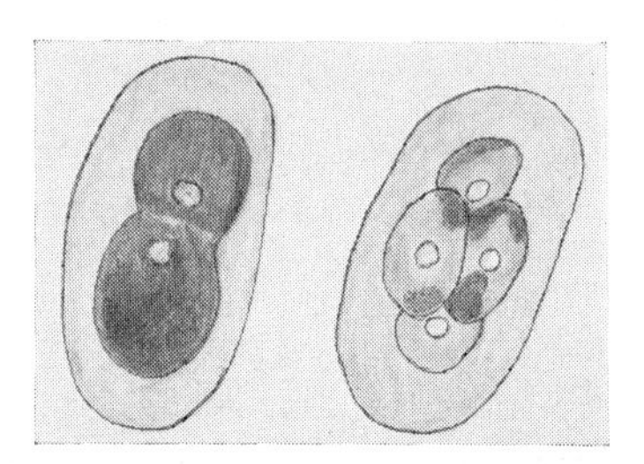

Occasionally eggs may be found in the several cell stages or containing a motile larva. They look like this:

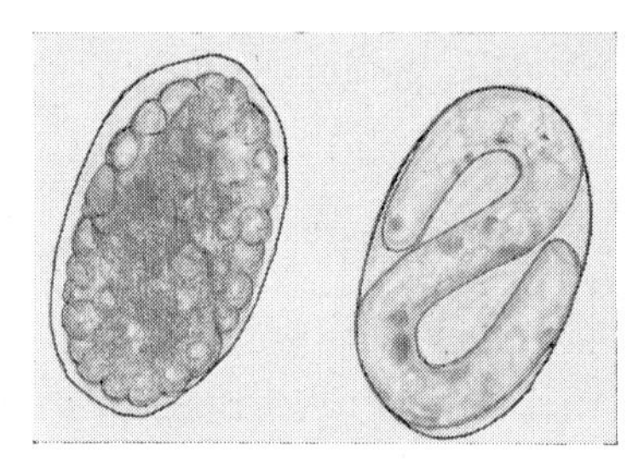

A good thing to do is to ask the parasitology department of the nearest medical school for sample slides and study them well.

Cestodes

Cestodes are the tapeworms. They are not particularly common in the United States because of the care used in producing our meat supply. When a human being ingests meat containing the unkilled larval forms, the worm takes up residence in the intestine and rapidly develops into the adult form.

Diagnosis is usually made by the patient when he passes a string of worm proglottids. Often he will bring these to the office. The important point for laboratory determination is to make certain that the worm has been completely killed.

Technique

The appearance of segments of the adult worm is entirely typical. They look like this:

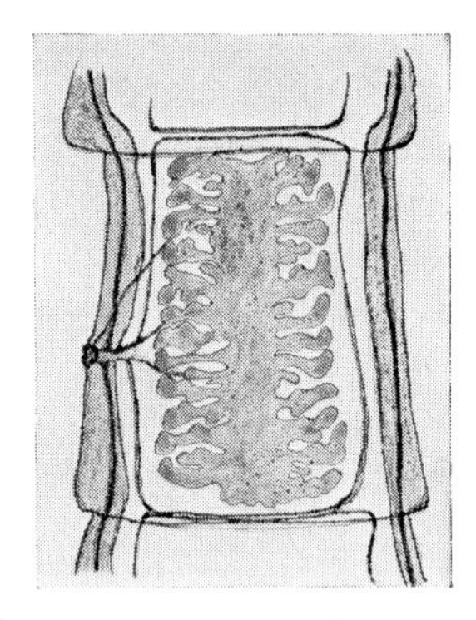

If the patient does not bring the worm in for identification, feces should be concentrated and checked for eggs which look like this:

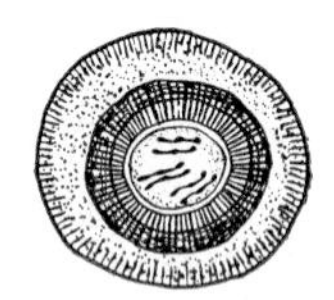

The problem, actually, is to determine when, under treatment, the scolex, or head, of the worm has been passed.

After treatment, feces may be liquefied with an equal amount of water and strained through a fine wire mesh strainer. The scolex is usually about the size of a pinhead and will be retained by proper-sized wire. Use of the hand lens will usually allow adequate identification. This, plus stool tests at monthly intervals for six months which show no eggs, is conclusive evidence of cure.

This is a typical scolex:

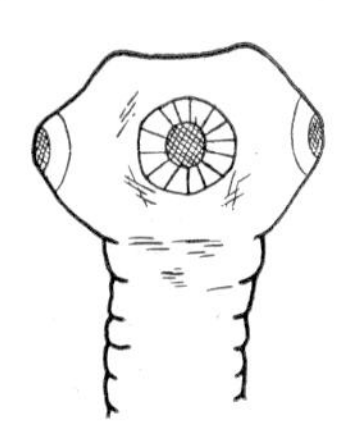

CHAPTER ELEVEN

Vaginal Content

The small office laboratory can give a great deal of information about gynecologic disorders and diseases. The most important point in obtaining this information probably is to make certain that specimens are taken from exactly the area one wishes and not in a haphazard manner.

Microscopic smear and moist preparation are the most important means of laboratory examination of vaginal content. I cannot caution the practitioner enough to be certain that these specimens are secured precisely. For example, suppose one wished to find out all the information available about an endocervicitis which is patently present on examination. A smear of the general vaginal discharge may be of no help whatsoever, but a carefully taken endocervical smear will give precise information as to what is occurring. Methods and techniques for taking these specialized specimens will be found throughout this chapter.

DÖDERLEIN BACILLUS

Döderlein bacillus is a member of the Lactobacillus group, capable of metabolizing carbohydrates to lactic acid. The bacillus lives best at body temperature and in a slightly acid medium which it will create for itself if given ample carbohydrates. The normal vaginal content contains an ample amount of carbohydrates. The Döderlein bacillus routinely invades and finds the vagina a perfect home.

One now encounters the question of the hen or the egg. Does the Döderlein bacillus cause the slight acidity which is normal in the human vagina or does the slight acidity allow the Döderlein bacillus to thrive? So far as I know, normal cervical secretions are slightly alkaline but contain an ample amount of carbohydrates. The bacillus probably has a great deal to do with changing the reaction and maintaining the slight acidity which is normal.

In the event of disease the Döderlein bacillus is simply thrown out by the invader which overgrows and kills it. One practically never finds Döderlein bacilli in association with any of the common pathogens. For this reason their presence may be taken as an indication of relative normalcy, although it is possible (but unlikely) to have a normal vagina in the absence of these bacteria.

Technique

A Gram stain is made of the vaginal discharge. The sample is taken from within the vagina, not at the forchette. The technique for Gram's stain will be found on page 155.

The Döderlein bacilli are large, pleomorphic, gram-positive organisms which usually look like this:

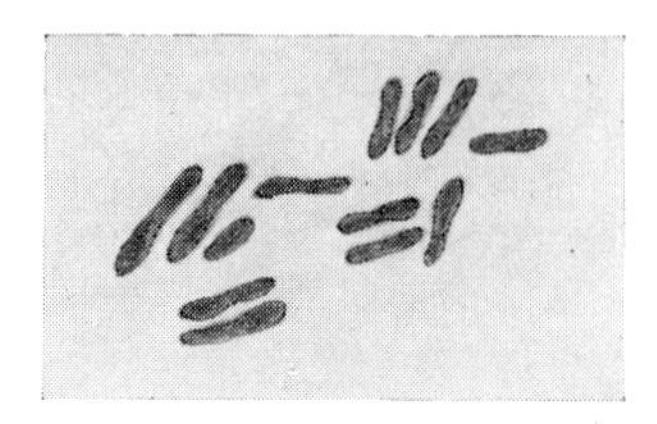

It is not often necessary to carry identification further than that which can be made by microscopic examination with the oil immersion lens. If such structures are present chances are overwhelming that one is dealing with a normal vaginal content.

Errors

This test is practically without error. One should remember, however, that the Döderlein bacillus is subject to great change in form and all members of the tribe may not be similar. They are usually plentiful in the normal vaginal smear and one does not have to search to find them. If only a rare gram-positive rod is seen this should not be taken to mean that a normal population of Döderlein bacilli exists. An entirely normal vagina will show many, many thousands of such bacilli in every smear. This fact, in itself, makes diagnosis easy.

Interpretation

The test is actually a valuable one in the physician's office. Many women believe they have some vaginal disease when what they actually have is a sexual psychoneurosis. There are normal variations in the amount of vaginal secretions and occasionally girls take a normal increase to mean a vaginal disease.

A normal pelvic examination, plus the finding of profuse growth of Döderlein bacilli, serves to point up the probable cause of the "discharge."

TRICHOMONAL DISCHARGES

Trichomonas vaginalis is the only important mastigophoran parasite of man. It is commonly found in the vagina, rarely in the urethra, and sometimes in the trigonal area of the bladder. No convincing proof exists that it has ever been found elsewhere.

Parasitologists and gynecologists have a distinctly differing view about these protozoa. There are other Mastigophora which normally live in the human intestine and in the mouth, and gynecologists have for years taught that infestation with *T. vaginalis* may result from rectal contamination of the vagina. If parasitologists are to be believed, the intestinal parasite and the vaginal parasite are entirely different. The intestinal flagellate will not live in the human vagina more than a day or two and will not cause symptoms. This, of course, leaves us in one position only. The disease we call *T. vaginalis* infestation must be of venereal origin.

The parasites are so delicate and die so quickly upon exposure to the vicissitudes of temperatures and light that the old theory of the infected toilet seat becomes almost ridiculous. A few outstanding gynecologists now believe that *Trichomonas vaginalis* vaginitis is a venereal disease and I am inclined to agree with them on the basis of clinical experience and some carefully taken, accurate, clinical histories. Without regard to this, the fact remains that this disease is one of the most frequent seen by the practitioner in his office.

Technique

If you wear a suit coat in the office, place 1 ml. of sterile normal saline in each of several test tubes and put them in your shirt pocket underneath your coat. Keep them there so that the normal saline solution will gradually assume body temperature.

When doing a gynecologic examination, if you suspect a Trichomonas vaginitis, use a cotton-tipped applicator to pick up some of the bubbly discharge and twirl the applicator in one of the test tubes of normal saline.

Remember that cooling destroys these organisms rapidly. Have the nurse clasp the test tube tightly in her hand so that the warmth of her palm will prevent the tube from cooling. Take it immediately to the laboratory. Heat a penny in the Bunsen flame and put it on one end of a microscopic slide, placing a drop or two of the normal saline-discharge mixture in the center. Add a cover glass and examine the preparation at once. *T. vaginalis* is usually profuse in the specimen.

The parasite looks like this:

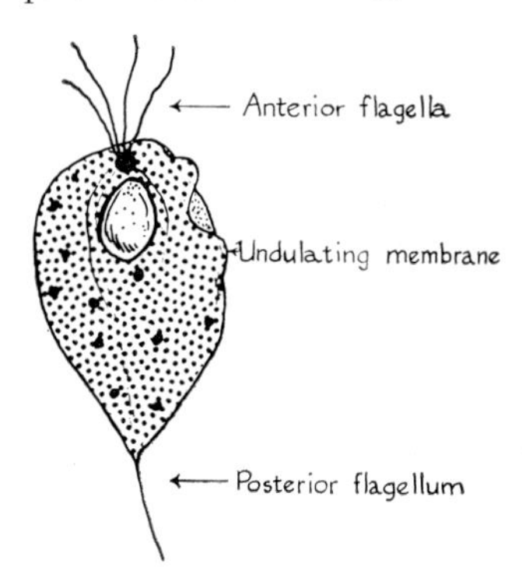

but what you will usually see is this:

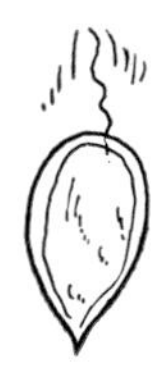

Be sure to stop the light down so that a minimum of light is used, and look for the motion of the flagella. This whiplike motion with undulations of ten to twenty per second is so characteristic that once seen it will never be forgotten.

In dying organisms the motion becomes progressively slower. If there is doubt about whether one actually sees flagellar motion or whether it is rapid enough to be *T. vaginalis,* it usually means that the preparation has been allowed to cool.

Errors

The most frequent error, of course, is to allow cooling. A preparation for trichomonads that has been allowed to cool even slightly is totally useless. Examination must be done quickly and the specimen must be kept warm. It is also possible to fry the trichomonads by getting the penny on the slide too hot, but this seldom, if ever, occurs in office practice.

Another error is to give up too soon. A single negative preparation means little. If you believe the disease is infestation with *T. vaginalis* and do not find the parasite the first time, treat the disease anyway. If the test has been done just before the patient's cycle, take another smear immediately after her menstruation when the trichomonads are usually more profuse than at other times.

Interpretation

Much ink may be spilled about the possibility of other mastigophoran infections of the vagina. In actual practice, if the "whip-bearing" organism is identified, one may assume that trichomonad infestation is present.

The Persistent Case

Trichomonads are easy to kill. At least a hundred routines have been devised for treating the disease and every one will eradicate it. When one persistently finds positive slides one must assume that reinfection from the male is taking place. Here, certain techniques come into play.

The male may harbor the parasite in the moist areas underneath the foreskin. It may even cause a slight irritation of this area, although this is not the usual thing. We have made repeated efforts to identify the parasites in this area, using smears, flushes with normal saline, and other techniques, all of which have worked out so poorly that we actually believe it to be a waste of time. This is a typical case where clinical assumption outweighs the value of the laboratory.

In other cases the male may harbor the parasite in the prostate. A smear is made as follows: Warm a slide and place a drop of the prostatic secretion upon it. Add a cover glass, place a warmed penny on one end of the slide and make the examination immediately. By careful examination, repeated several times, we have often been able to demonstrate the parasite in prostatic secretion and sometimes believe that it may have been responsible for a mild prostatitis, although this is certainly not a proved fact.

INFLAMMATORY DISCHARGES

The most common cause of minor vaginal discharges is probably the application of chemicals to a vaginal wall through improper douching and excessive vaginal manipulation. Excellent personal hygiene can be obtained by plain washing and an occasional douch of mildly acidified water.

In a surprising number of cases of vaginal discharge one will find nothing but signs of mild irritation on the vaginal walls and an overplus of polymorphonuclear cells along with a few Döderlein bacilli. Such a finding is an excellent diagnostic tip-off.

Technique

The ordinary Gram stain as mentioned on page 155 will serve to show both the polymorphonuclear cells and the remaining Döderlein bacilli. The smear, of course, should be taken from the area of greatest irritation or redness.

Errors

These cases are often interpreted as infections and so treated. It is certainly true that they are excellent breeding grounds for bacterial invasion, but in actuality they remain in the category of irritation.

Interpretation

The finding of leukocytes in some profusion, along with remaining Döderlein bacilli and no other bacterial invasion, should make one suspicious that he is dealing with a purely irritative phenomenon not related to the acute infections.

INFECTIOUS DISCHARGES

Occasionally we see what we might call a nonspecific infection of the vagina (i.e., an infection with staphylococci, streptococci, even with diphtheroids), but for all practical purposes an obvious vaginal infection is gonorrhea until proved otherwise.*

I must clarify the fact that I am talking about vaginal infections—not about cervical infections. In the conditions of which we speak, the vaginal walls are red, edematous, irritated, and show every sign of an acute infection. Such cases should have a Gram stain of the purulent discharge at once. In addition to making a smear of the vaginal discharge itself, one should gently milk Skene's gland and the distal urethra like this:

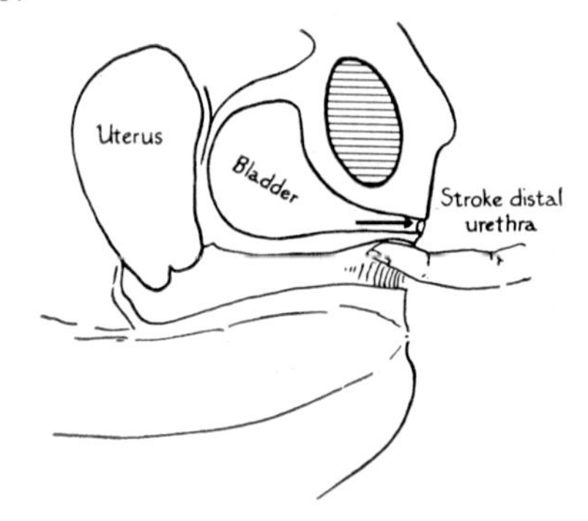

for a bead of pus. If pus is found a separate smear should be made of it.

*For many years we have had a concept of specificity with regard to vaginal infection. A great many physicians still refuse to recognize the entity called "nonspecific vaginitis." Maybe they are right in their contention that nonspecific vaginitis is just a polite term for a condition due to poor feminine hygiene. Even so, the fact is that such a condition is extremely irritating to the patient. Let's use the polite term.

Technique

Use the routine Gram stain technique as specified on page 155. There are no special aspects to the technique.

Errors

One should always try to obtain a drop of fresh pus rather than pus that has been in the vagina for a period of time. Both the leukocytes and the contained Neisserian organisms will degenerate over a period of time and will become more difficult to identify. Of course, in the vagina it is somewhat difficult to decide which pus is fresh and which is not, but if one can milk a drop from Skene's gland, it is the preferred material from which to make a stain.

Interpretation

One does not see acute vaginal infections in which the invading organism is excessively rare. The simplest of identification technique learned in premedical biology courses will serve to clarify the acute case. The Neisserian organism may be found both intracellularly and extracellularly and usually looks like this:

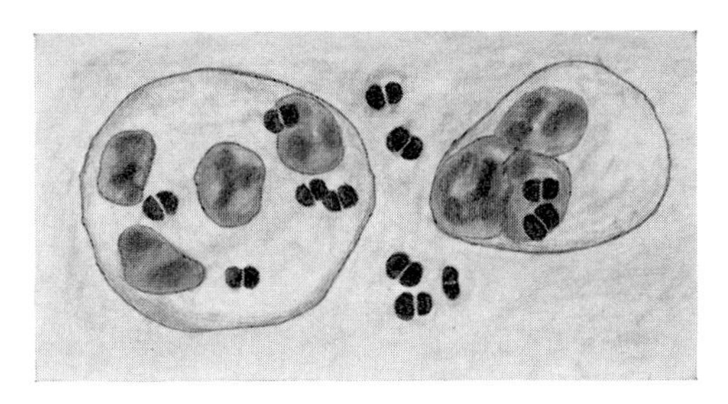

Diphtheroids are gram-negative as is *Neisseria gonorrhoeae,* and look like this:

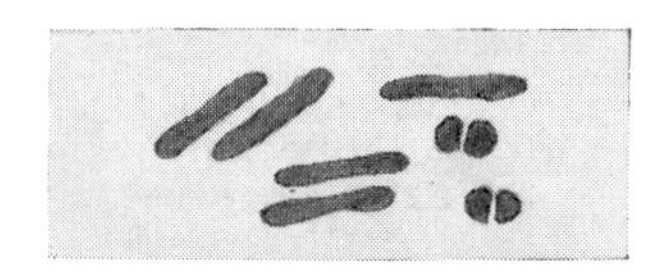

Staphylococci and streptococci are just as characteristic vaginally as in any other area.

The Chronic Case of Gonococcal Infection

It is true that gonorrhea burns itself out. Over a period of months a spontaneous cure will occur in most cases. After the acute phase is over, identification of the organism is a perilous business, using smears alone.

When the acute stage is passed, the organisms become progressively more rare and, therefore, one does not have the overwhelming weight of numbers as one has in the acute disease. Identification of gonorrhea after it has become quiescent is a matter for culture and usually for culture under carbon dioxide tension, which does not come within the purview of the office laboratory. That does not mean one should not try, but be extremely chary about making any diagnostic pronouncement as to the nature of the infecting organism.

FUNGOUS INFESTATIONS

The Monilia group are the common invaders of the human vagina. These seem to overgrow when there is an excess of carbohydrate material in the vaginal canal. This condition is most often met in pregnancy and in the presence of diabetes mellitus.

One distinctive point should always be remembered and that is that monilial organisms can be present as contaminates in the presence of other infections and may add to the symptomatology. They should be searched for in any case presenting the typical clinical findings of myocologic infection and also as a contaminate in any patient who does not seem to be responding readily to treatment.

Technique

Mix a drop of vaginal discharge with a drop of 10 per cent potassium hydroxide on a microscopic slide, add a cover glass, and warm the preparation gently. Typical Monilia organisms look like this:

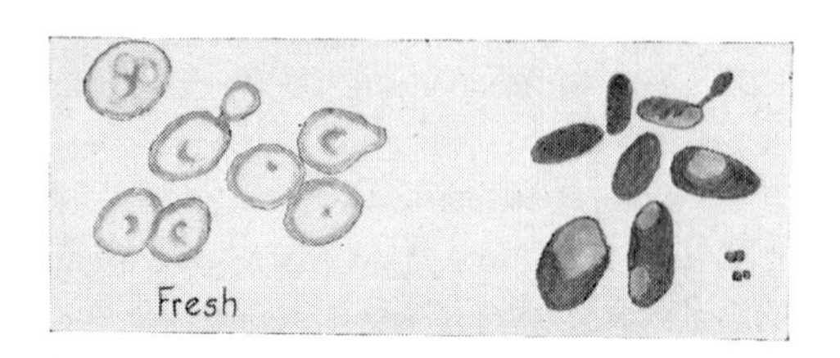

Errors

See section on office mycology on page 164.

Interpretation

The various fungi are not normal inhabitants of the vaginal canal, but their presence is not proof that they are causing the symptoms unless typical clinical findings are also present. Their *exclusive,* or almost exclusive, presence has a different connotation altogether.

Fortunately, treatment is so simple that one need seldom go into more extensive procedures for identification. If mycelial elements are present to the exclusion of any obvious bacterial invader, treat the disease as monilial infection.

SPERMATOZOA

Living spermatozoa are normally found in the human vagina for as long as twenty-four hours (and sometimes more) following intercourse. They have only the obvious significance, but their identification may be important in medicolegal cases.

It is also possible to achieve an estimation of the total sperm count by collecting sperm from the posterior vaginal pool shortly after it is deposited. This procedure actually serves two purposes. It gives a good estimation of the total and shows whether the sperm actually continue to live after having been deposited in the female vaginal secretion so that one actually does two tests in one by following this procedure.

Technique

To identify the sperm place a drop of the suspected fluid from the vagina on a warm microscopic slide, add a cover glass, and examine without stain. They look like this:

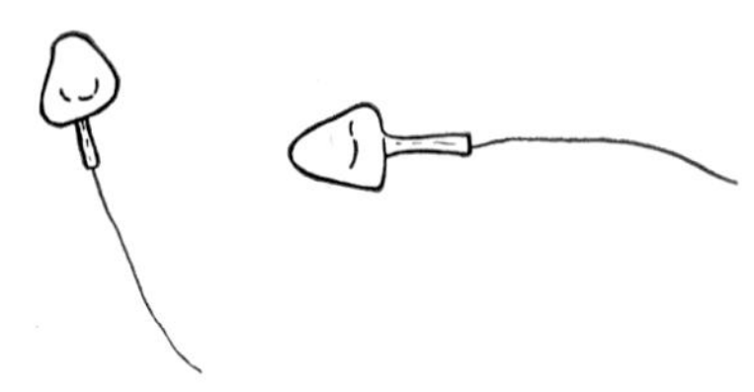

Even after many hours most sperm should be actively motile when obtained from the posterior fornix, and a rough estimation of the number of inactive sperm can be made by observing a hundred specimens on the warm, moist slide preparation.

Sperm may be counted by using 0.5 per cent Chlorazene as a diluent. Use the white blood cell pipette and draw the semen to the 0.5 mark. Then draw 0.5 per cent Chlorazene to the 11 mark. Shake thoroughly and place a drop in the counting chamber.

Count the sperm in two square chambers diagonally across from each other. Use the same squares that are used for the white blood count. To the figure obtained by adding the number in both squares add five zeros.

Stain the sperm by gently heat-fixing the specimen, applying a 0.2 per cent basic fuchsin for five minutes, then washing, drying, and examining. Check the stain by examining one sperm in the "collar" area.

Errors

Errors are practically unheard of in the identification of sperm, but errors in the identification of abnormal sperm are quite common. The series of illustrations in this section may help clarify the point.

Interpretation

The presence of sperm in the vagina in any quantity is almost incontrovertible evidence that the woman involved has had intercourse. I once heard a lawyer try to argue a jury into believing otherwise. It was worth the price of a show.

There is great variation in the normal sperm count, but as an arbitrary figure one may say that anything less than 60 million per cubic millimeter is distinctly low, and pregnancy may not occur unless the count is higher.

The normal stained sperm looks like this:

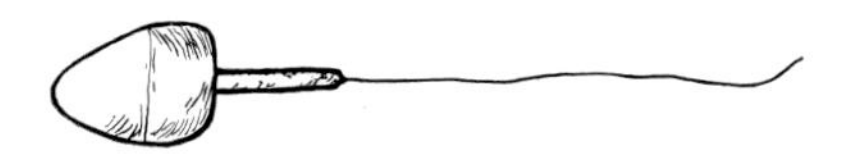

When checking for abnormalities one should always check the head, the neck, and the tail of each sperm for possible changes. Following are some typical abnormalities:

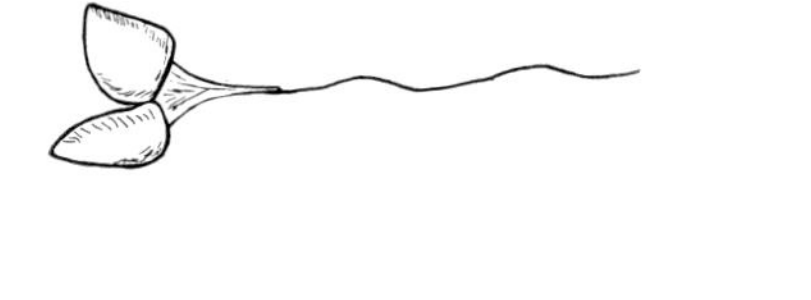

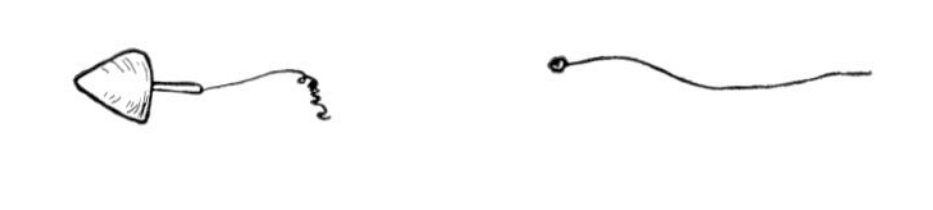

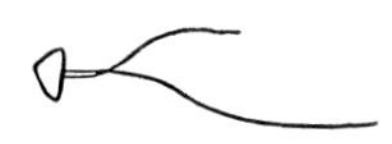

When more than 20 per cent of the spermatozoa are of abnormal form one may infer some abnormality of spermatogenesis and also may infer that pregnancy is at least unlikely. The perfectly normal male will show 1 to 2 per cent abnormalities at times.

CERVICITIS

It is sometimes of interest to the physician to know what organisms are involved in disease of the cervix. Particularly is this true when a previous examination has shown that Döderlein bacilli are absent, even though no organisms appear in the routine vaginal smear.

A typical smear is taken like this: A dry surgical sponge which has been dipped in Caroid powder is placed firmly against the cervix and held for five seconds or so. This is removed and the cervix gently sponged dry with another bit of gauze. The Caroid powder serves to dissolve the thick ropy mucus which is often on the surface of such lesions and allows both visualization of the cervix itself and the taking of an adequate smear.

One now uses a dry cotton-tipped applicator which is pushed gently into the cervical canal about a quarter of an inch like this:

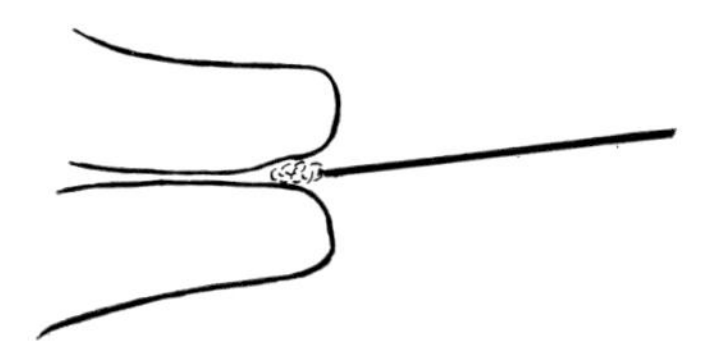

and firmly but gently raked around the mucous membrane. This material is used for a smear.

Technique

Apply ordinary Gram's stain as specified on page 155.

Errors

Errors in technique are rare. Most of them arise in interpretation.

Interpretation

The grossly irritated cervix has usually been invaded by bacteria and numbers of them are found in the exudate. Döderlein bacilli are conspicuous by their absence in most cases.

A typical exudate of mixed infection will look like this:

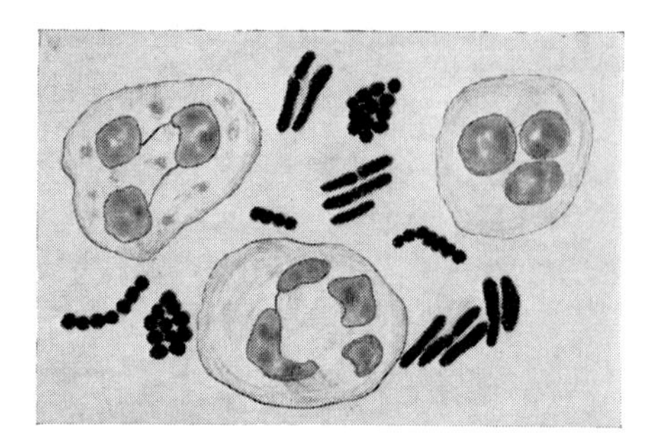

When one finds an exudate containing pus cells but apparently no organisms, one thinks first of the possibility of gonorrheal infection which is distinctly on the wane. Gonorrhea usually overgrows other organisms and there are seldom any other germs in the exudate until the Neisserian invader is almost entirely gone. In such a case one should probably resort to cultural methods.

EXFOLIATED CELLS

The cells exfoliated by the vaginal epithelium of the normal female give some clue to the existence of an estrogen deficiency. This finding is particularly valuable at the time of the menopause or when premature menopause is suspected. It is also valuable in guiding the treatment of senile vaginitis.

As estrogen effect becomes less and less pronounced, the vaginal cells become smaller and tend to be more round. The nucleus is slightly more dense and more central than in typical cells showing full estrogen effect.

Technique

Place a small drop of normal saline in the center of a microscopic slide. Use a cotton-tipped applicator to take a smear from the vaginal wall. Mix this with the normal saline solution and add a cover glass. No stain is necessary although a small drop of methylene blue placed at one side of the cover glass will stain the nuclei and make the cells more readily apparent.

Errors

Errors are largely in the field of interpretation and seldom in preparation of the specimen.

Interpretation

Cells showing full estrogen effect look like this:

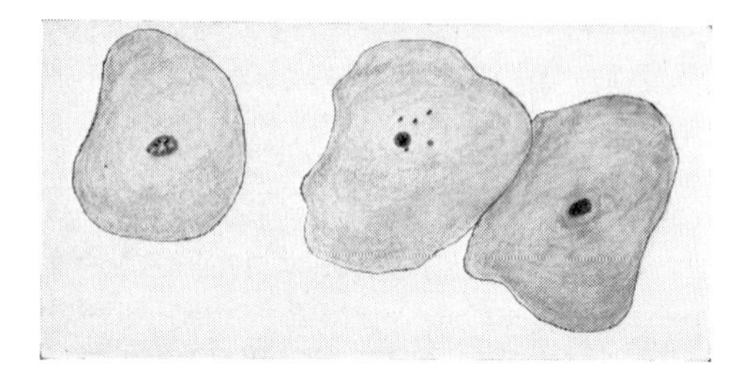

As the estrogen effect diminishes they become somewhat smaller and more irregular in outline. They look like this:

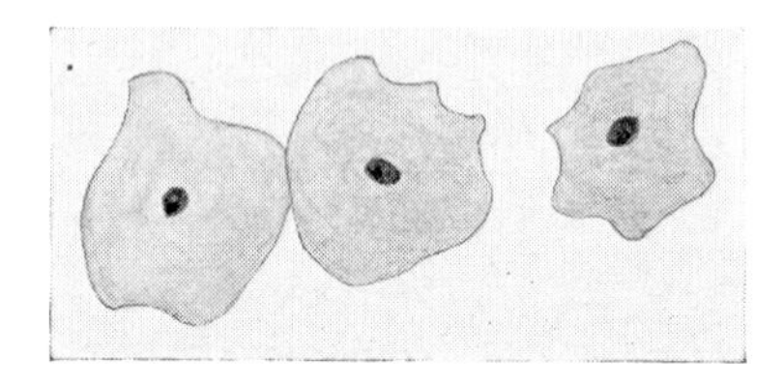

Part of the advanced estrogen deficiency shows a further change toward roundness of the cells and nuclei which are somewhat larger. Usually the epithelial cells are admixed with polymorphonuclear cells and the result looks like this:

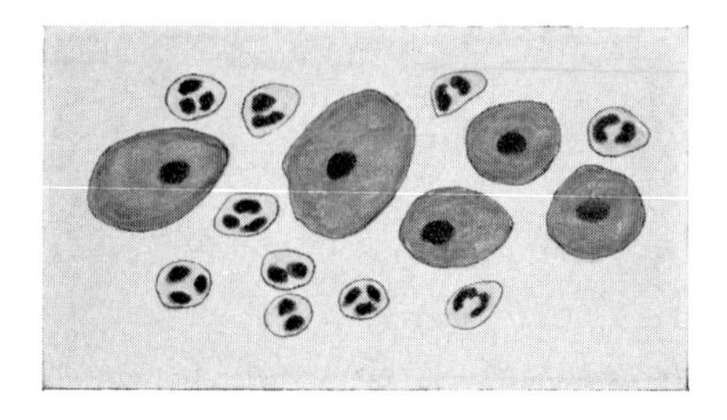

A case of far-advanced estrogen deficiency shows only small round cells with relatively large nuclei and many polymorphonuclear cells like this:

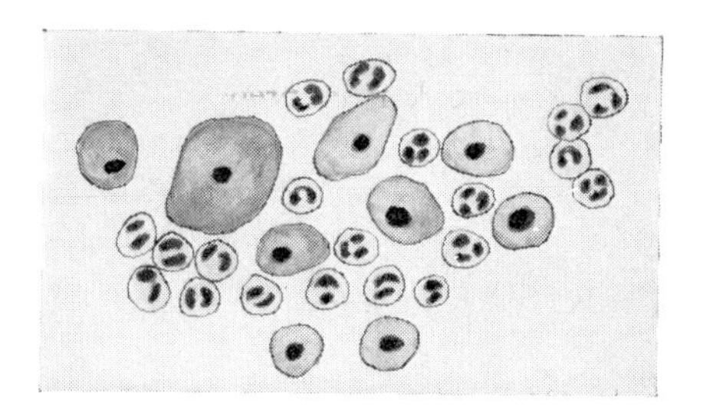

During the treatment of senile vaginitis the process is usually gradually reversed, but no effort should be made to carry it back until the cells show full estrogen effect. Relief of symptoms—not establishment of a normal reproductive vagina—is the criterion in senile vaginitis. Periodic smears, however, will often serve to establish the need for mild doses of estrogen before the patient becomes aware of symptoms.

In questionable cases of premature menopause this test may be of extreme value in illustrating whether or not a natural deficiency of the estrogenic hormones does exist.

The average physician, unless he has special training in cytology, should not attempt to read a Papanicolaou smear. It must, however, be taken in the office and prepared for shipment to a pathologist in the office laboratory.

Prepare a small jar, just large enough to contain the slides, and fill it with a mixture of half alcohol and half ether. The slides should then be held together, back to back, with either a rubber band or a paper clip and immersed in the mixture. The whole setup should be sent to the pathologist.

OTHER BIOPSIES

Other biopsies of gynecologic lesions should be fixed in 10 per cent formalin solution and sent in this solution to the pathologic laboratory of your choice.

CHAPTER TWELVE

Office Bacteriology

The problem in office bacteriology is to get the maximum information with the minimum of equipment. No office laboratory should attempt extensive bacteriologic studies. On the other hand, the average practitioner sees several cases weekly which could be made clearer by exercise of simple bacteriologic procedures.

In this chapter I will outline the simple bacteriologic determinations which we have used in a small laboratory for many years and which have proved satisfactory. I recommend that you consider seriously this matter of minor smear-and-culture techniques in the office.

EQUIPMENT

A small incubator can be purchased for about $60. A perfectly adequate home-made incubator can be constructed for a bit more than $10. One of the little portable iceboxes used on camping trips may be mounted on its side and a shelf or two installed. A covered electric light bulb provides ample heat and a sensitive thermostat and relay completes the installation.

Petri dishes, platinum loops, and media (which will be mentioned later) make up the necessary equipment. We use a pressure cooker for sterilization.

STAINS

For ordinary work done in the office only three stains are needed: methylene blue, carbolfuchsin, and Gram's stain.

Methylene Blue

Make up methylene blue stain by dissolving 0.3 Gm. of methylene blue in 30 ml. of 95 per cent ethyl alcohol. Add the resulting solution to 100 ml. of 0.01 per cent potassium hydroxide in distilled water.

Material for staining with methylene blue is usually heat-fixed. Apply the stain for one minute although the time may vary slightly with different batches. This is probably unimportant, for it is almost impossible to overstain with methylene blue. Wash the slide in water and dry for examination.

Carbolfuchsin

Make up carbolfuchsin by adding the following three ingredients to 90 ml. of distilled water: basic fuchsin, 1 Gm.; carbolic acid (phenol crystals), 5 Gm.; absolute ethyl alcohol, 10 ml.

Its use for acid-fast bacilli is described in the section on sputum, page 126.

Gram's Stain

Gram's stain is the standard stain for bacteriologic work. It separates microorganisms into two great classes: those that stain violet and are called gram-positive and those that stain pink or faint red which are called gram-negative.

The stains may be made up as follows:

In 20 ml. of ethyl alcohol dissolve 4 Gm. of crystal violet.

Next dissolve 0.8 Gm. of ammonium oxalate in 80 ml. of distilled water. Make the crystal violet stain. Mix the two solutions —20 ml. of the first and 80 ml. of the second.

Make Lugol's iodine solution by dissolving 1 Gm. of iodine crystals and 2 Gm. of potassium iodide in 300 ml. of water.

Then make the safranine counterstain by dissolving 0.25 Gm. of safranine in 10 ml. of ethyl alcohol and add the resultant solution to 90 ml. of water.

First air-dry the smear to be stained and then fix with heat. This is accomplished by gently passing the slide, smear side down, immediately above the flame of a Bunsen burner three or four times.

Then apply the crystal violet solution, leaving it in place for one minute. Wash off the stain and wash the slide in tap water. Apply Lugol's solution and allow it to remain in place one minute. Then wash it away and gently blot the slide until dry.

Then pour ethyl alcohol on the slide and gently agitate until no more color is seen to flow away from the tiny visible particles on the slide. Usually this will take from fifteen to thirty seconds. Once again wash the slide, pour away the excess water, and apply the safranine counterstain for ten to fifteen seconds. Then wash, dry, and examine.

Gram's stain is rather like a friend. On first acquaintance you are not sure just what to make of it for it does not always work out as it should. As your acquaintance ripens you know exactly what to expect and the behavior of your friend becomes nearly a mathematical certainty.

When a technician new at the job starts using the stain, things will not decolorize just right, areas will be overstained, some slides will not seem to stain, and every kind of trouble you can imagine will happen. Usually in a few weeks the stain is an old friend and results are excellent.

MEDIA

The real problem with media is to keep on hand the smallest number that will do the job. Literally hundreds of media and variations are available. Four or five are all that need be stocked.

The small office cannot well afford to keep plates and broths sterile and in stock. We usually make them up as needed. Media are obtained in dehydrated form from Difco Laboratories in Detroit or from regional dealers. They are supplied in one-pound cans. We calculate the amount of media needed for one or two flasks of broth or plates and have our drug room weigh out the amount and package it in individual papers like medicinal powders.

When media need to be made we dissolve the contents of the proper number of powder papers, pour the resulting solution into flasks or Petri dishes, and sterilize immediately. We cool the resultant flasks or dishes in the icebox for a few minutes and then use when the proper temperature is reached. If you follow this technique it is wise always to incubate a blank to make as sure as possible that the media are sterile before inoculation.

This is not good bacteriologic technique, but it is the only feasible technique for office use. If there is sufficient time or it is necessary that the technique be more exacting (for example, a blood culture), be more leisurely and more accurate. Any good text on bacteriology will supply details.

Nutritive Broth

We use the Difco brain-heart infusion. This is made up in our drug room in packages containing 3.7 Gm. of dehydrated medium and 0.1 Gm. of agar. When prepared for actual use the contents of one paper are dissolved in 100 ml. of distilled water and the resultant solution put in a 500 ml. Erlenmeyer flask. It is sterilized for fifteen minutes at 15 pounds pressure.

Although the broth will grow most pathogens, even some anaerobes, it is seldom used except for blood work. For a blood culture we add 10 ml. of blood and incubate for twenty-four hours.

Agar Base

For slants or Petri dish agars we use as a base the Difco blood agar base. This is put up in papers containing 0.8 Gm. of the dehydrated medium which is added to 20 ml. of distilled water. This amount will make two slants or fill two Petri dishes.

To make blood agar the medium is cooled to about 45° C. and 0.5 ml. of citrated fresh blood is added. We supply the blood ourselves except when *Hemophilus influenzae* is under consideration, in which case rabbit blood is preferable.

Chocolate agar is prepared by adding 1.0 ml. of citrated blood per 10 ml. of media while still hot (70° to 75° C.). The blood should immediately turn dark brown. If it does not, then reheat.

Slants and plain agar plates may also be made up from the Difco heart infusion agar which has the same composition as the product mentioned above but which is slightly alkaline. Preparation is the same, 0.8 Gm. to 20 ml. We do not often add blood to this medium.

Technique

In the office, practically all bacteriology begins with a streak-plate inoculation. Use sterile cotton-tipped applicators to obtain a specimen of the material to be cultured. Elevate one side of the Petri dish cover an inch or slightly more and lightly streak the applicator over the surface of the medium.

Then close the Petri dish, invert it, and incubate overnight. In almost half the cases —particularly in the acute infections—the pathogen will be obtained in almost pure culture. If microscopic examination does not suffice, it may be transferred to other plates.

When there are several suspicious cultures of differing appearance on the plate, examine each microscopically. Begin by placing a small drop of physiologic saline solution on a microscopic slide. Using the platinum wire loop, pick up a tiny bit of a suspicious colony and mix it thoroughly with the drop of normal saline.

Next, spread the drop widely over the slide and allow to air-dry. Obvious contaminants can usually be differentiated from the obvious pathogens by this examination. If there is any question be sure to follow up the supposed contaminant until you are sure.

Be sure to sterilize the loop of platinum wire both before and after touching the plate or slide. When one is relatively certain that the pathogen has been separated from any contaminant, use the wire loop to pick up a bit of a colony of pathogens and smear it on a new plate or slant.

If carefully done this will result in a plate of pure cultures of the pathogen in twenty-four hours. These can then be used for whatever tests seem applicable. Actually one seldom needs to go this far. Microscopic examination of the first plate of colonies usually suffices for office bacteriology.

SYSTEMIC DISEASES

Tuberculosis

The technique for staining smears for acid-fast organisms has been mentioned on page 126.

Just recently we have become interested in a quick culture method which looks promising but which by no means has been proved. I pass it along to you as an idea but not as an established technique. As a medium we use Difco's TB broth base enriched with their TB medium albumin as instructed in the Difco manual.

This medium, although a liquid, is put in Petri dishes and sterilized. Throughout the rest of this technique the most rigid precautions as to sterility must be observed.

Thick smears of suspected sputum are made on two *sterile* slides and these are completely immersed in 6 per cent sulfuric acid for twenty minutes. The acid is removed by gently dipping the slides in sterile water two or three times.

The slides, which should have been so treated that they remain sterile, are then put in the Petri dish, smear side up so that they are completely immersed in the broth.

After two days of incubation one slide is removed and stained with carbofuchsin and picric acid as mentioned on page 126. The next slide is examined at four days. The characteristic acid-fast "pile of sticks" indicates *Mycobacterium tuberculosis.*

Each slide should be gone over thoroughly. Frequently there will be only one or two small cultures and they are easily missed.

Rheumatic Fever

Throat cultures should be taken periodically and plated on blood agar. After twenty-four hours the plate should be examined for the presence of beta hemolytic streptococci.

Such organisms show sharply defined rings of complete hemolysis around the colonies, like this:

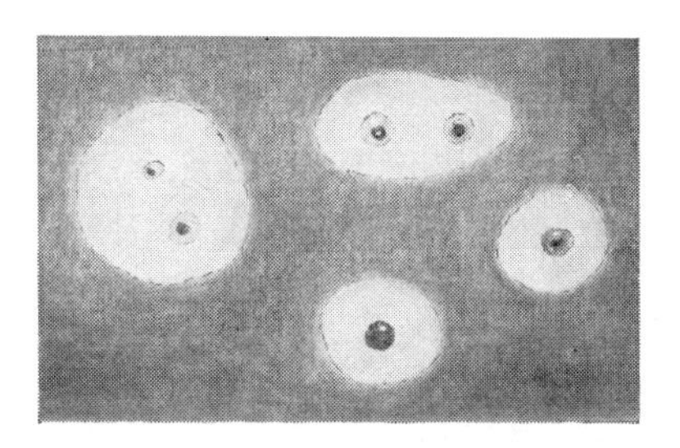

If there is question, examine the hemolytic area with the low power of the microscope. No blood cells will be seen if the colony is of the beta hemolytic type.

When smeared and examined microscopically the streptococcus is a gram-positive organism that forms chains, like this:

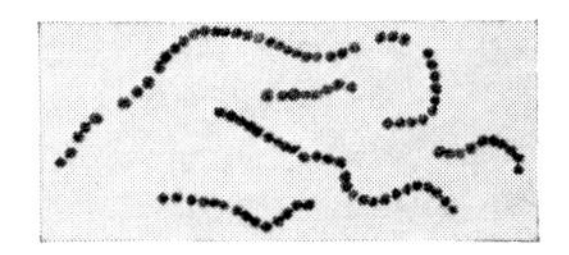

Actually there are always a few individuals that decolorize and appear gram-negative. Apparently these individuals are more numerous in the hemolytic strains.

Septicemic Diseases

Few patients with acute septicemias will be seen in the office laboratory and they certainly will not stay for examination. There are, however, two conditions involving the septicemic process which are occasionally seen in office patients. They are endocarditis and staphylococcal septicemia.

When the course of a disease makes one suspect the presence of one of the more chronic coccemias, a blood culture should be taken. Prepare 100 ml. of nutrient broth as specified on page 156. Using sterile technique through each minor detail, withdraw 10 ml. of blood from the patient and deposit it in the broth. Incubate overnight.

Cultures of the organisms will usually be apparent. Remove an area of growth from the broth, using the platinum loop, and plate on blood agar. If no growth is present incubate the culture for another twenty-four hours before discarding.

While it would seem that they should grow out readily, blood cultures do not always do so. Organisms are not always present in the peripheral blood, and repeated tests may have to be made before one gets a positive result. If two cultures at the office have not given any information, we ask the patient to be hospitalized if symptoms and signs still indicate septicemia.

When growth occurs we look for two principal offenders. The first is *Streptococcus viridans,* which may produce hazy hemolysis and a greenish cast on blood plates. It is gram-positive. The second is *Staphylococcus aureus.* It produces round, smooth colonies of the rich, golden-yellow color of natural butter. It is a gram-positive organism.

Staph. aureus is often a contaminant. One should certainly never make a diagnosis of staphylococcal septicemia on the basis of a single positive blood culture unless every clinical sign points in the same direction. Staphylococcal septicemia is practically never seen at the blood culture stage without secondary abscess formation.

Another point to remember is that young infants (1 to 10 weeks of age) may have a virulent septicemia with little in the way of clinical evidence except the obvious fact that they are ill. When a child in such an age group has an obscure illness not readily diagnosed, a blood culture may be of service.

Should you find some unusual bacterium in the blood culture (for example, say, *Escherichia coli*), do not believe it but take another culture. If the unusual organism is still present, hospitalize the patient. Office bacteriologic technique is seldom reliable enough for us to base a rare diagnosis on the findings.

Typhoid Fever

Isolation of the typhoid bacillus from the feces is hardly within the purview of the office laboratory. However, during the first week or ten days of the disease the bacillus may be cultured from the blood. Take the cultures in the routine way (page 157) and incubate for twenty-four hours.

Then transfer the broth to plain agar plates and to the surface of a slice of potato. On plain agar *Eberthella typhosa* grows luxuriantly, while the other microorganisms commonly found in the blood stream do not.

On potato the bacillus presents no readily apparent growth, but there are areas where the potato surface appears slick and glassy. Coliforms show exuberant growth of gray-brown colonies on potato.

When stained, *E. typhosa* shows no distinguishing characteristics. It is a large, gram-negative rod.

LOCALIZED DISEASES

There are four diseases not previously discussed which are sharply localized and in which office bacteriology may play an important part. Other important localized diseases need bacteriologic diagnosis but, for the most part, patients are far too ill to tarry in the office and the necessary procedures are best done in the hospital.

Chronic Osteomyelitis

No one should undertake the treatment of a draining osteomyelitis until he knows for certain what bacteria are causing the process. If smears fail to reveal the organism at fault, streak plates should be made on both blood agar and plain agar.

In most cases the organism identified will be *Staphylococcus aureus*. Rarely other bacteria will be found. No matter what the organism, it should be isolated in pure culture and tested for sensitivity to the various antibiotics as outlined on page 163. Not to do this in chronic osteomyelitis is to court sudden and complete disaster.

Meningitis

Surprisingly enough, a number of patients with meningitis are office diagnostic problems, particularly in rural practice. When spinal fluid is secured it may be smeared, fixed with heat, and stained with Gram's stain.

In adults, the most common cause of bacterial meningitis is *Neisseria intracellularis*. It is a gram-negative diplococcus which looks like this:

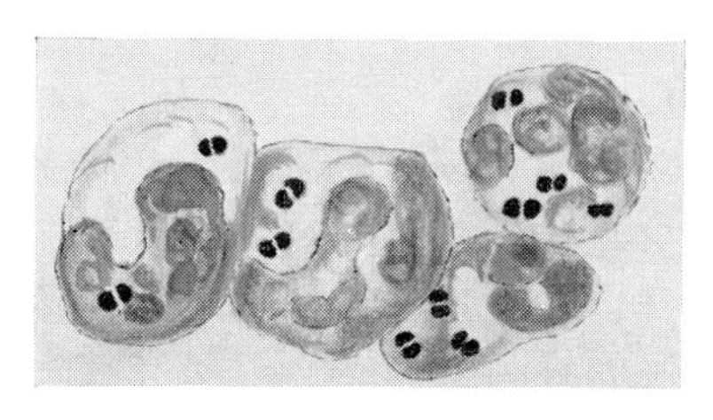

Unfortunately the organisms degenerate quickly and may be either absent or unidentifiable in the fluid obtained. Cultural methods may be used but are by no means certain in the office laboratory, for the meningococcus grows best under increased carbon dioxide tension. Spinal fluid may be streaked on blood agar plates and incubated for twenty-four hours.

In a significant percentage of cases (but not in all) the meningococcus will appear on the plates.

Recent information would seem to indicate that *Hemophilus influenzae* is the most frequent cause of meningitis in young children. The organisms are small gram-negative rods which do not stain well. With methylene blue they are somewhat better visualized. This is a typical field from spinal fluid:

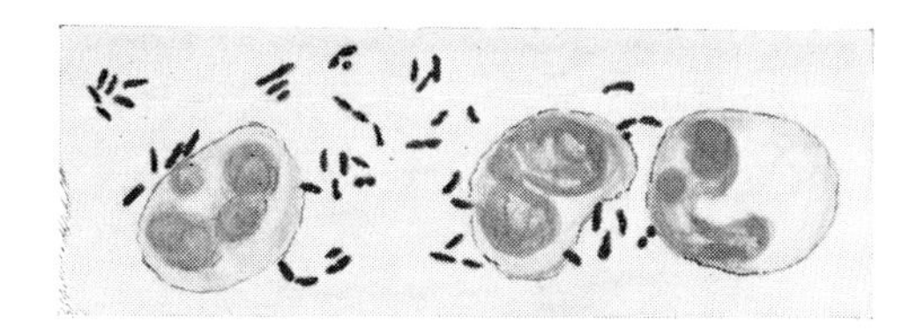

They will grow reasonably well on blood agar or chocolate agar and specimens of the suspected spinal fluid may be plated in the office. Within eighteen to twenty-four hours colonies will appear which are dome-shaped and transparent and look much like small drops of water.

Actually, because of the difficult problems of isolation involved, we prefer to take most patients with meningitis to the hospital before performing a spinal tap.

Chancroid

The bacillus of Ducrey is often easily seen in scrapings from chancroidal lesions, rendering cultural methods unnecessary. Secretions taken from the bottom of the ulcer or from underneath the overhanging sides are most satisfactory for this purpose. The organism is gram-negative, very small, and sometimes forms chains. It looks like this:

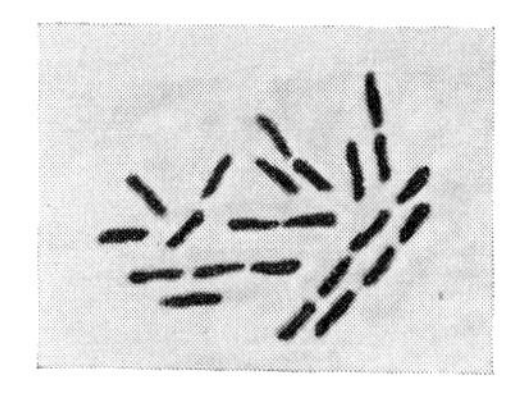

If the clinical findings are those of chancroid and nothing is seen in a smear, the platinum loop should be used to scrape the depths of the lesion and the material obtained plated on blood agar. Colonies are slow to appear and are usually not seen until after forty-eight hours of incubation.

They are small and of a dull, opalescent, gray-white color.

So many contaminant colonies are often present that it may be wise to smear a typical colony and replate if it seems to show typical *Hemophilus ducreyi.*

Diphtheria

Rarely we see a case in the office that has all the characteristics of diphtheria. The suspected area should be wiped with a cotton-tipped applicator and both direct smears and chocolate agar plates made.

Smears should be stained with methylene blue. *Corynebacterium diphtheriae* show irregular transverse bands which stain lightly, alternating with heavier staining areas, and look like this:

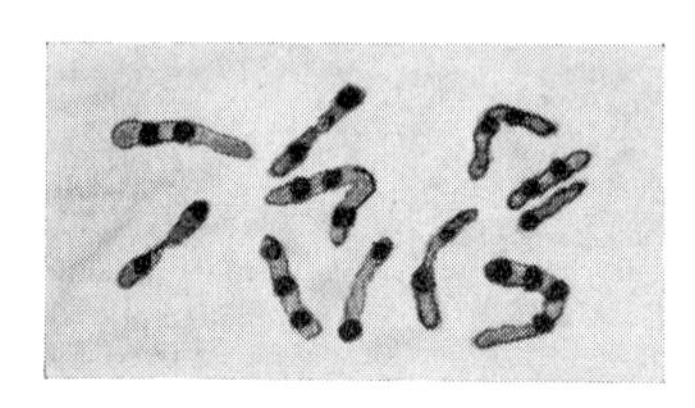

On any kind of blood-enriched medium, colonies are usually sufficiently well developed in twenty-four hours to allow smear and staining. Bacilli from such colonies usually show an enlargement near one end. They have been described as club-shaped. This is a typical appearance:

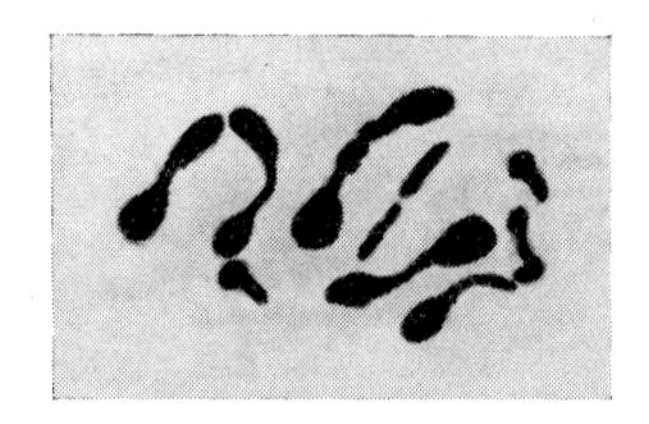

There is a series of bacteria that strongly resembles *C. diphtheriae* in staining reaction and cultural characteristics. For lack of a better name, they are called the diphtheroids. Seemingly they are principally saprophytes, normally being found in the body orifices but seldom in profusion.

When one isolates a pure culture of diphtheroids from a lesion, a real problem presents itself. Are these organisms causing or doing anything to prolong the pathologic process? The answer is by no means clear. Being a typical middle-of-the-road thinker, I usually assume that the diphtheroids are incapable of primary invasion but are capable of prolonging a process once it has been initiated.

They are probably best eradicated.

DISCHARGES

Here is where the office laboratory can really be of great service to the practitioner. In both acute and chronic disease (more often in chronic) a bacteriologic determination often avoids a costly mistake or needless treatment.

The determinations involved are simple and require no great bacteriologic skill. Tentative identification is often all that is necessary, and a test for sensitivity to antibiotics sometimes renders even this needless.

By these statements I mean no condonement of slipshod medicine. On the other hand, the practitioner cannot be a highly skilled bacteriologist along with all his other duties. He must make practical use of bacteriology and leave advanced techniques in the hands of the experts.

The Ear

Chronic discharges from the ear are a common problem in practice. The possible invaders are legion.

We use a sterile medicine dropper to suck up a drop or two of the discharge from deep in the canal. This is mixed with 1.0 ml. of warm sterile physiologic saline solution in a test tube. An applicator is dipped in the resulting solution and streak plates made on chocolate agar.

In twenty-four hours the plates are checked and smears made of the predominating organism. A test for sensitivity to the antibiotics is run as specified on page 163.

Common findings on the original chocolate agar plate are as follows:

1. *Staphylococcus aureus.* The organism has the typical appearance already described. When it is the cause of the trouble as is often the case, one usually obtains a plate with dozens of *Staph. aureus* colonies and practically nothing else. A significant number of these organisms seem highly resistant to penicillin.

2. *Streptococcus viridans.* The growth is exactly as previously described for this organism.

3. Coliforms. Short, gram-negative rods that grow out well on plain nutrient agar. The fecal odor of the discharge from the ear is usually characteristic.

4. *Pseudomonas aeruginosa (pyocyanea).* A small gram-negative rod, irregularly staining. Colonies usually exhibit a blue-green pigment. If there is question, inoculate a test tube containing 5 ml. of fresh milk with bacteria from a typical colony. It will coagulate and turn yellowish green.

5. Diphtheroids. Appear as described above. Treatment in such a case is probably not wise until one knows the antibiotics to which the organism will respond.

The Eye

There is a particularly vicious form of corneal ulcer which is caused by the pneumococcus and which sometimes results in corneal opacities. Smear and culture sometimes help in establishing treatment, although one should not await the results before taking some action. As a matter of self-protection, these laboratory procedures are probably wise.

Seldom does one see a conjunctivitis that will not respond adequately to routine treatment. Bacteriologic study is seldom indicated.

The Mouth

It does not seem as if it should be so, but there are occasional cases of Vincent's angina which cause a great deal of confusion. Pus can usually be expressed by rolling an applicator firmly from low on the gum toward the gum margin.

Smear the drop of pus so obtained and stain with methylene blue. *Borrelia vincentii* looks like this:

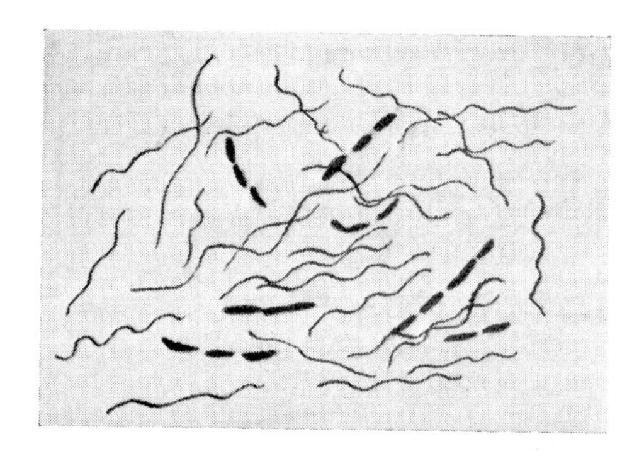

It has been said many times that the fusiform organisms shown in the illustration must be present as well as the spirillum in order to make a diagnosis of Vincent's angina. Our experience has certainly not indicated that this is so. We feel that the diagnosis is positive when the great majority of organisms present are made up of typical spirochetes.

The Pharynx

With our present antibiotic techniques, there are few, if any, acute pharyngeal infections that need culture or smear. Often in children and rarely in adults we see persistent postnasal drip due to chronic infection in the posterior nasopharynx.

These patients are better treated when one knows the germ with which he must deal and has determined to which antibiotic it will best respond.

Mixed infections are exceedingly common in this area and must be treated adequately. In our experience little of permanent value can be accomplished unless one either shrinks with drugs or removes the swollen, boggy lymphoid tissue which is usually most involved.

The Sputum

The sputum has been discussed, beginning on page 124.

The Urine

Urine culture is an extremely important part of office bacteriology. We all see many patients with mild or moderate infection of the urinary tract who can be well handled without hospitalization.

Probably all culture specimens should be obtained by catheterization. In the male the distal urethra would seem to contain, of necessity, some contaminant organisms. In the female it is difficult to avoid some vaginal contamination.

For ordinary work, techniques designed to concentrate the urine are not necessary. If the infection is grossly obvious a small bit of urine may be used to make streak plates on plain nutritive agar and chocolate agar.

If there is a question about the existence of infection place 10 ml. of urine into an Erlenmeyer flask containing 100 ml. of broth and incubate for twenty-four hours or more. Then make streak plates. A single negative result by no means proves the absence of infection.

The Genitalia

The procedures to be used on the female genitalia are discussed, beginning on page 145.

The only really important procedure upon the male genitalia is the smear of urethral discharge. In practice now we see not nearly as many cases of gonorrhea as we did years ago. About half the cases of urethral discharge are now classified as nonspecific urethritis which is, of course, a nice way of saying we do not have any idea what causes them.

A smear from the typical case of gonorrhea usually looks like this:

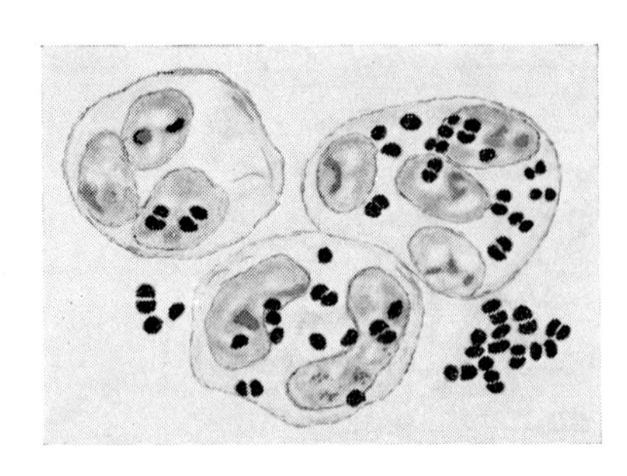

Nonspecific urethritis looks like this:

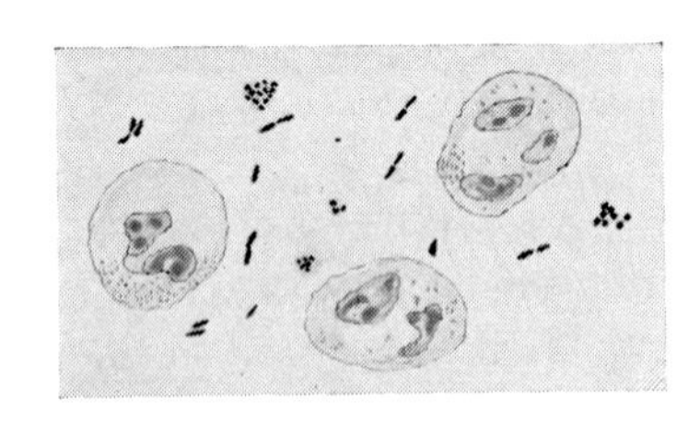

Gonococci are conspicuous by their absence and there is much more debris than is usually seen in the typical smear with Neisseria. There may be a wide range of organisms or none at all. Our cases have been divided about half and half.

Abscesses and Infection

Needless to say, any persistent and puzzling infection should be examined bacteriologically. One particular kind of abscess suggests itself immediately.

The deep perirectal infection is often caused by coliforms and may not respond well to the treatment applied to acute infections elsewhere. Just smelling the drainage is sometimes enough to identify the organism, but smear and culture may be necessary.

ANTIBIOTIC SENSITIVITY

Our range of antibiotics is now so great that one has difficulty choosing among them. Bacteriologic techniques designed to determine the proper antibiotic are in widespread use and can be applied with facility to the office laboratory.

Through the various surgical supply houses one can obtain proper disks saturated with the various antibiotics. Place these on a blood agar plate.

Next, obtain a sterile test tube containing 0.5 ml. of sterile physiologic saline solution. Pick one of the cultures of the pathogen from the original plate by means of the platinum loop and thoroughly disperse in the saline.

Then dip a sterile cotton-tipped applicator in the saline solution and use it to streak the plate with the sensitivity disks in place. Also inoculate another plate without sensitivity disks so as to provide a pure culture of the pathogen.

In twenty-four hours read the sensitivity test. If the bacterium responds to a drug it will not grow in the area immediately surrounding it.

Such a simple subcultural device will serve to delineate basic sensitivities. Now, suppose we wish to know *how sensitive* the particular germ is to Aureomycin. One can buy the same type of paper rosette which has various dilutions of Aureomycin impregnated on the different disks. Follow the same technique to make a streak plate and read the results in twenty-four hours. The disks look like this:

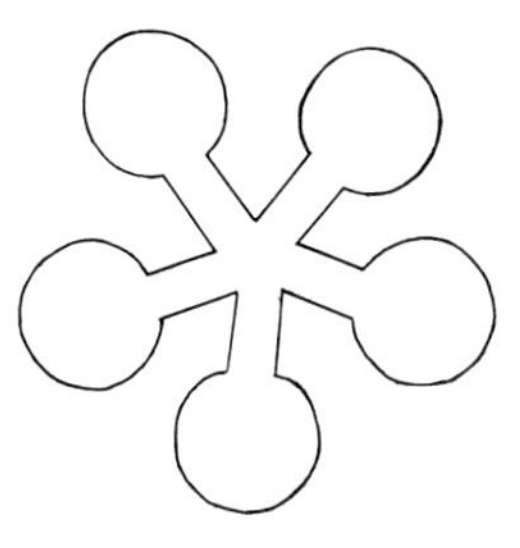

This chapter has been a sketchy outline of minor office bacteriology. If you are interested in delving further into the subject, refer to one of the standard texts such as *Textbook of Microbiology** or *Clinical Laboratory Methods and Diagnosis*.†

*Burrows, W.: Textbook of Microbiology, Philadelphia, 1954, W. B. Saunders Co.

†Gradwohl, R. B. H.: Clinical Laboratory Methods and Diagnosis, St. Louis, 1956, The C. V. Mosby Co.

CHAPTER THIRTEEN

Office Mycology

Most practitioners see mycologic disease with some frequency, but it is only in recent years that the simple laboratory techniques of mycologic diagnosis have become available. There is no reason for the physician to try the advanced techniques in the office laboratory, but the minor procedures are often of great value.

Techniques

Slides are ordinarily examined unstained. They are best mounted in a drop of 10 per cent potassium hydroxide, after which the slide is gently warmed over a Bunsen flame.

Two culture media are all that are usually needed. As in the preparation of bacteriologic media, we use the ready-prepared dehydrated product prepared by Difco. Proper quantities are measured out into papers and diluted as needed.

The most commonly used medium is the Sabouraud dextrose agar. It is measured into papers containing 1 Gm. of the medium. For dilution put the contents of one paper in a standard one-ounce medicine bottle and dilute with 15 ml. of sterile water.

We keep a solution on hand in a dropper bottle containing 3.385 Gm. of copper sulfate dissolved in one ounce of water. One drop of this solution is added to the medium before sterilization, resulting in a concentration of copper sulfate of about 0.05 per cent. This effectively suppresses the growth of most bacteria. After sterilization for fifteen minutes at 15 pounds' pressure cap the bottle tightly to prevent dehydration of the medium and slant.

After solidification place the medium in the refrigerator. It will keep for a week or more when so treated. When taken out for use, the technician should use pliers to loosen the bottle cap for it will usually be tightly stuck.

The Littman oxgall agar is also of value for isolation of fungi, although the colonies are slower to appear. To prepare this, suspend 1.1 Gm. of the dehydrated medium in 20 ml. of sterile water and autoclave for fifteen minutes at 15 pounds' pressure. Then pour this amount into a Petri dish and, when the medium is about cool, add 100 mg. of streptomycin.

One stain is of some use in examining cultures. It is the lactophenolic cotton blue which is made up as follows:

Phenol crystals	20 Gm.
Lactic acid	20 ml.
Glycerol	40 ml.
Distilled water	20 ml.

Dissolve this mixture by heating it in a water bath and then add 0.05 Gm. of cotton blue.

THE DERMATOPHYTOSES

Skin lesions caused by the three genera of dermatophytes are extremely common. Probably at least once a day every practitioner sees a case caused by these organisms which attack the skin, hair, and nails and nothing else.

In the ordinary case it may not even be necessary to make a microscopic examination, for the lesions are entirely typical. Perhaps one case out of ten will not be so clear-cut, but microscopic observation, if properly done, will usually reveal fungi.

Without using cultural methods it is not easily possible to separate the three genera. In only the rare and persistent case will culture be necessary, but the procedure is so simple and satisfactory that it should be used if any doubt exists.

The lesions caused by the dermatophytes are so protean and so similar that it is best to consider them by area rather than to attempt etiologic differentiation.

Tinea Capitis

Ringworm of the scalp is usually diagnosed on sight or by examination in Wood's light. If there is any doubt, pull several infected hairs and examine microscopically after mounting in 10 per cent potassium hydroxide. A typical hair infested with fungi looks like this:

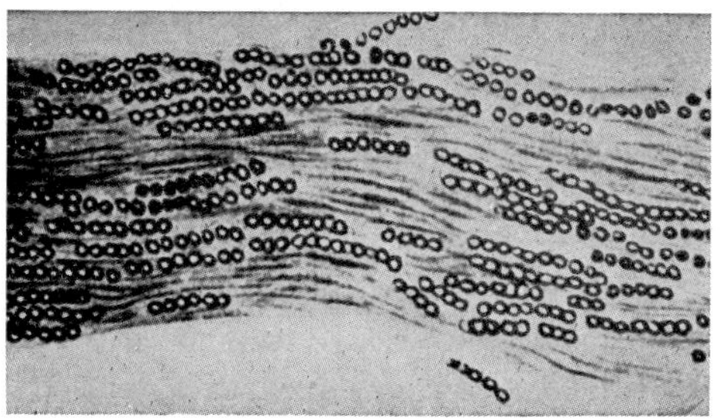

(Bruhns-Alexander: Grundriss der mykologischen Diagnostik, Julius Springer, Berlin.)

The real problem is to determine whether the animal type, *Microsporum canis,* or *Microsporum gypseum* or the human type, most usually *Microsporum audouini,* is present. Clinical differentiation is often possible because of the increased inflammatory reaction which accompanies the animal types.

If there is any question, a Sabouraud culture should be planted by placing two or three infected hairs on the surface of the medium. Should there be a question of severe bacterial contamination (and there usually will not be), place the hairs to be cultured between two sterile slides pressed firmly together and wrap in waxed paper. Leave undisturbed for from five to seven days and then culture on the fungous media.

M. audouini can usually be identified by its growth characteristics without resort to the microscope. It is much slower growing than either *M. canis* or *M. gypseum,* taking approximately twice as long to appear and to cover the surface of the medium.

The aerial part of the colony is closely matted and shows furrows radiating spokewise from the center like this:

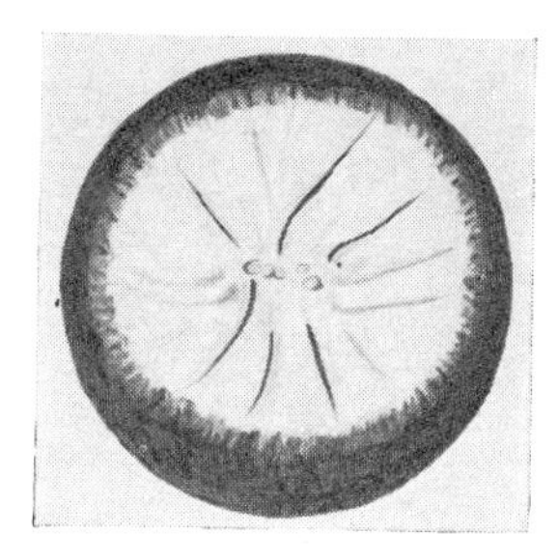

M. canis is fast-growing, with a cottony appearance and feathery streaks radiating outward from the edge of the colony.

M. gypseum appears much the same as *M. canis* but does not show the extensive radiating spicules of aerial growth.

Since *M. audouini* often requires x-ray therapy in order to obtain adequate results, it is probably better to plant a culture at the first visit if there is any doubt as to the infectious agent.

Tinea Corporis

Ringworm of the body is a common disease in children. It may be necessary to make smears for diagnostic purposes, but cultures are actually seldom indicated. There is no particular dermatophyte that is a great deal more persistent than the others.

I cannot, however, urge too strongly that mycologic studies be made if there is any doubt about the diagnosis. Both the physician and his laboratory technician should be familiar with basic mycology. One of the standard textbooks is a good investment to make. This book is only introductory.

Take scrapings from the advancing edge of the lesions after washing with 70 per cent alcohol. We use the sharp blade of a scapel to scrape away, not cut away, a few bits of the superficial skin layers. Mount these in 10 per cent potassium hydroxide and heat the slide gently in a Bunsen flame.

Typical fungous filaments look like this:

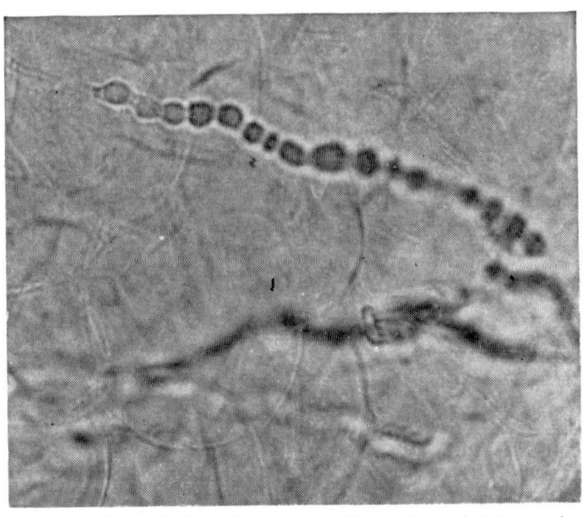

(Gradwohl: Clinical Laboratory Methods and Diagnosis, 1956, The C. V. Mosby Co.)

The most frequent error is to mistake an artifact for true fungous elements. This common mistake is made by both beginners and mycologists of some experience. One artifact causes the most difficulty. It is the "mosaic fungus" sometimes seen in potassium hydroxide preparations of the skin. The branching elements look like this:

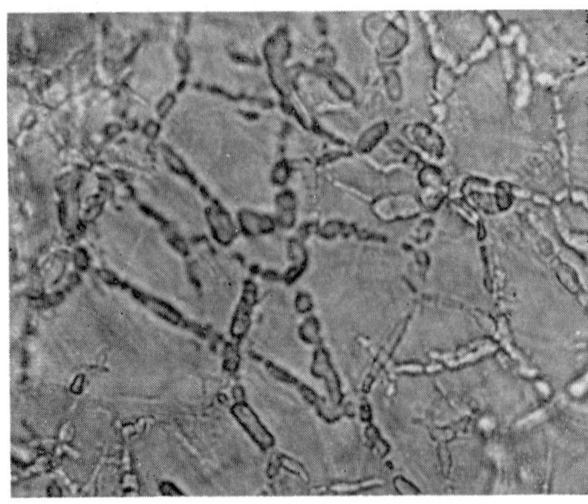

(Gradwohl: Clinical Laboratory Methods and Diagnosis, 1956, The C. V. Mosby Co.)

The irregularity of organization is the key point in differentiation. It is an artifact, not a living growth.

If small vesicles are present in the advancing edge of the lesion, the tops of one or two should be snipped off with manicure scissors and subjected to examination in potassium hydroxide.

Tinea Cruris

The dhobie itch (jockey-strap itch, gym itch, ringworm of the groin, etc.) is a disease that practically never requires any diagnostic procedure other than inspection. If any question should exist scrapings taken from the margin of the lesion and mounted in potassium hydroxide should clarify the problem.

If the condition does not respond readily to treatment, one should suspect infection with *Trichophyton rubrum.* On Sabouraud's medium the culture characteristically develops a deep red to purple pigmentation on the underside. This may extend to the aerial part of the growth as a faint pink to blood red discoloration.

Other Trichophyton cultures show a depression or humping of the colony center, with infolding about the edges. Rubrum and gypseum groups of the genus Trichophyton do not show this characteristic and this serves as a primary differentiating method.

Microscopic evidence must be used to separate the gypseum and rubrum groups unless pigmentation is unmistakable. Characteristics present in the genus are:

1. Microconidia borne in clusters along the hyphae, like this:

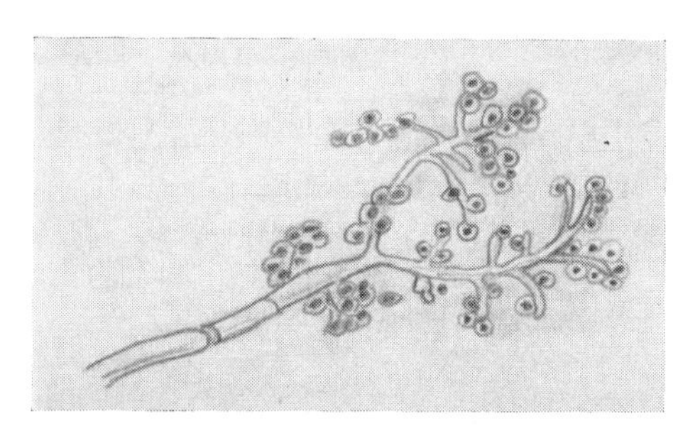

Both *T. rubrum* and *T. gypseum* have this characteristic.

2. Spiral hyphae, like this:

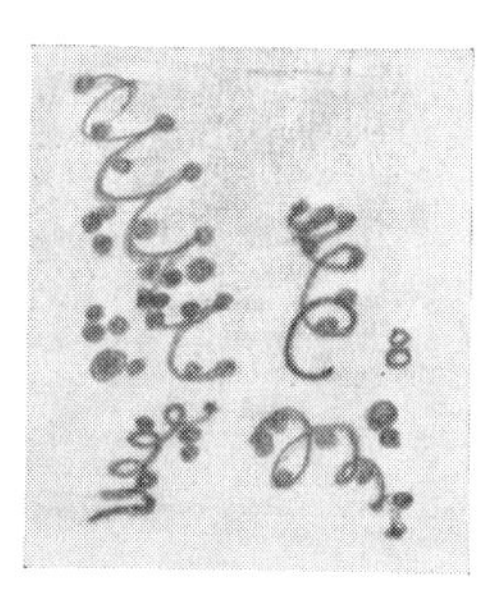

These are rarely found in rubrum but are often seen in gypseum.

3. Racquet hyphae, like this:

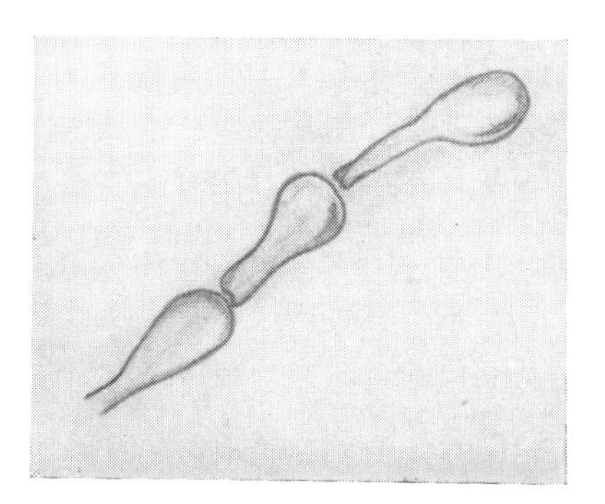

These are seldom seen in the rubrum group but are found in gypseum.

Tinea Unguium

Take scrapings from the friable portion of the nails and mount in potassium hydroxide. The fungus is usually apparent. Also subject detritus from underneath the nail to the same examination.

The infection rarely may be due to *Candida albicans,* but differentiation can usually be made clinically because detritus beneath the nail is usually not seen in *C. albicans* infection.

Tinea Pedis

Tinea pedis is the most common of all the dermatophytoses. If microscopic examination is needed for diagnosis and it frequently is, scrape away a few scales from the side of a typical lesion and mount in potassium hydroxide. Do not attempt to get material from macerated areas.

Most persistent cases are the result of reinfection from shoes, the gym, etc. If one feels that a case is not responding as it should, the possibility of this reinfection should be thought of first. If a careful check seems to indicate that this is not so, culture for *Trichophyton rubrum* as mentioned on page 166.

Tinea Versicolor

Every time somebody develops a good rule in medicine, something or someone comes along to invalidate it. As we have said previously, there are only three dermatophytic genera which show great similarity in the diseases they produce. Now comes along a completely different fungus called *Malassezia furfur* to produce the typical lesions of tinea versicolor.

Diagnosis is easy. Scrape some scales from a typical lesion and mount them in 10 per cent potassium hydroxide. Heat gently and then place a small drop of methylene blue stain at one edge of the cover slip. *M. furfur* looks like this:

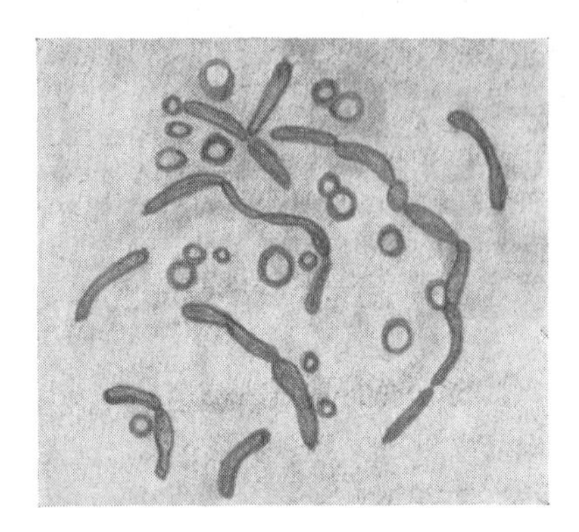

MONILIASIS

Infections with *Candida albicans* are relatively common. Fortunately the bronchopulmonary types and the more serious cutaneous types are rare.

Ordinary thrush is the most common monilial infection seen in the practitioner's office. It consists of patches of pale white membrane sometimes pinhead-sized and sometimes forming large plaques as big as a dime on the mucous membrane. These patches are lightly stuck to the membrane but may be removed by gentle manipulation. Underneath them is a light red inflammatory base. There is usually little or no bleeding from the area beneath the patches.

The newborn infant and young children are most often affected, although the disease is occasionally seen in the healthy adult and is seen with some frequency in debilitated people or in cachectic states.

Vulvovaginitis with the monilial organism is seen most often in patients who are pregnant or who have diabetes. It is rarely observed in perfectly normal adult women and is practically never seen when adequate vaginal hygiene is accomplished.

One important factor to remember in the cases of vulvovaginitis is that the typical white patches do not always occur. Sometimes the vaginal or vulva lesions resemble those of a typical infectious dermatitis. A smear should probably be taken of any vaginal or vulva lesion that does not give a clue to its diagnosis by its appearance.

Paronychia is caused more frequently by the monilial organism than many physicians realize. Such a lesion appears in no way different from the ordinary pyogenic paronychia, except that it does not contain pus. In cases where the nails, too, are infected, one may expect typical unguinal changes like this:

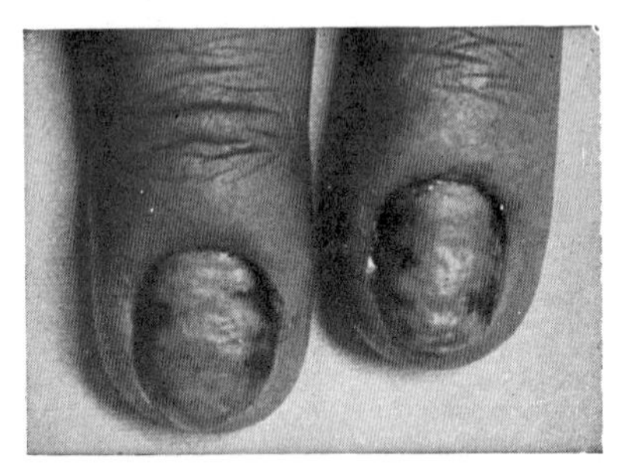

(Sutton: Diseases of the Skin, 1956, The C. V. Mosby Co.; courtesy Dr. W. Herbert Brown.)

When the perianal skin becomes soggy and macerated, *C. albicans* may sometimes invade and serve to further the process. Often the appearance is typical, the white boggy membrane being surrounded by a faint halo of red inflammatory reaction. Any cases of pruritus ani which do not clear up rapidly under simple treatment or in which the etiology is obscure should be checked for the presence of monilia.

Intertriginous lesions of moniliasis are relatively rare in practice. They consist of red exudative patches usually in areas where the skin is moist, such as the axillae, the groin, or beneath the breasts. On first glance they offer superficial resemblance to lesions of psoriasis often found on the body. The lesions have papulosquamous borders, immediately outside of which there are often small vesicles or pustules.

Technique

Mount scrapings from the suspected lesions in 10 per cent potassium hydroxide and gently warm the slide. Usually only the oval budding cells are seen like this:

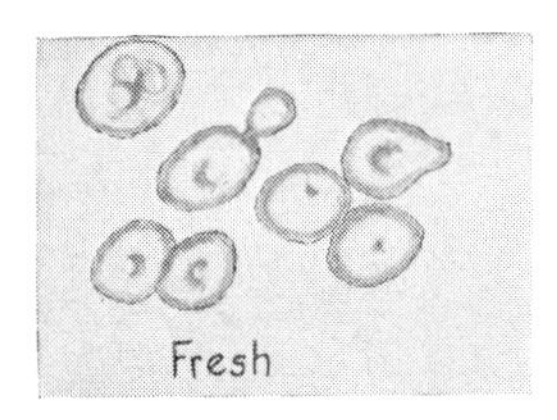

A Gram's stain will occasionally be of some help in making the diagnosis. Typical stained cells look like this:

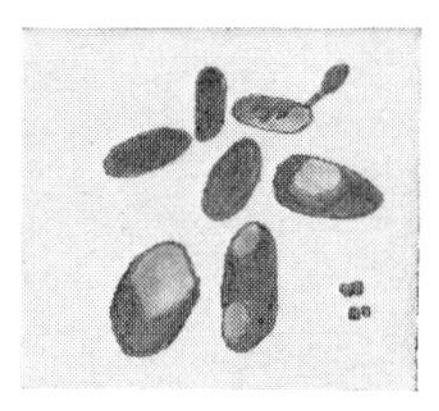

The hyphae are ordinarily not found in such preparations but rarely we see one showing points of constriction to which the budding cells are attached like this:

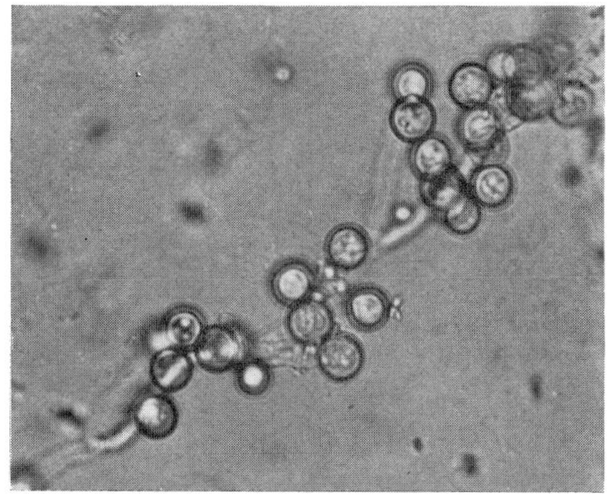

(Gradwohl: Clinical Laboratory Methods and Diagnosis, 1956, The C. V. Mosby Co.)

Place material from white patches on a slide and gently tease apart with dissecting needles. Then mount it in either potassium hydroxide or stain with Gram's stain and examine.

Culture is ordinarily not necessary for proper differentiation.

Errors

In examining a typical slide various artifacts may be mistaken for the *C. albicans.* If there is any doubt, Gram's stain will certainly serve to settle the question.

One should always remember that members of the Candida species are sometimes found in the human mouth, vaginal canal, gastrointestinal tract, and occasionally on the skin. The fact that a few organisms are present means nothing and the fact that organisms can be cultured from the mouth, vagina, or perirectal area also has little meaning. It is only when one finds these organisms in great number along with clinical symptoms expected from monilial infection that one should make a positive diagnosis.

Just recently I saw a woman in my office who was quite excited because a physician had taken a culture from her vagina and isolated *C. albicans.* She had no symptoms, no discharge, no difficulty of any kind, but was certain that she was about to die because of the presence of the organism. Certainly no mistake is implied on the physician's part because he did not tell her that these organisms indicated something wrong. It was simply a case of her asking in a tremulous voice, "What did my culture show?" and his saying quite offhand, "Oh, it showed a fungus, one we call *Candida albicans.*"

Remember always that any physician or any laboratory anywhere can culture members of the Candida species from various orifices.

Interpretation

This is a simple matter. If the organisms are present in large number along with typical clinical findings, one is usually safe to make a diagnosis of moniliasis. If these criteria are not met—if the organisms are scarce and the clinical symptoms not typical —it is best to reserve judgment.

It is worth repeating again: the presence of a few monilial organisms means nothing.

One other point: this book is written to apply to the average American practice. In hot, humid climates *no* fungous infection is rare.

ACTINOMYCOSIS

Actinomycosis is a disease caused by one of several varieties of primitive fungi. Office identification of the various organisms involved is not usually a profitable undertaking. This should be left for the bigger laboratories.

In about 60 per cent of the cases infected teeth or tonsils are the cause of the disease. It has been conclusively demonstrated that at least some of the pathogenic organisms live in the human mouth and apparently infection is of endogenous origin.

The clinical picture begins with a soft but not painful swelling usually about the angle of the jaw. This gradually becomes more marked and then assumes a rocky hardness. The overlying skin gradually discolors, being first bright red, then dark red, and finally purple. At this stage the lumps are clearly felt.

The skin then breaks down and multiple draining sinuses appear. Most people are not seen by the physician until at least one abscess is clearly formed or is draining.

Technique

In order to identify the fungus expel onto a slide or into a small test tube a bit of the pus which is draining from one of the sinuses. Use the platinum loop to pick up one of the tiny granules which are usually clearly seen in such fluid and place it on another microscopic slide. Fix and stain with Gram's stain.

The presence of branching mycelial elements, varying greatly in length and about the width of an ordinary bacterium, is diagnostic. This is the edge of a typical granule stained with Gram's stain and visualized under the high power:

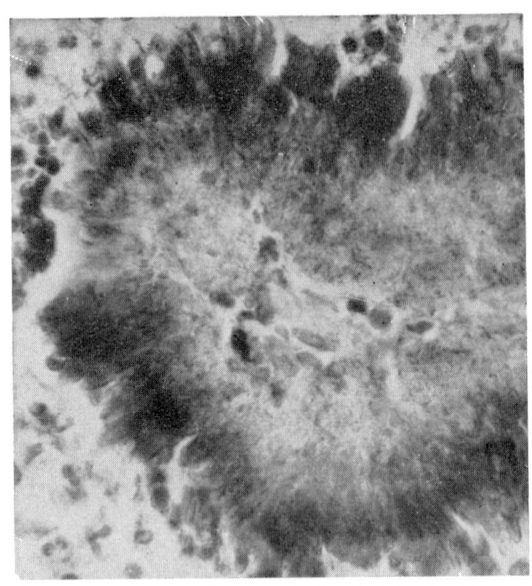

(Emmons, C. W.: Mycologia 24: 377, 1937.)

If no granules are present it is probably wise to curette the walls of the sinus and look for them in the curettings, or place a small piece of gauze over the opening of the sinus and leave it in place for twenty-four hours. Granules will become entangled in the gauze and can usually be clearly identified.

If all these techniques are performed and no granules are apparent and yet the disease seems very like actinomycosis, make repeated smears of the ordinary pus stained with Gram's stain and look for the branching mycelia.

Errors

Occasionally this organism will be seen in long filaments which look like chains of bacteria. Careful examination, however, will reveal that branches like this:

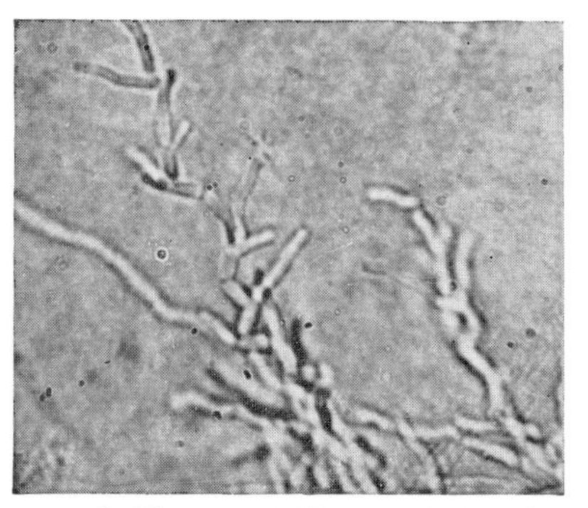

(Emmons, C. W.: Puerto Rico J. Pub. Health Trop. Med. 11: 63, 1935.)

do occur and, since we know of no pathogenic branching bacteria, this makes the diagnosis certain.

Methods of cultural identification are so subject to error that they are not within the purview of the office laboratory. If there is any doubt, refer the patient to a large commercial laboratory.

BLASTOMYCOSIS

Blastomycosis is not a common disease. In endemic areas perhaps the practitioner may see one or two cases a year but seldom more.

The disease occurs in two forms, the systemic in which the port of entrance is usually through the mouth, and the cutaneous in which skin lesions are usually the only manifestations of the disease. Both types are apparently caused by the same organism.

In the systemic type the illness usually begins as a persistent subacute respiratory infection and there is wide dissemination throughout the body involving bones and sometimes abdominal organs, kidneys, and prostate.

In a number of these systemic cases the correct diagnosis is not suspected until a small subcutaneous abscess appears. This drains and either heals, leaving a deeply tinted scar, or forms a spreading serpiginous ulcer.

The skin lesions of the cutaneous type usually consist of ulceration with extensive granulomatous overgrowth. Often they can be identified by inspection, but laboratory confirmation should be sought.

Technique

Examine sputum and scrapings from the undermined edges of skin ulcers by direct smear. Mount the material in 10 per cent potassium hydroxide and gently heat the slide and subject it to direct microscopic examination.

The organism is round or budding and is normally about twice the size of a red blood cell. It is thick walled and this heavy wall often gives the appearance of a double outline. Typical organisms look like this:

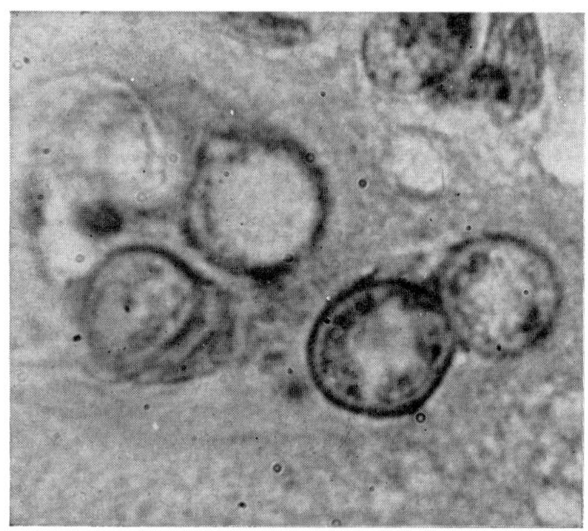

(Gradwohl: Clinical Laboratory Methods and Diagnosis, 1956, The C. V. Mosby Co.)

When these are found or the disease is suspected, inoculate cultures of urine, sputum, or material from skin lesions on Sabouraud's medium. A white cottonlike mycelial growth usually rapidly becomes apparent on this medium. As the colony progresses the surface of the plate becomes overgrown with a typical aerial mycelium.

When such culture develops, inoculate a bit of the growth onto blood agar. It will once again develop a typical yeastlike form which looks like this:

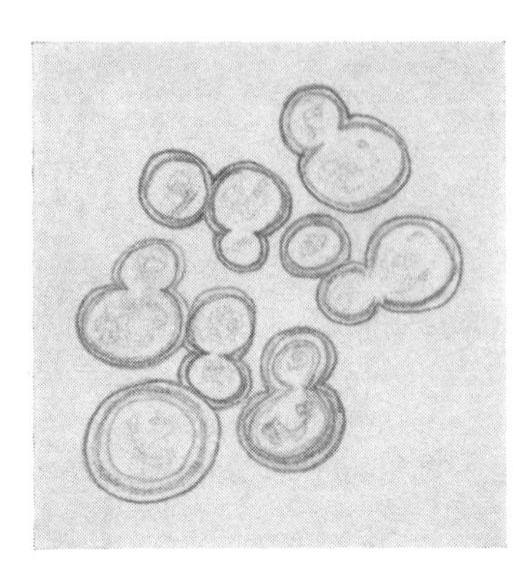

Such cases are usually not matters for further handling by either the office laboratory or the practitioner.

Errors

The principal error is not to suspect the disease. Methods of identification are usually easy and the technique described will make specific and accurate identification to allow referral of the patient to a medical center.

OTOMYCOSIS

Otomycosis is frequently seen in practice and actually rates a separate heading because of the confusion which the laboratory may cause in its diagnosis and treatment. The external otic canal is subject to a variety of insults, including mild staphylococcal infections and an occasional infection with the less virulent forms of streptococci. It is also subject to the eczematoid dermatoses.

In such a case fungus may appear as a contaminant without actually being the true etiologic agent. Many of the saphrophytic fungi have been accused of a causative role in otomycosis when their presence actually prolongs rather than causes the difficulty.

It is possible to culture from a perfectly normal ear at least a dozen of the common saphrophytes.

Techniques

Mount a portion of the cellular debris from the infected ear in potassium hydroxide and gently warm the slide. Examination for fungous elements should be meticulous. When present in profusion, mycelial elements are easily seen. Occasionally one sees the spore-bearing structures.

Errors

The presence of fungus in the debris from the external otic canal does not necessarily mean that the fungus is the root of the difficulty. One must make a relative judgment in assessing the slides from such a lesion, for a few fungous elements mean nothing.

If the clinical picture is consistent with that usually found in fungous infection, and, in addition, mycelial elements or other characteristic fungous bodies are found in profusion, it is probable that the fungus at least has enough etiologic association that it should be eliminated. An occasional mycelium probably means only secondary invasion of the debris by saphrophytic organisms.

Interpretation

Any time there is a large amount of fungus in the ear canal it should be eradicated. One must not, however, fall into the interpretative error of saying that the presence of any mycotic elements proves fungous infection.

CHAPTER FOURTEEN

Immunologic Procedures

In this chapter a group of only casually related tests are considered. Actually the same general principle is involved in all the tests but admittedly sometimes the relationship is a little bit difficult to see.

These tests are not often required in the practitioner's office, but since they are not particularly complicated they should be in the armamentarium of the office laboratory. Sometimes they give information of the utmost utility and value.

PATHOGENICITY OF STAPHYLOCOCCI

Many strains of staphylococci are essentially saphrophytic and do not readily attack the human organism. When one is searching out the causative agent of some particular infection, staphylococci are often found growing upon the culture media. Then the physician must answer the question: Are these harmless saprophytes that have gotten into the culture by the usual procedures of contamination or are they the true pathogens involved?

One way to answer this question is to take advantage of the fact that the pathogenic strains of staphylococci produce the enzyme, coagulase, which will cause plasma to clot.

Technique

Make a suspension from the suspected culture in 0.5 normal saline solution. Obtain a specimen of blood from some laboratory animal, usually a rabbit, and citrate. Centrifuge and place 0.5 ml. of the supernatant plasma in a small test tube. Add two drops of the saline suspension of culture and incubate the whole at 37° C.

In three hours examine the tube. If the staphylococci are pathogenic a clot will usually have formed in the plasma and will be quite apparent when the tube is moved about.

Errors

Other than those inherent in bacteriologic technique, there are practically no errors to which the test is subject.

Interpretation

So far as we know most of the pathogenic staphylococci produce coagulases while most of the saprophytic staphylococci do not. In all probability this is one reason for the pathogenicity of the virulent organisms. If the organism you test coagulates the plasma, chances are it is a virulent organism. The test is not certain, only indicative.

TYPHOID FEVER

Typhoid fever is becoming so rare that the office laboratory practically never has occasion to perform the test. In the rare occasion where an unhospitalized patient may be suspected of having typhoid fever, it is better to use the facilities of a more complete laboratory than it is to attempt to stock materials for the test.

BRUCELLOSIS

Agglutination reactions for the brucella are comparatively easy to perform but are so completely uncertain of interpretation that they are not recommended as an office procedure.

THE COLD HEMAGGLUTININS

After seven to ten days, the serum of patients with virus pneumonia contains certain agglutinins which will affect red blood cells at low temperatures, 0 to 5° C., but not at room temperature.

In an occasional puzzling case this test may be of great value and should be in the armamentarium of the office laboratory.

Technique

Use ten test tubes. In the first place 0.8 ml. of physiologic saline solution and in each of the remaining test tubes, 0.5 ml. of saline solution.

Obtain sample of the patient's blood, allowing it to clot. When the serum is clear, place 0.2 ml. in the first test tube containing 0.8 ml. of normal saline solution. Thoroughly mix this and withdraw 0.5 ml., placing it into test tube 2. Then thoroughly mix these two and withdraw 0.5 ml., placing the mixture into tube 3. Continue this process through the ten tubes.

Ask someone around the office who has type O blood to denote 0.5 ml. of his blood and mix this with 10 ml. of normal saline solution in a test tube. Invert the tube several times to ensure complete mixture and then place 0.2 ml. in each of the ten test tubes.

Then you have:

TUBE NUMBER	TITER
No. 1	1:7
No. 2	1:14
No. 3	1:28
No. 4	1.56
No. 5	1:112
No. 6	1:224
No. 7	1:448
No. 8	1:896
No. 9	1:1792
No. 10	1:3584

Then place the tubes in the refrigerator near the refrigerating unit itself for twelve hours. Agglutination is sometimes not visible grossly but may usually be made out with a powerful hand lens. If not, refrigerate microscopic slides for a moment and spread a drop of the various dilutions microscopically on a cold slide.

Errors

Other than those common to the usual serologic techniques, there are no specific errors.

Interpretation

Agglutinations through the first three tubes, up to 1:28, are sometimes found in normal people. Higher agglutinations in the presence of indefinite pulmonary symptoms or out-and-out pneumonitis usually indicate the entity known as virus pneumonia.

It must be emphasized that this test is not positive in the early days of the disease. Quite often its main value is to diagnose a puzzling case in a patient who is getting well anyway.

BLOOD TYPING

The four blood types and their physiology are far too well known to need explanation here.

Technique

Obtain a drop or two of blood from a finger prick, placing it in a test tube containing from 3 to 5 ml. of normal saline solution. No specific dilution is necessary but the resultant solution should be of only a faint pink color.

Make two circles on a glass slide with a wax pencil and label them, respectively, A and B. Then place serum A in the circle labeled A, and B in its own circle. Add two drops of the blood dilution to each.

After thirty minutes examine the slide and read the blood type as follows:

BLOOD TYPE	SERUM A	SERUM B
AB	Agg.	Agg.
A	Agg.	O
B	O	Agg.
O	O	O

Errors

The most frequent error is to mix the serum or to make a mistake in reading and confuse type A and type B blood. This is carelessness, of course, and since it means potential death to the patient it should not be condoned.

Rarely may there be some confusion about whether a slight agglutination has taken place in one of the sera. Let the specimen set another fifteen minutes and re-examine. If there is still any confusion, repeat the test.

Interpretation

This is self-apparent.

Cross-matching should not be a matter for the office laboratory, for it is probably better never to transfuse the patient at home or in the office when a hospital is nearby.

Rh FACTOR

Obtain a vial of any Rh serum from one of the biological manufacturers and follow the directions exactly. The test is practically not subject to error if carefully done.

CHAPTER FIFTEEN

Miscellaneous Procedures

The miscellaneous procedures that can be done in the laboratory are, in actuality, limited only by the genius for improvisation which the physician brings to his office. If one remembers well the physiologic principles involved in the various tests and the rigid limitations of accuracy faced by the laboratory, the information to be provided by these miscellaneous tests sometimes assumes importance even greater than that usually provided by the various "routine" procedures.

It would be impossible in this chapter to list all the miscellaneous applications of the office laboratory. Instead of attempting to do so I am going to list only those tests which are in the "routine" range and leave to the expertness of the reader all the special applications.*

SPINAL FLUID

The spinal fluid is formed by the choroid plexes in the ventricles of the brain. There is a gradual circulation of the fluid throughout the channels within the nervous system. Then it passes through the foramina of Luschka and Magendie to the subarachnoid space, so that the total extent of the fluid may be represented diagrammatically like this:

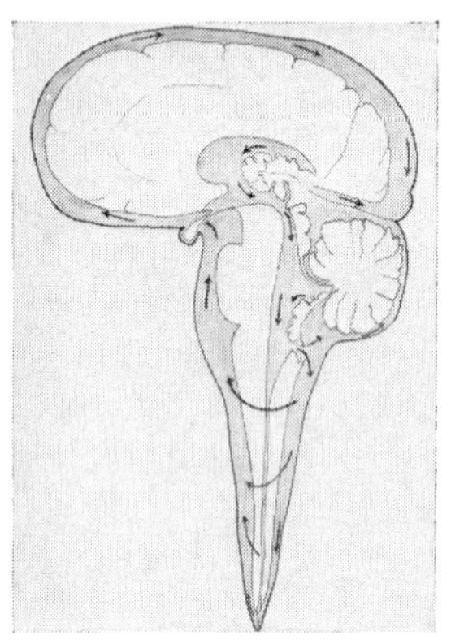

Since there is some circulation of fluid from the channels within the central nervous system to the channels surrounding the central nervous system, it might reasonably be suspected that any lesion near enough to the fluid tract to cause alteration in the fluid itself could ultimately be detected through a simple spinal tap.

This statement presupposes two important facts which every practitioner should know. The first is that abnormal findings in spinal fluid may represent a lesion any place along the tract of the fluid itself. The second and by far the most important is that lesions of the nervous system may engender no changes at all in the spinal fluid unless they approach the fluid tract.

*As you devise special applications please write and tell me about them. I will be most interested.

In ordinary office work one does not usually attempt to make pressure determinations. This probably should not be done except upon the hospitalized patient.

Gross inspection of the fluid should be done to determine the color and cloudiness. Normal spinal fluid is watery and transparent. Sometimes a slight haziness can be detected with 50 or 60 cells per cubic millimeter, although this is more often apparent if the cell count approaches 150 or more.

When there are 300 to 500 cells per cubic millimeter the fluid has a limpid opalescent appearance like greatly diluted milk. By the time the cell count tops 500 there is usually a marked pearly translucency.

Fresh blood, of course, is easily apparent upon examination, and unless well admixed with all portions of the fluid may usually be taken to have originated from trauma at the time of the spinal tap.

As blood ages in the spinal canal, the pigments gradually degenerate until there is a light, dirty yellow discoloration of the fluid, which is known as xanthochromia. When one sees xanthochromic fluid one may presuppose that whatever lesion there is has been present for several days, for it takes this long to develop a full-blown xanthochromia. There have been rare cases where no historic reason for the occurrence of xanthochromia has been demonstrated but wherein it is present. Autopsy technique could demonstrate no lesion to be held accountable.

These cases are exceedingly rare and in office practice one may certainly presume that xanthochromia indicates a bleeding lesion in the central nervous system until proved otherwise.

Simple tests for spinal fluid sugar and proteins furnish a great deal of information in differentiating the various infections. Pyogenic bacteria apparently use the spinal fluid sugar in their nutritive processes. For this reason, in pyogenic infections the spinal fluid sugar is lowered, markedly so in coccic and less markedly so in bacillary infections.

The mildest of the infectious processes from the standpoint of lowering spinal fluid sugar is tuberculous meningitis, although there may be some lowering in this disease.

The various viral meningitides, such as poliomyelitis, usually engender no change in spinal fluid sugar. This is an important diagnostic point and may be of great service in the office. Detailed tests are not necessary but one of the minor screening tests should be done on any suspect fluid.

Place 5 ml. of ordinary Benedict's solution (that used to test the urine for sugar) in a test tube and bring to the boiling point. While it is still hot add ten drops of the spinal fluid and reheat to boiling. In normal or relatively normal spinal fluids a reduction will occur, and results are reported as a positive test for sugar.

In pyogenic processes, on the other hand, the sugar in the spinal fluid is usually lowered enough so that no reduction will occur, and the test is reported as negative. When sugar is negative one should consider a pyogenic process present until proved otherwise.

Proteins in the cerebral spinal fluid are increased in all inflammatory conditions. This would include syphilis and tuberculosis, as well as the pyogenic infections and the viral diseases. It is notable, however, that the increase in the viral condition is not nearly so great as that found in the diseases caused by bacteria.

A simple office test serves to point out the presence of excess proteins. Use a saturated aqueous solution of phenol. Put approximately 1 ml. of this solution in a test tube and add a drop of spinal fluid. If excess proteins are present, a bluish white cloud will form.

The test is subject to one gross error which must always be ruled out before putting any dependence at all in the result. If there is any leakage of blood into the spinal fluid there is likely to be leakage of plasma protein as well, and a positive test will be obtained. If there is gross or microscopic evidence of more than a tiny trace of blood in the fluid, one should not depend upon the results obtained from this test.

In rare cases one may suspect tuberculous meningitis, particularly in a child. There is a simple test to determine the presence of tryptophan in the fluid, which is an almost specific indication that the mycobacterium is the etiologic agent.

Use a 25 ml. test tube and begin by putting in 2 ml. of the spinal fluid. Add 16 ml. of concentrated hydrochloric acid and then two or three drops of 2 per cent formaldehyde solution. Allow this preparation to set for at least five minutes.

Make up a solution of 0.06 sodium nitrite and layer 2 ml. of this on top of the material in the test tube. If tryptophan is present a purple ring will form at the junction of the two fluids. Occasionally a brown ring will form in the presence of nontuberculous fluid, but usually no ring at all appears unless tryptophans be present, in which case the color is a brilliant purple.

UNUSUAL FLUIDS

Rarely in the office one may wish to tell the difference between a transudate and an exudate. This may be simply done by taking the specific gravity of the fluid. A typical inflammatory transudate has a specific gravity of less than 1.018, usually in the range of 1.008 to 1.010. Exudates, on the other hand, are almost always of a specific gravity above 1.018. As a matter of fact, most of the time one can tell by observing, without bothering to measure the specific gravity, but an occasional case may be somewhat puzzling.

If there is too little fluid to allow use of the urinometer to determine specific gravity, dilute the fluid with its own volume of distilled water and take the specific gravity of the mixture. The necessary mathematics will suggest themselves.

Occasionally cytologic study of these fluids is of some benefit. If cells are plentiful a bit of the fluid should be mixed with some citrate and normal saline solution, several smears made quickly, and both dried and fixed by application of heat. One or two of the smears should be fixed in an alcohol-ether mixture (half of each) and sent to the nearest pathologic laboratory if there is any question of malignancy.

The heat-fixed slides are then stained with Giemsa's stain and examined for cellular content. Acute inflammatory processes, of course, show a preponderance of polymorphonuclear leukocytes, whereas convalescent processes or the less acute inflammations, such as tuberculosis, usually show a preponderance of lymphocytes.

Sometimes transudates will show groups of mesothelial cells which may easily be mistaken for malignant cells. This differentiation should never be attempted in the office laboratory. Typical mesothelial elements look like this:

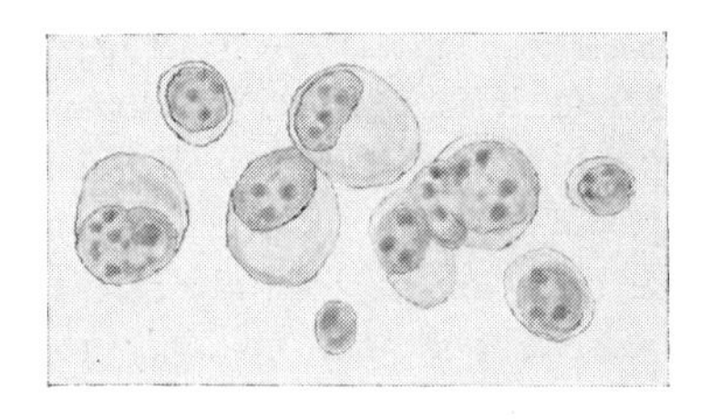

If you are in doubt, send the slide to a good cytologist.

ARTHROPODS AND INSECTS

Arthropods and insects are often found, particularly in patients who are less delightfully clean than usual. Such parasites should be identifiable by the office laboratory if not grossly identified by the physician.

Sarcoptes Scabiei

Sarcoptes scabiei is the typical itch mite which lives in a burrow formed in the deep layers of the skin. Often if there is any question, a fleck of skin containing a burrow may be picked up and snipped away without causing the patient more than a tiny twinge of pain. Mount this fleck of skin in a drop of normal saline solution and examine with the lowest power of the microscope. A typical burrow looks like this:

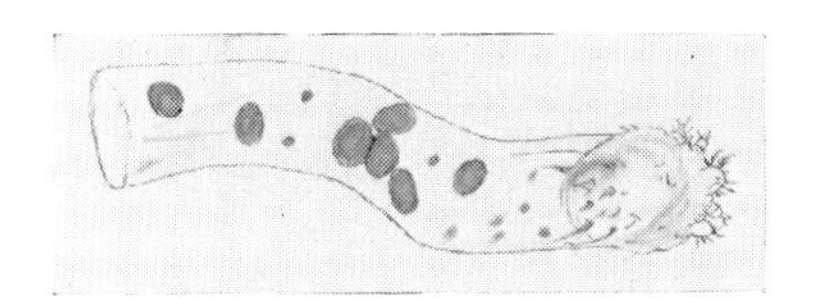

The parasite itself looks like this:

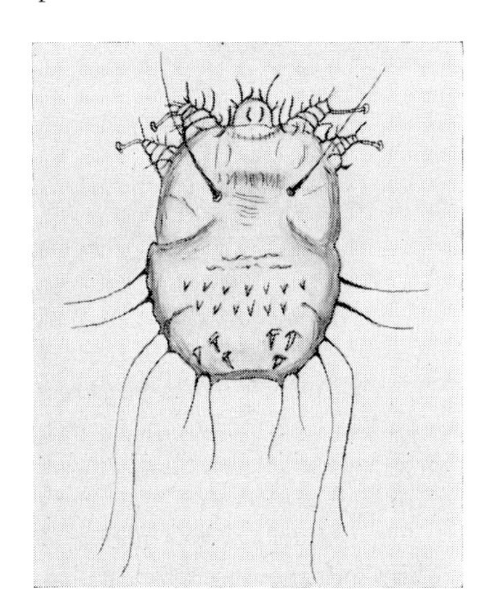

Sometimes a mild folliculitis may be caused by a similar parasite which lives in the hair follicles and sebaceous glands. It may be seen by squeezing out the secretion of the glands and examining in a saline mounting.

Ticks

I will not insult the intelligence of the average physician by drawing pictures of a typical tick, but I must tell you this story. Not too long ago a young lady was referred to the particular department in which I worked, with the statement that there was a small gray tumor of the scalp which should be removed. Upon the application of a little Cresatin to its backside this tumor loosed its grip and backed out and was promptly thrown away. I suppose it is unnecessary to mention in a textbook to beware of tumors that have legs.

LICE

Louse infestation is becoming progressively more rare, but the physician may still see an occasional case. A specimen of the parasite may be mounted between a cover glass and slide and identified quite easily.

They are typical insects. The body is divided into three distinct regions, the head, thorax, and abdomen, there being one pair of antennae and three pairs of legs. The body louse is somewhat bigger than the other two common parasites and has an abdomen approximately twice the width of its thorax like this:

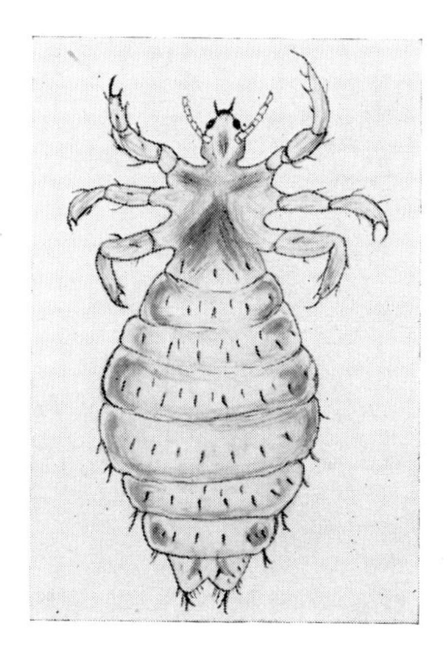

The head louse is not as big and the thorax and abdomen are approximately of equal width like this:

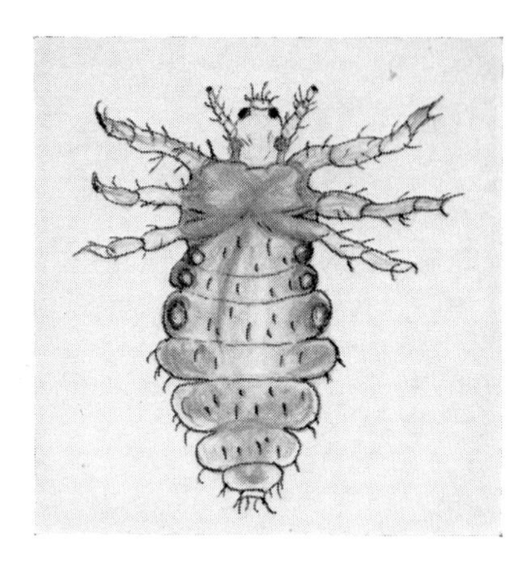

The pubic louse does not have nearly as clear a distinction between thorax and abdomen. It looks like this:

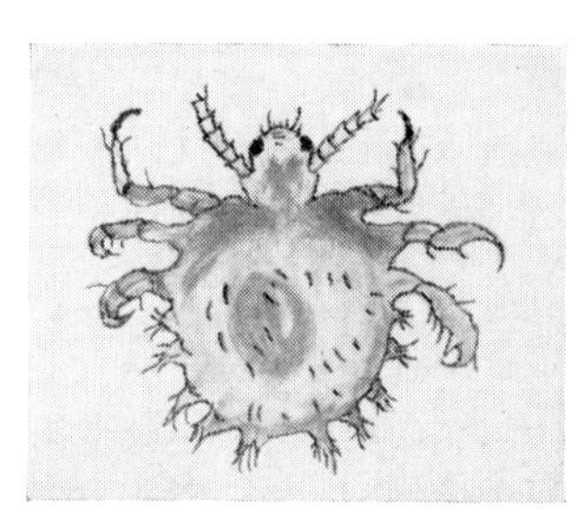

Under the microscope typical egg sacs or nits may be seen attached to the hair. They look like this:

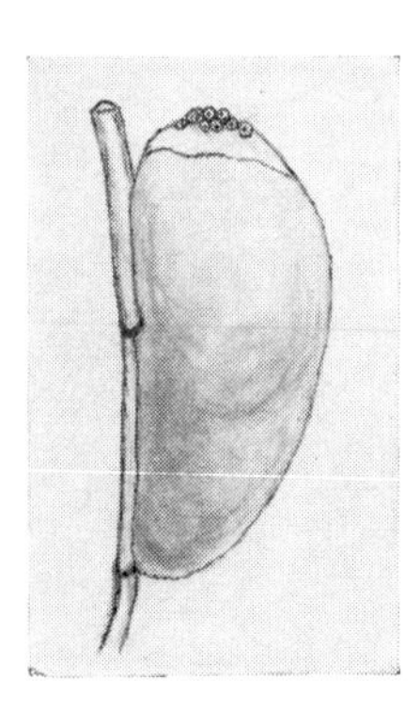

Ordinarily the nits can be seen with the naked eye. They are usually attached about ¼ inch from the skin and are seen as little white dots. With the hand lens it is possible to make out gross structure.

BEDBUGS

Occasionally typical bedbugs may be found in the clothing or on the skin of the patient. They are somewhat larger than the common body louse and look like this:

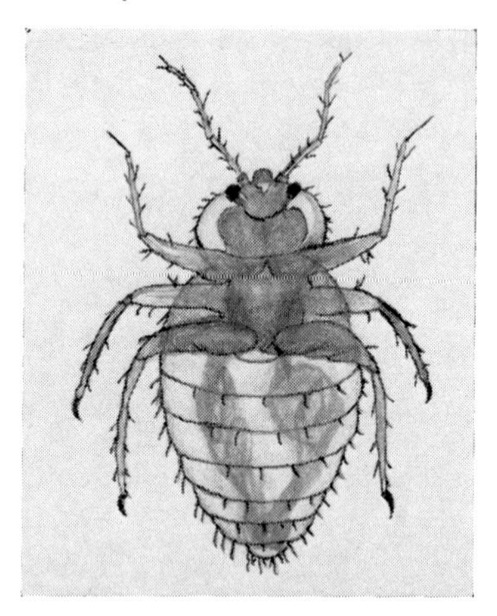

Notice particularly the difference in the legs as shown in the illustration.

The common error is failure to examine with sufficient attention to visualize the parasite. A casual glance is not enough. Even a painstaking examination may at times fail.

When you find a parasite be sure to examine it under the microscope unless gross examination provides certain identification.

Bedbug bites are not as rare as you might think. Their distribution is not at all like that of the lesions associated with louse infestation. When you see typical papules on the skin be sure to examine the patient's clothing, particularly around the seams. If there is a suspicious insect, put it under the microscope and compare with the illustration above.

CHAPTER SIXTEEN

General Comment on the Office Laboratory

There are two means by which one may judge the skill of a physician in the use of his laboratory. First, does he routinize tests and "get in a rut" in using the laboratory or does he improvise? The object of the laboratory is to give the physician the information he wants, not to furnish beautifully typed reports.

A urinalysis or a blood culture has no intrinsic worth from the standpoint of the patient. Only as it provides *usable* information to the physician has it any value. The ideal office laboratory is one designed to provide the answers to specific questions from the physician, not the request for a specific test.

May I cite a personal example?

For a time my laboratory was run by a fine and scholarly man. We reached the point where we would exchange "notes." This is an example:

Lab: I think this woman has a chronic pyelitis, probably with coliforms. (1) Does lab confirm infec.? (2) What about urine? (3) Is there much tissue destruction?

Dr.: (1) White and diff. normal. Polys look good. No decrease in eos. (2) Sed. rate normal. (3) Urine cultures *Staph. aureus* but am not satisfied. This tests virulent. Probably a contaminant. Will repeat on nutrient agar. Lab. Imp.: Can't confirm diagnosis. Do you want further check?

We had a wonderful time with the laboratory. We used it not to make reports but to answer specific questions designed to confirm or deny my impressions. I admit that such a plan would never work in a large hospital but that is the beauty of the office laboratory. Improvisation to answer specific questions and narrative reports extend its value.

The second way to tell the skill with which a physician uses his laboratory is to note whether he overuses it and whether he relies on himself or the laboratory reports. If there are specific questions to be answered the laboratory should be asked to furnish specific answers but no more.

If, when a young woman comes in to complain, "Doctor, I just feel so weak all the time," that is an excuse for blood sugar, a nonprotein nitrogen, complete blood count, urinalysis, and many other tests, the doctor is wasting time and the patient's money. It is foolish to worry about 17-ketosteroids when the patient has an imperfect airway, but I have seen it done.

Should the laboratory disagree with your findings, check your work, and if it seems all right, believe yourself. Chances are much in favor of you over the laboratory. Sometimes young physicians seem to have great difficulty learning to believe this fact.

COSTS

There are, of course, two aspects to this problem of cost: one from the standpoint of the physician and the other from the standpoint of the patient. It is easy to dispose of the problem of laboratory cost to the physician. In the ordinary office a perfectly adequate laboratory may be established for less than $2,000. This includes all equipment, even a fine microscope.

One point is perhaps worth emphasizing: There is absolutely no percentage in buying inferior laboratory equipment at less cost. An inadequate microscope, for example, is worse than useless, for it will be the source of many costly errors. You should not take this to mean that one has to have a $3,000 research microscope for the office laboratory, but I have seen some physicians buy a $50 used model at the pawnshop or an old and completely beaten-to-pieces student model and expect it to do adequate work. This is a fallacy.

The problem of cost from the patient's aspect is a much more major item. Too many doctors and too many patients try to use the laboratory as a substitute for the physician's common sense. Extensive tests are ordered where a few simple questions would have settled the problem just as well.

A good question the doctor should pose about laboratory work is this: The proposed test is going to cost the patient $5. If I had his trouble, would the test result be worth $5 to me? In a surprising number of cases the answer will be "No."

The laboratory, if properly used, can furnish information of incalculable value and few patients resent paying for it, but it must be properly used and used with judiciousness and caution. Do not allow your laboratory to become a routine.

It seems almost foolish to say this, but we must also protect the patient's pocketbook against his excess of faith in laboratory determinations.

ACCURACY

The office laboratory in a busy practice is not often as accurate as the hospital laboratory, although it certainly could be. From a practical standpoint it is necessary to take this into account. Attempts are often made in small laboratories to do procedures beyond their competence, which simply results in trouble.

Of course, one cannot expect complete accuracy from the hospital laboratory, for the tests have inherent error and then there is the human element to be considered.

There is certainly no way that we can set an exact figure, but if I were estimating I would say that a good office laboratory obtains results of approximately 80 per cent accuracy (not 102 per cent accuracy as so many patients and physicians think). To expect more is excellent perfectionalism but poor judgment.

SHOULD YOU HAVE A LABORATORY?

The physician reading this book unquestionably has a laboratory or he would not have bought the book. But there is a group in American medicine that follows the contention that the practitioner has no reason at all to depend on his own local laboratory facilities. They claim that laboratory work is a specialized job and should be left entirely in the hands of regional clinical laboratories. The statement is made that the practitioner should perhaps do urinalyses and an occasional blood count, although this is best done in the local hospital. I do not agree, but believe the physician has an obligation to do everything *within* his power to aid his patient. If his small laboratory will provide information of definite value in diagnosis and treatment, then he should have it and use it.

There is a point beyond which the small laboratory cannot go and should not try to go. That point varies, depending upon several factors:

The first is the skill of the technician, which will be discussed in the next section.

The second is the physical equipment at hand. Most office laboratories are simply not equipped to do the finer biochemical or bacteriologic procedures. To attempt them is to invite gross and dangerous error. Not to do the simple procedures is only a way of making medical care more expensive by forcing the patient to seek other facilities and often pay more for them than would be required at home. Average medical care is already too expensive.

The third limiting factor is the type of practice in which one engages. In isolated areas it may be wise to attempt more than one would try in metropolitan areas, but this is a point which must be decided by the practitioner and cannot be discussed in a book.

THE TECHNICIAN

In the small office, I would recommend that the physician train his own technician, since school-trained technicians are experts on advanced techniques.

Here are a few details on two technicians we trained:

The first was my secretary who from sheer necessity was taught the simpler and then the more complex laboratory tests. From the first, the point was emphasized that the laboratory was to answer questions —not to make out reports. She did not become an expert technician but over a few months was entirely adequate for the small office laboratory.

There are many men who have had an adequate prescientific education in chemistry, biology, and other sciences who did not go on to medical school. Such a man would be a fine choice as he can be a tremendous asset to a practice.

One began working in my clinic when he was nearly 40 years old. He had the mental capacity to grasp the importance of the laboratory and enough scientific background to be able to understand and read about it. In a matter of months this man was practically indispensable not only in the laboratory, but also in many other aspects of the practice.

Perhaps because he had no set limitations or formal training, he quickly grasped the concept that he must answer specific questions. After a little more than a year he was an expert in x-ray technique, laboratory work, physiotherapy, and in the practical problems of the patient, which is most important. He did not have the background to grasp the more complex biochemical procedures but they were not used in the office anyway.

In the average big office practice, such a man is more valuable than any other personnel I have been able to obtain. He should be paid $400 to $800 a month and, if anything, he is probably worth more. I would certainly recommend to your attention the possibility of turning your office laboratory over to such an individual. Without regard to other advantages, the improvement in public relations will pay the bill.

CHAPTER SEVENTEEN

Office Electrocardiography

One can find many statements pro and con as to whether the practitioner should own an electrocardiograph. Certainly the more difficult interpretations are far beyond the skill of the office electrocardiographer, but then one must remember that the more difficult conditions make up a tiny minority of medical practice. In general, one may list many easily interpreted conditions amenable to the office electrocardiograph, all of which are important.

1. Diagnosis of conduction difficulties. There are many patients with changes in the conduction mechanism of the heart that are perfectly apparent upon examination with the electrocardiograph. Since there is nothing difficult about the interpretation of these changes, there is no reason why the practitioner should not have his own equipment to secure the tracing and make the interpretation.

2. Abnormalities in rhythm. These, too, are often seen in practice, are easy to interpret, and should be well within the competence of any practitioner.

3. Diagnosis of rheumatic carditis. In actuality, this perhaps should be considered with No. 1 above because changes in conduction are usually the principal diagnostic signs. Nonetheless, this is such a valuable use for the office electrocardiograph that I cannot recommend study of this point too highly.

4. Reassurance of cardiac psychoneurotics. We all see a tremendous number of persons who are thoroughly convinced that they have heart disease when it is perfectly obvious that they do not. Some of these individuals will not be persuaded without an electrocardiogram. Upon this point there are various beliefs. My stand is that the patient should be told something like this: "There are absolutely no findings here warranting an ECG. On the other hand, you will probably be more satisfied if we took one. Therefore, I tell you frankly that you are wasting $10 but we will certainly waste it if you wish." Patients soon learn to appreciate this truthfulness.

5. The diagnosis of vascular diseases affecting the myocardium. Myocardial ischemia and infraction, while not often problems for the office, still may be diagnosed on the basis of ECG tracings. We have found the portable electrocardiograph particularly valuable since it can be used in the home as a means of preliminary diagnosis before subjecting the patient to the strain of movement. Obviously, in most of these cases the diagnosis is clinical, but there are times when a bedside ECG may settle a difficult problem.

In summary, it is my belief that the practitioner most assuredly should have an electrocardiograph and should make at least a preliminary reading on his own tracings. It is decidedly unfair to take a tracing and refer it to a cardiologist for interpretation with no further information.

If the case is not clear-cut after office examination and office interpretation of an ECG, it is probably best to refer the ECG *and the patient* to a cardiologist for diagnosis and recommendations.

THE MACHINE

There can be no question but that the string galvanometer machine reproducing the motions of the string photographically is more accurate than the direct writing machine. It is also much more fragile and, in general, is unsatisfactory for the rough-and-tumble office practice.

Most manufacturers now make excellent direct writing machines that are accurate enough for all practical purposes even though they may not be adequate for research.

For the last several years we have used a Beck-Lee Cardi-all direct writer. Although there is a difference of opinion regarding this machine, we have obtained consistently good tracings with sufficient accuracy to record anything within our ability to diagnose. No doubt any of the standard-brand direct writing electrocardiographs will do an equivalent job.

TECHNIQUE

Actual instructions for mechanical use of the machine, application of electrodes, etc., are always included with the machine itself and need not be repeated here. Certain points, however, are important enough to bear some emphasis.

One of the most frequent sources of error is failure to standardize the machine. In a properly standardized machine a current of 1 millivolt should cause deflection of 1 centimeter in the base line, like this:

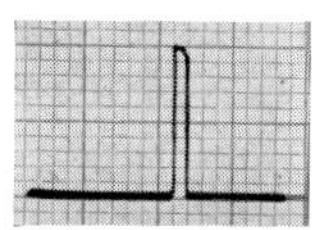

In occasional cases where the heartbeat causes extreme deflection of the stylus, it may be necessary to reduce the sensitivity so that 1 millivolt causes a deflection of 0.5 cm. If one leaves the standardization markings on the record as a part of the final record the interpretation is obvious.

Be sure that the patient is comfortable and the electrodes are firmly but not tightly applied. When the electrodes are applied too tightly or the patient is uncomfortable, tiny somatic tremors may be induced in the base of the ECG, like this:

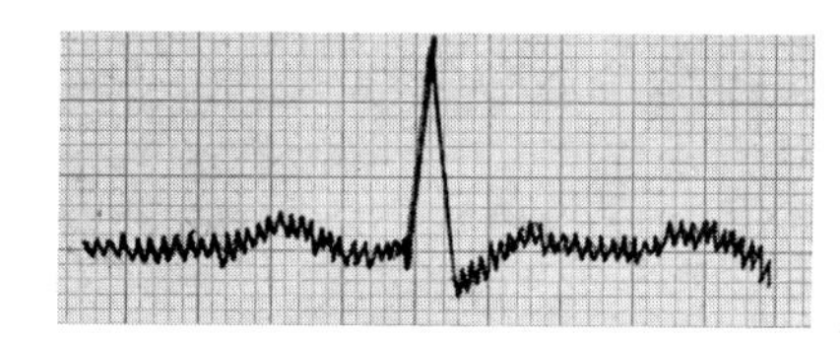

Occasionally the base line of an ECG will wander around like this:

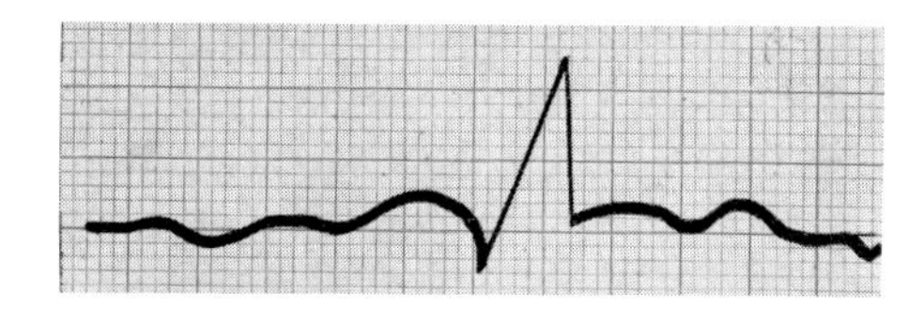

It is most often due to movement of the patient but may be due to pull on one of the lead cables caught under the patient or to the weight of the cable and connector itself, which may tend to pull the electrode away from the skin. Rarely, change in the line voltage may cause the difficulty.

For the office electrocardiogram the standard three leads plus a single chest lead are entirely adequate. The chest lead should be a V_4 taken in the mid-clavicular line and in the fifth interspace as shown:

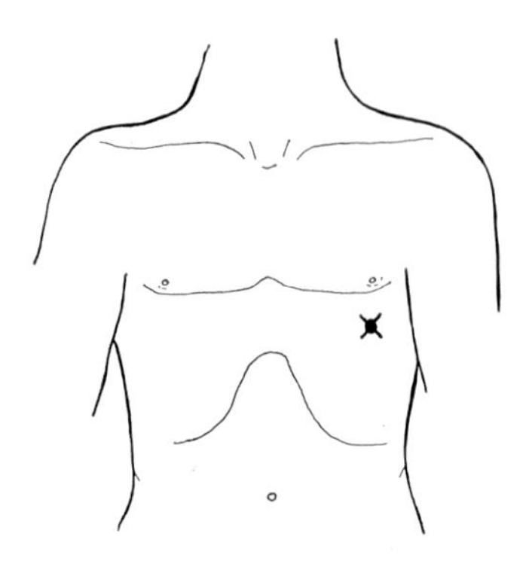

If you expect to send an occasional electrocardiogram to a cardiologist for interpretation, ask him the exact technique he wishes to have followed in recording the various leads so that your technician may provide as nearly as possible an electrocardiogram standardized to the particular physician's desires. This is extremely important. No cardiologist can interpret an ECG unless he knows exactly how it was taken. Often you will find it a good idea to send your technician to the cardiologist's office for a few days. Such instruction will benefit both you and the consultant.

READING THE ELECTROCARDIOGRAM

This chapter can do little more than provide a basic introduction to the problems of electrocardiographic interpretation. An excellent little book to study is *Cardiography.**

There are usually six factors regarding which notes should be made on every electrocardiographic interpretation. At least in the beginning you should consider all six in routine fashion, never varying the order in which they are entered into the record.

*Evans, William: Cardiography, St. Louis, The C. V. Mosby Co.

The Rate

Ordinary cardiographic paper has heavy vertical lines representing 1/5 of a second, like this:

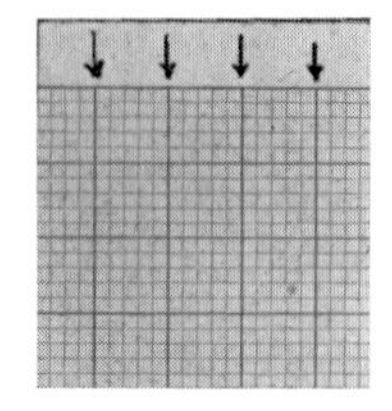

Lighter lines separate the paper into spaces representing 1/25 of a second.

The following table gives an approximation of the heart rate; this information is accurate enough for clinical purposes. Begin by taking two typical QRS complexes and measuring the number of 1/5-second spaces between them. Now refer to the table.

NO. OF 1/5-SECOND SPACES	RATE PER MINUTE
1.0	300
1.5	200
2	150
2.5	120
3	100
3.5	85
4	75
4.5	66
5	60
5.5	55
6	50
6.5	46
7	43
7.5	40
8	37
8.5	35
9	33
9.5	31
10	30

I would suggest that you have your secretary type this table on some durable material and keep it in the desk drawer.

The Rhythm

A note should be made regarding the regularity in, or the absence of, the spacing of QRS complexes. The same should be noted regarding P and T waves. If there is a lack of regular relationship between the P waves and the QRS complexes, this, too, should be noted.

Duration of P-R

Each small square of the ECG paper represents 0.04 second. Five squares, or one interval between heavy lines, represent 0.20 second. A measurement should be made from the beginning of the P wave to the crest of the R, as follows, and noted:

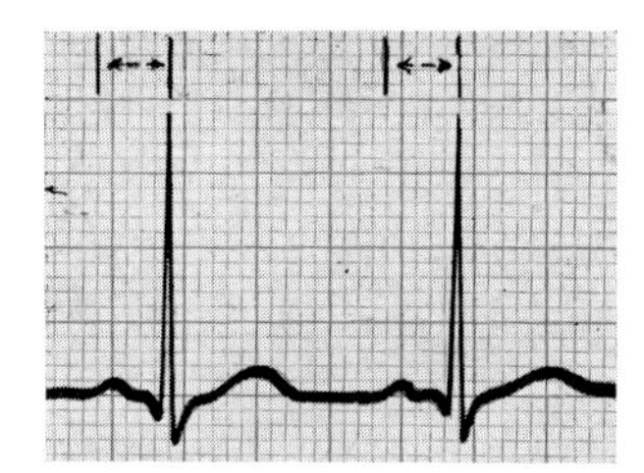

Electrical Axis

Note should be made of the direction taken by the electrical axis. It is not necessary to plot the complicated Einthoven triangle, but gross abnormalities should be noted. This will be discussed more fully, beginning on page 205.

Configuration

A note must be made about any deviation in direction, amplitude, or form of the P, QRS, or T waves. To avoid extensive writing we often simply circle the abnormal wave with red pencil and leave the mounted ECG in the patient's file.

The R-T Segment

As mentioned above, any abnormalities are circled and often noted.

THE NORMAL ELECTROCARDIOGRAM

Sometimes the most difficult problem in electrocardiography is to determine just what is a normal ECG. Variations are legion and some of these verge upon pathologic tracings. Another point that seems well proved is that many types of tracing which we have been taught are positive indicators of pathology can be brought about by functional disease.

This adds up to the conclusion that the ECG, like many other laboratory tests, is not reliable if not backed up by the sound clinical judgment of the physician following careful history and physical examination.

To say this another way: rely on yourself for a diagnosis. Use the electrocardiograph only to substantiate. When such is done, better cardiology results.

The P Wave

The electrical excitation of muscle is well proved. In the heart a sufficient change in potential is encountered when the myocardial fibers contract to register on a sensitive instrument. One must remember that the nodal impulses and the currents set up in the conducting system are far too faint to appear in the ECG. It is the actual contraction of muscle fibers that produces the current we record.

Impulses for normal cardiac contraction originate in the sino-auricular node and spread directly, through the muscles of the atria for there is no special conducting system in these chambers. Muscular contraction produces a change in potential registered as typical P waves, like this:

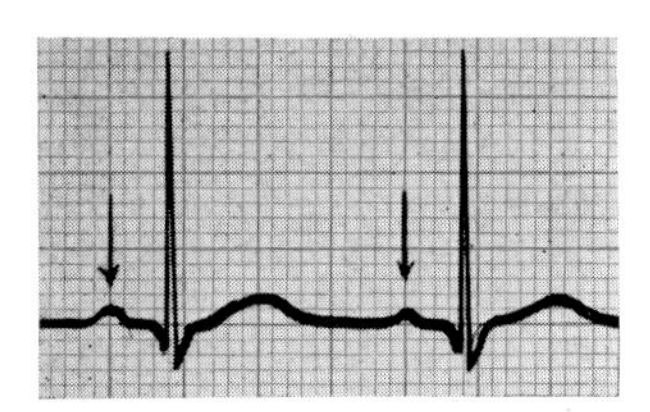

Occasionally the restoration of normal potential in the atria results in a second, much smaller deviation called P_1. It looks like this:

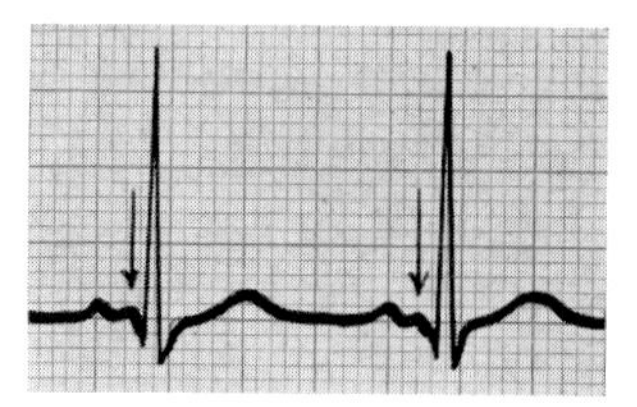

but is usually covered up by the QRS complex.

The time lapse between the earliest change in the atria (i.e., the beginning of the P wave) and a definite potential change in the ventricular muscle is usually about 0.14 to 0.20 second. This represents the P-R interval.

The QRS Complex

The electrical impulse generating the heartbeat originates in the sino-auricular node. Diagrammatically the process may be represented like this:

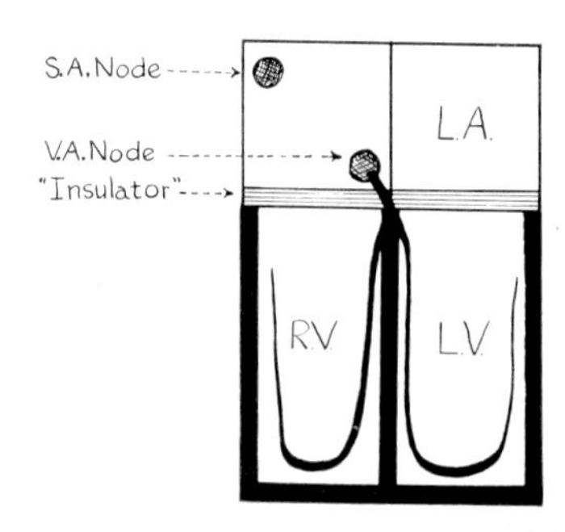

If the A-V node is slightly delayed (or maybe there is a "trigger level," a certain total stimulation from the various atrial fibers required to set it off), the impulse ultimately is "fired" from the A-V nodes and travels downward along the Purkinje fibers which lie in the wall of the interventricular septum.

There is some arborization of these fibers and from them the wave of depolarization (and consequent muscular contraction) passes through the ventricular muscle. The electrocardiographic result of this ventricular depolarization is the QRS complex. It usually looks like this:

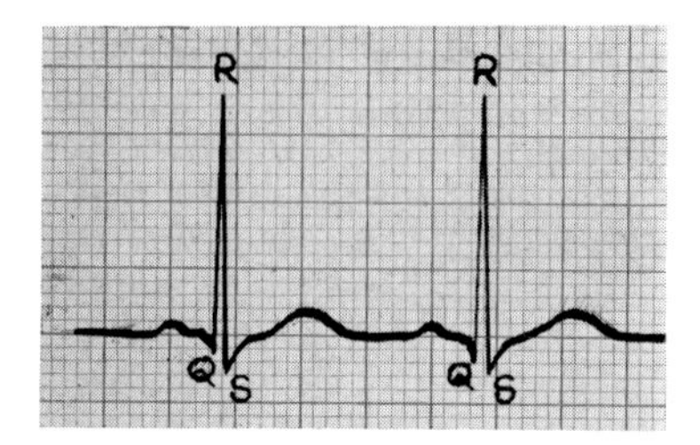

Normally the process of ventricular depolarization takes about 0.08 second.

The T Wave

You will remember that the repolarization of the atria is represented by a wave known as P_1 which is usually not seen, for it is covered up by the QRS complex. A similar repolarization of the ventricular musculature takes place. It is represented by the T wave.

The complete electrocardiographic tracing with corresponding normal time values looks like this:

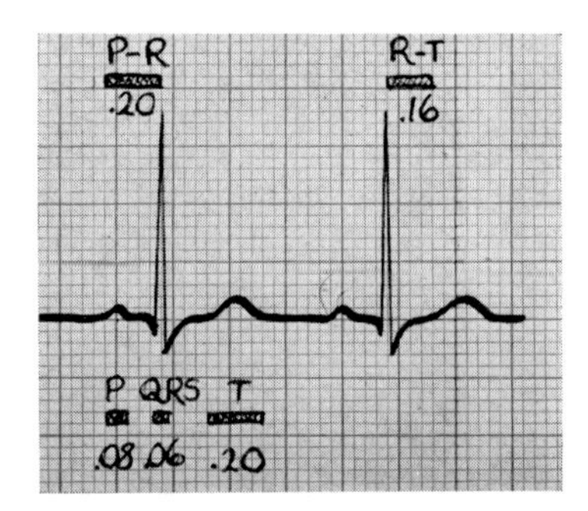

Following are the six points previously mentioned on page 186 as necessary in every electrocardiographic interpretation:

"1. The rate is neither too slow nor too rapid (60 to 100 a minute).

"2. The rhythm is normal, the impulse arising in the sino-auricular node (sinus rhythm).

"3. The P-R period (measured from the start of the P wave to the start of the R wave) is neither too short nor prolonged (0.10 to 0.22 second).

"4. There is no abnormal deviation of the electrical axis.

"5. The P wave, QRS complex, and the T wave are upright in the limb leads, and of normal amplitude and form. In CR_1 there is never a Q wave and the S wave is greater than the R wave, and in young subjects the T wave may be inverted; in CR_4 or IVR the S wave may be deep; in CR_7 the S wave is small.

"6. There is neither undue elevation nor depression (greater than 1 millimeter) of the R-T segment."*

SINUS TACHYCARDIA

The existence of sinus tachycardia does not imply disease of the heart. It is an increase in heart rate, usually to between 100 and 160, due to imbalance of the sympathetic accelerator and parasympathetic inhibitor fibers.

It is probably most often seen in the fevers and in cardiac psychoneurosis. The fevers present little diagnostic problem, but the cardiac psychoneurosis with sinus tachycardia may be difficult to separate from paroxysmal auricular flutter. Clinically this may be surmised from the rate which, in flutter, is usually greater than 160.

Various drugs, exercise, emotion, hyperthyroidism, and even digestion of a large meal may cause sinus tachycardia.

The ECG

A typical tracing looks like this:

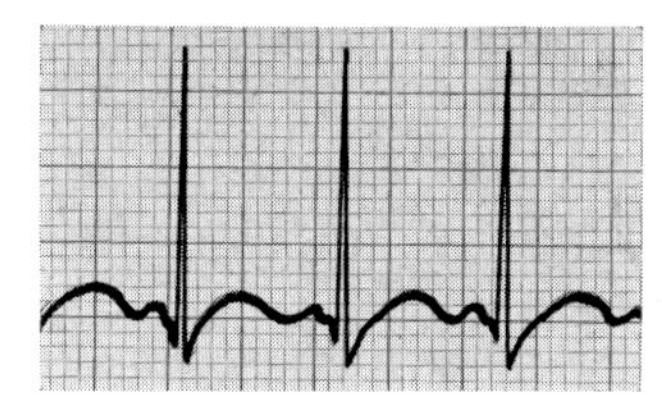

The rate is about 120 but the configuration of the tracing is entirely normal.

*From Evans, William: Cardiography, St. Louis, The C. V. Mosby Co.

Notice that the impulse begins, as would be expected, in the S-A node and there follows normal depolarization of the atria as they contract. Simply, the P wave is of normal size, shape, and placement.

The P-R interval is toward the lower range of normal. The QRS complex is of normal configuration and T waves appear as expected.

Now look carefully at the tracing and notice that the whole complex, the PQRST, is essentially normal. Rather than great speeding up of the complex itself with consequent shortening of P-R and R-T intervals, there is an increased number of PQRST complexes at the expense of diastole.

Here is a comparison of normal and sinus tachycardia tracings, showing the PQRST complex as solid lines and diastole stippled:

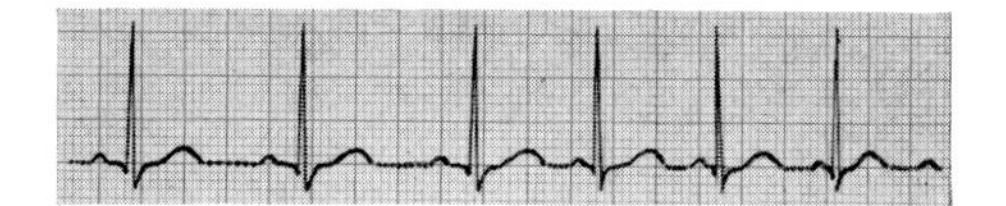

Errors

If one notices the perfectly normal configuration of the various waves and their normal relationship one to the other within the complex there is no reason for error. Probably the most frequent mistake is to assume that sinus tachycardia indicates some organic disease of the heart. Actually, it indicates just the opposite.

In the presence of this finding the practitioner should be warned to seek the extracardiac origin of the difficulty.

SINUS ARRHYTHMIA

Sinus arrhythmia is a change in cardiac rate seen almost constantly in children and often in adults. Most often it is related to the respiratory cycle, the heart speeding up upon inspiration and slowing down upon expiration. This is seemingly mediated by the vagus, a burst of vagal impulses occurring as inspiration nears its end. These are, of course, efferent impulses, but they coincide properly in time to initiate efferent impulses which slow the heart. Impulses arising in the great veins of the thorax are probably also responsible in part.

Be that as it may, the sinus arrhythmia engendered is a physiologic phenomenon initiated by impulses arising from extra-cardiac sources.

The ECG

The PQRST complexes are usually normal, although notching of the P waves may sometimes occur, like this:

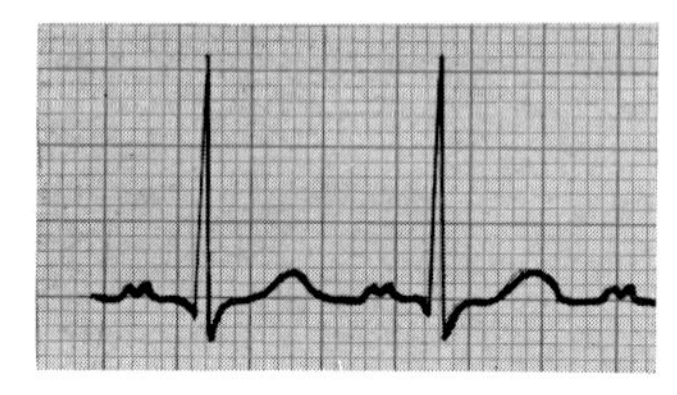

The striking changes occur in the duration of diastole. Notice that the T-P interval is variable but that the rest of the tracing remains normal.

Errors

There is little need to use the ECG to diagnose this entity. It can be easily picked up clinically, even without a stethoscope. Palpating the radial pulse while observing respiration is sufficient.

Again, one must remember that such a tracing is *not* indicative of organic heart disease. Most often it is physiologic.

SINO-ATRIAL BLOCK

Sino-atrial block is a generic term that actually indicates several entities. The S-A node has an inherent rhythmicity of its own, but this rhythm may be profoundly altered by changes in the balance of sympathetic and parasympathetic impulses.

Visualize this control as a teeter-totter. So long as the weights on each end are equal, balance is maintained and the heart rate is normal. When the sympathetic side is in control, whether by more weight on the sympathetic side or less on the parasympathetic, the heart rate increases. Now suppose a burst of parasympathetic impulses arises, say from gagging. This sudden overbalancing may so influence the S-A node that it will miss a beat altogether.

Rarely, arteriosclerotic heart disease may completely knock out the S-A node and atrial standstill will result.

Such conditions are rare in practice. The common cause of sino-atrial malfunction is exuberant administration of the digitalis and quinidine group of drugs.

Three stages are apparent. The first evidence of difficulty is sinus bradycardia. In this the auricular rate is slow, sometimes 30 to 35 per minute. Occasionally it is slower.

The physician should remember that the A-V node has a rhythmic tendency of its own. If the atria contract infrequently enough, the A-V node may escape and set up a rhythm independent of atrial contraction.

As sinus bradycardia becomes more pronounced, occasional beats are altogether lost and the ventricle shows more and more tendency to escape into its own rhythm. Finally the S-A node is completely eliminated as a pacemaker and the atria fail to contract. When this happens the ventricles establish an independent rhythm as dictated by the A-V node.

Sometimes careful observation will allow demonstration of all three stages in the same patient. Such serial tracings are valuable for study.

The ECG

The first of the above stages, that of sinus bradycardia, shows a normal tracing except for greatly extended diastole. A typical Lead I looks like this:

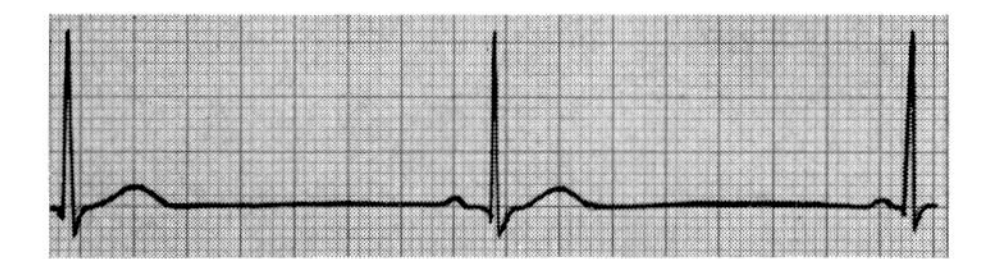

Notice that the PQRST complexes are essentially normal. Next, beats begin to be lost altogether or the ventricles show a tendency to escape. This is a lost beat:

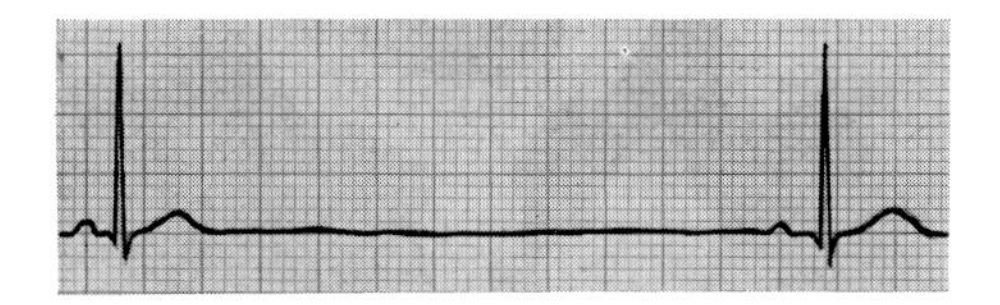

This is a ventricular escape:

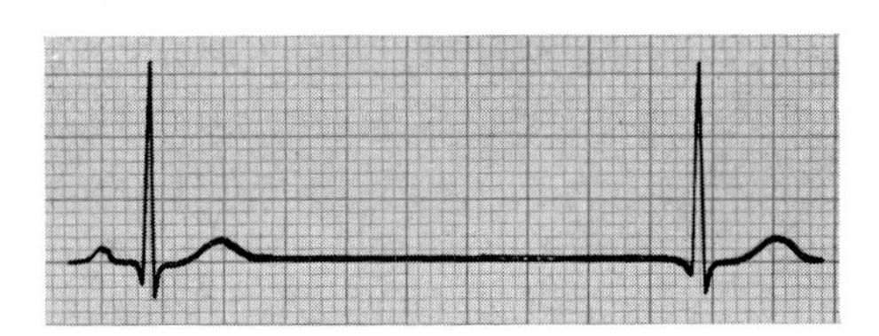

The final stage, that of atrial standstill, looks like this:

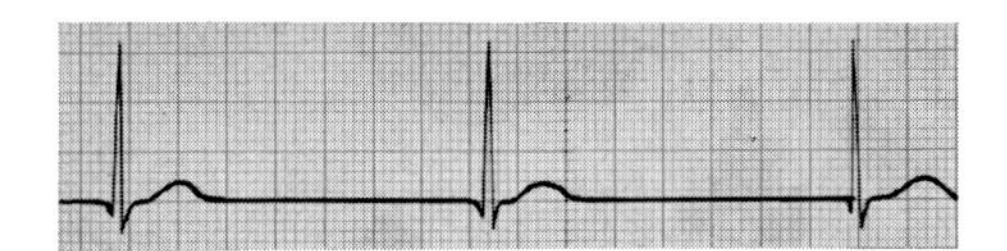

Notice that there are no P waves.

Errors

When these findings appear, chances are better than 500 to 1 that some extracardiac cause is operative. It is possible, but highly improbable, that atherosclerotic disease might knock out the S-A node.

EXTRASYSTOLES

Premature beats are the commonest cardiac arrhythmia to which the human being is subject. They are, in fact, so frequent that one might almost class them as a normal phenomenon of the heart. Certainly it is difficult to find any adult who has not had them.

While much has been written about the exact mechanism of their causation, we actually do not know why they occur. It is apparent that an impulse for these beats arises some place in the heart which ordinarily does not furnish the impulse. Why this should occur we do not know.

The relationship of these ectopic beats to heart disease also poses a difficult question. The vast majority of persons who show such phenomena have no evidence of organic heart disease and long-term surveys indicate that they are no more likely to develop heart disease than the normal person. On the other hand, the presence of organic disease definitely increases the number of ectopic beats.

In other words, the chances are that a person showing extrasystoles does not have organic heart disease. The actual figures are 10 to 1 against organic disease being present. On the other hand, when a person has pathologic changes in the heart he may have ectopic beats as a result of these changes.

From a clinical standpoint this simply means that extrasystoles are insignificant. One should base his diagnosis of heart disease upon other findings and realize that the added beats are incidents rather than a basic cause.

The impulse for extrasystoles apparently may arise from any part of the cardiac structure and the electrocardiogram will be altered, depending upon what part is involved. In perhaps 90 per cent of patients seen by the practitioner these beats arise in the ventricular conductive mechanism. A smaller percentage arise in the area of the A-V node and almost a trivial percentage arise in the area of the S-A node.

The ECG

The typical ventricular extrasystoles show a widened aberrant QRS complex appearing earlier in the cycle than would normally be expected. Bizzarity of form is one of the principal characteristics of a tracing showing such a beat. A typical one looks like this:

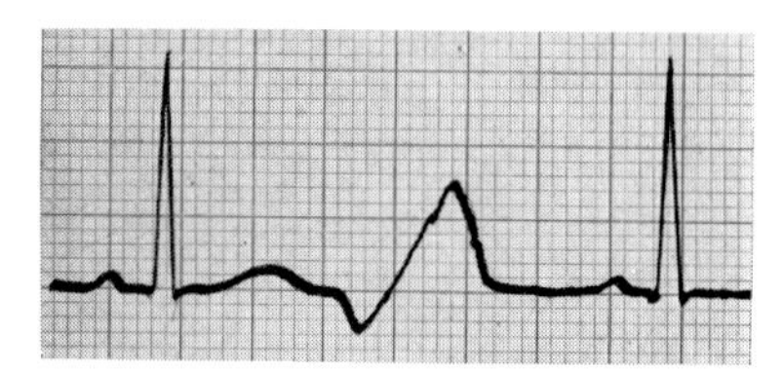

This beat probably originates before the refractory period of the heart muscle is entirely past so that conduction of the impulse is slower (making the QRS complex wider) and distinctly aberrant. Repolarization is abnormal as well and the T wave usually partakes of the bizarre form found in the QRS. It is often written in the opposite direction from the main QRS and may look like this:

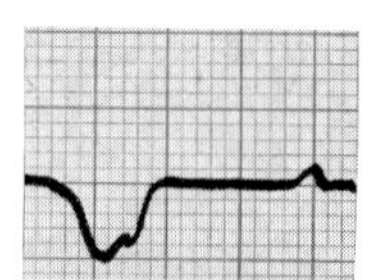

Notice particularly that there is no sign of a P wave initiating the contraction and that the pause following the contraction is somewhat longer than would be expected. This is probably so because the normal impulse for the next contraction arises during the absolutely refractory period of the heart muscle and no response is obtained.

Why a sudden fright or startle reaction should elicit one or several extrasystoles, we do not know. That such a thing occurs is a matter of common knowledge. Why the aberrant impulse is not explained.

Occasionally these extrasystoles will occur at regular intervals. Why, we do not know. In some cases each normal beat is followed by an extrasystole like this:

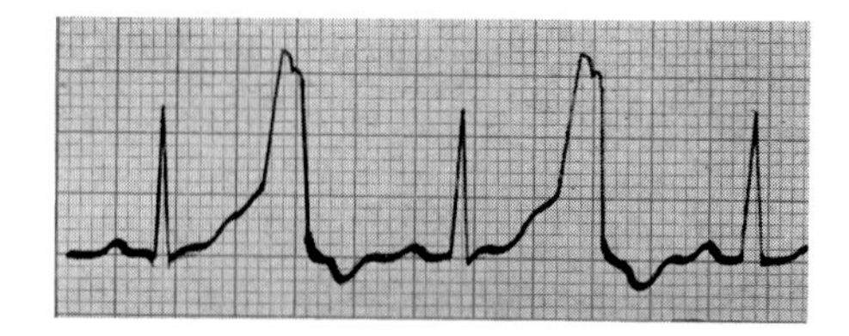

and the beats are said to be coupled.

In a few cases extrasystoles will arise in the area of the A-V node. In these the excitatory current spreads normally to the ventricular muscle and in retrograde fashion to the auricular muscle. The P wave may be swallowed up in the QRS complex but sometimes it occurs a fraction of a second before.

Since the impulse is spreading in retrograde fashion, the P wave is usually inverted and may be of bizarre shape and the P-R interval is greatly shortened. A typical example might look like this:

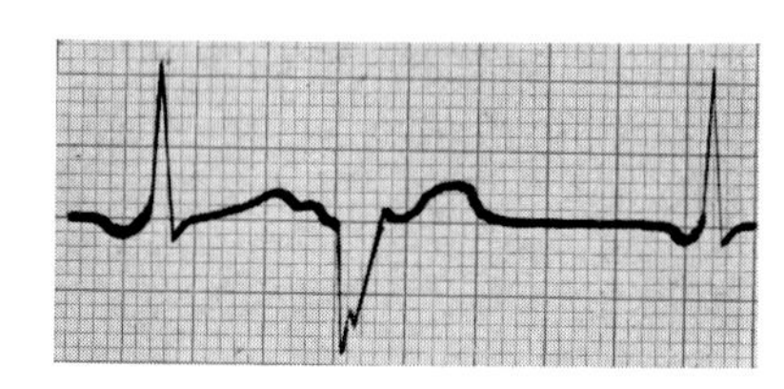

Even more rarely, the ectopic focus may be near the S-A node, in which case the PQRST complex will be relatively normal but displaced in point of time. This is a typical ECG:

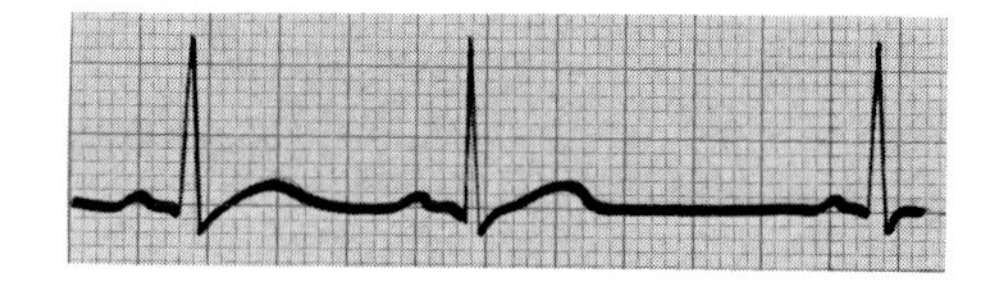

Errors

Errors in interpretation of the ECG are legion. In actuality these abnormalities mean nothing except what is shown on the face of the tracing—that ectopic beats are occurring. When they arise in the area of the S-A node they are usually associated with some type of disease; when they arise low in the conductive system (as most of them do) they are significant only in the light of the other cardiac findings.

Coupled beats may arise in the presence of overdigitalization but, from this single standpoint, clinical findings are probably more valuable than the ECG.

Interpretation

One must begin by repeating once again that the common ventricular extrasystole has no definitive meaning in and of itself. One should inquire historically about excessive use of tobacco or alcohol because these beats sometimes occur in the presence of such indulgence and disappear when it is interdicted. Probably the most frequent cause is nervous tension, and we practitioners see many cases in which mild sedation or exhibition of the tranquilizing drugs promptly stop the occurrence of extrasystoles. Even in the presence of mild organic heart disease these ectopic beats mean little or nothing.

In the presence of severe organic heart disease the sudden institution of ectopic beats and their gradual increase in number is a bad prognostic sign.

At the risk of being repetitious, it must be said again that extrasystoles in general *have no meaning* unless associated with other positive cardiac signs and symptoms.

PAROXYSMAL AURICULAR TACHYCARDIA

Paroxysmal auricular tachycardia is another relatively frequent arrhythmia which apparently is not often associated with severe organic heart disease. The etiology is not exactly known but it is assumed to be somewhat different from the typical circus-movement etiology of auricular flutter.

The condition is different from auricular flutter in that paroxysmal tachycardia usually lasts from a few minutes to one hour; the attacks are initiated suddenly and cease with equal suddenness, often spontaneously. Flutters, on the other hand, may continue for weeks, months, or years unless adequately treated.

Regardless of the exact etiology, the fact remains that something in the atria initiates extremely rapid impulses so that the rate of apial contractions often is 200 per minute. Standard texts make the statement that the ventricle usually responds to every auricular impulse, but this is not necessarily so. We have seen a few cases where the atria were contracting at the rate of almost 300 per minute and the ventricles showing a typical two-to-one block.

In the usual case, however, the pattern of heart action remains relatively normal except for its extreme speed.

Various nervous and toxic conditions have been blamed for the presence of paroxysmal auricular tachycardia but there has been no convincing proof that any one entity is peculiarly at fault.

The ECG

The electrocardiographic tracings remain relatively normal except for the extreme speed which is attained, usually at the expense of the T-P interval. Often P waves are partially obscured by impingement on the T waves, like this:

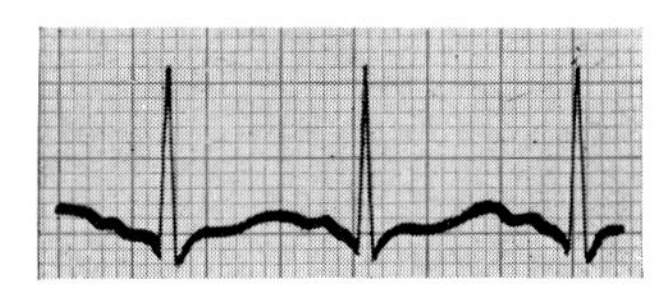

It is instructive to take an electrocardiogram while applying the usual clinical methods for relief and notice the sudden cessation of the rapid action.

If there is a question about A-V dissociation, take a right pectoral lead at the point shown here:

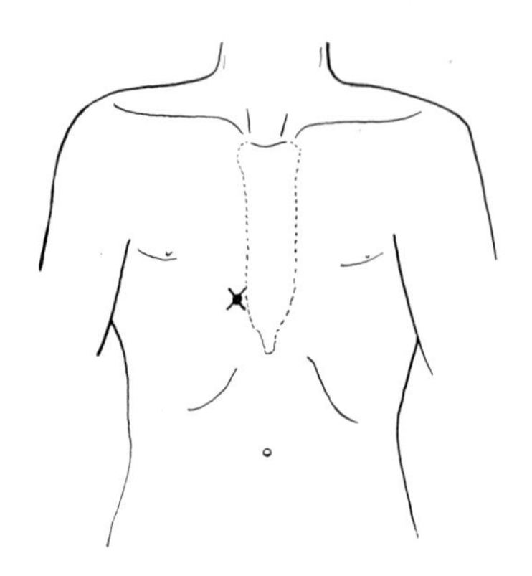

T waves are usually much more clearly shown in such a lead and may clarify the degree of dissociation should there be any.

Errors

There are practically no errors in the diagnosis of paroxysmal auricular tachycardia. The only condition with which it might be confused is typical auricular flutter and this may be distinguished both electrocardiographically, in most instances, and historically.

Interpretation

The presence of paroxysmal auricular tachycardia, is an indication for careful search leading to extracardiac causes. Only in rare cases does this disturbance occur in the presence of serious organic heart disease. Like a number of the other arrhythmias it is probably more often caused by nervous tension than by other entities. As a matter of fact I have never seen a case with proved organic cause.

AURICULAR FLUTTER

Auricular flutter is an arrhythmia seldom seen by the practitioner. It is due to a circus movement of the impulse. Diagrammatically the impulse may originate and proceed like this:

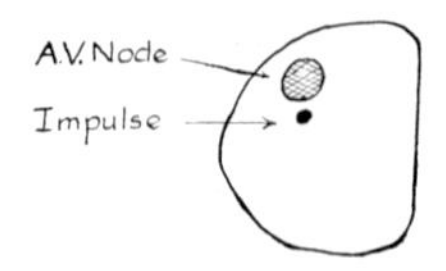

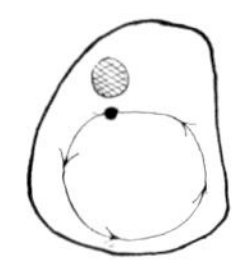

reaching its point of origin just as the muscle in that area has recovered from its refractory period and, therefore, continuing in its circular path. In almost all instances there is a degree of A-V block, usually either two to one or three to one. The atria may contract from 200 to 350 times a minute and the ventricles may vary from 100 to 250 per minute.

The ECG

Characteristic of this disorder is the rapidity and absolute regularity of P waves observed from the tracing. They frequently show a short, sharp upstroke and a sliding downstroke, like this:

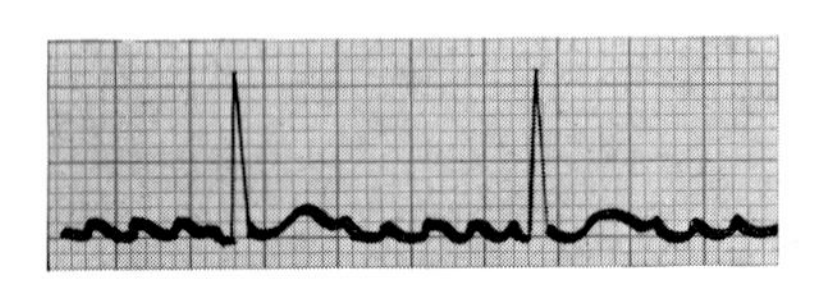

In most cases Lead II will adequately delineate these P waves; however, rarely, they may be partially covered by a rapid ventricular rate. When this happens the right pectoral lead taken here:

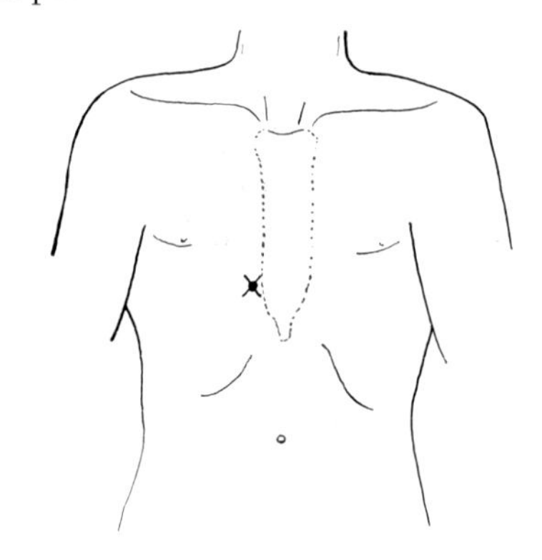

should be employed. Following is a typical illustration from the right pectoral lead:

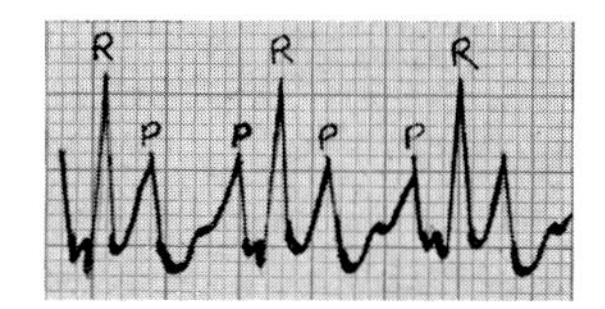

Errors

The only error of consequence is to confuse atrial flutter with paroxysmal auricular tachycardia. Here are some differences to keep in mind:

(1) The P wave.

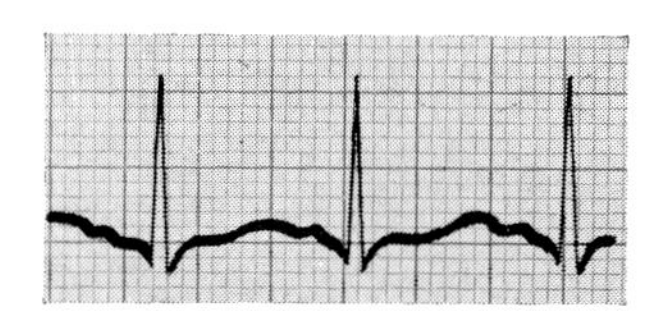

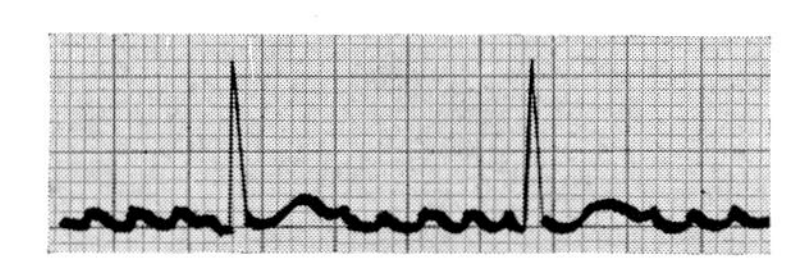

Notice that the P wave is essentially normal in paroxysmal auricular tachycardia or that it may be fused with the preceding T. Now notice its peculiar shape in flutter.

(2) Ventricular dissociation.

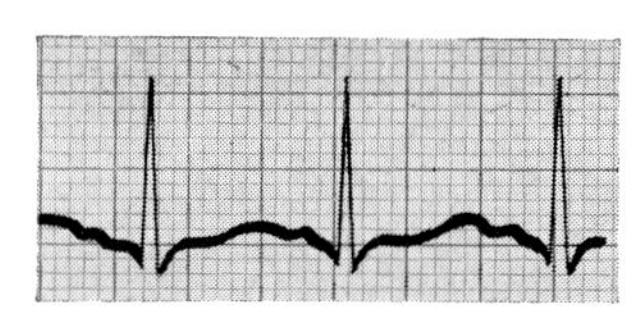

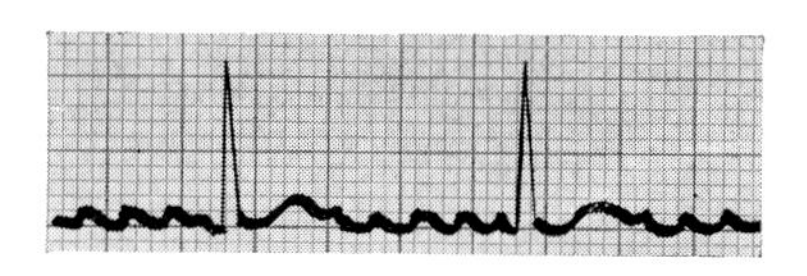

Notice that the PQRST complex is relatively normal in auricular tachycardia except for the impingement of the following P on the preceding T. Now notice the fact that there are several P waves for one QRS complex in flutter. Clinically the differentiation between the two is even easier.

Interpretation

Auricular flutter is usually an accompaniment of organic heart disease. Exactly what changes occur in the conductive system to bring on this arrhythmia, we do not know.

It is, however, most often seen in rheumatic heart disease and hyperthyroidism, and the presence of atrial flutter should make one give serious consideration to these possibilities.

AURICULAR FIBRILLATION

Next to extrasystoles auricular fibrillation is probably the commonest arrhythmia seen by the practitioner. It is a frequent accompaniment of organic heart disease and is usually seen in the presence of decompensation.

Apparently it results from an extremely rapid circus movement in the atrial musculature, the current making its complete circuit 400 to 600 times a minute. Because such rapidity almost always impinges upon muscle not completely recovered from its refractory period, conduction of the current in some areas is slow or ineffectual and in other more recovered areas, of almost normal rapidity. This makes for irregular, ineffectual contraction of the atrial musculature which actually shows twitching vermiform movements rather than really active and efficient contractions.

During these irregular circuits a certain number of the currents stimulate the A-V node and are followed by a ventricular contraction. Since the stimulants reach the A-V node in all stages of strength and timing, the ventricular impulses that are generated are totally irregular, sometimes striking the ventricle itself in the stage of relative refractoriness.

For these reasons ventricular contraction is completely irregular in terms of strength and timing. This irregularity of ventricular contraction is what gives rise to the clear-cut clinical signs by which auricular fibrillation may almost always be diagnosed.

The ECG

True P waves are characteristically absent. They are replaced by F waves (fibrillation waves) and actually consist of trivial deviations on the base line, like this:

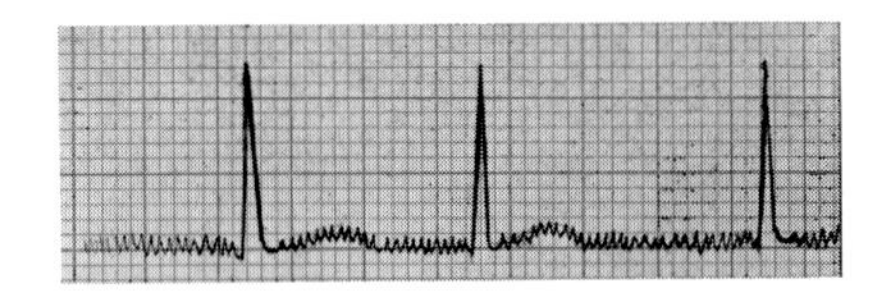

In a right pectoral lead taken at this point:

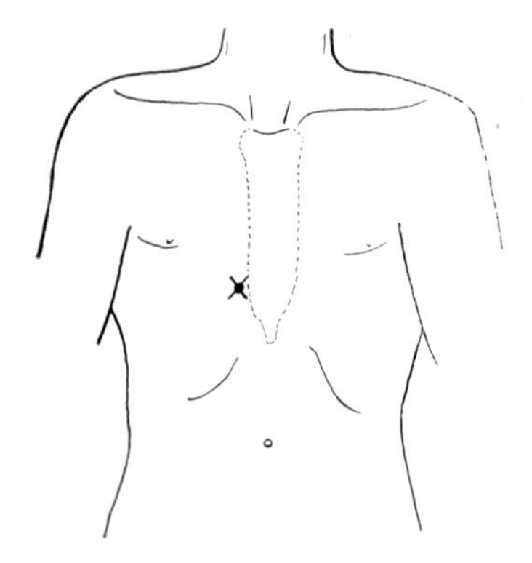

the auricular contractions are much more clearly delineated, but in none of the leads are there entirely typical T waves.

The irregularity of ventricular contraction is appreciable both clinically and on the ECG. A typical tracing from Lead II looks like this:

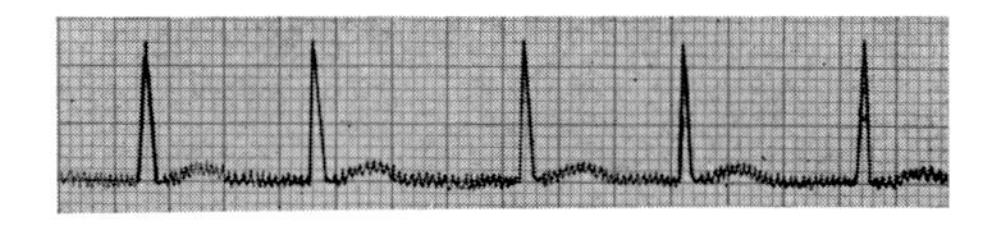

Errors

In a typical case of well-established atrial fibrillation there is practically no reason for error. Actually the basic error is having to use the ECG for diagnosis, for the entity is usually clinically clear-cut and entirely easy to distinguish.

Interpretation

Auricular fibrillation is usually associated with organic heart disease but there are certain cases in which it seems purely functional. These amount to perhaps 5 per cent of the total number of cases seen. Most often it is seen in arteriosclerotic heart disease with failure, in rheumatic myocarditis with failure, and in hyperthyroidism.

One point that the practitioner should keep in mind is that atrial fibrillation practically never occurs in the absence of failure if organic heart disease is present. Why this is so we do not know, but the percentage of cases in which it is proved untrue is very small.

One should remember that fibrillation probably increases the burden on an already overloaded heart and should be controlled if possible. In essentiality, the atria have no functional ability while fibrillating.

PROLONGATION OF THE P-R INTERVAL

It has been amply proved that many of the infectious diseases may cause prolongation of the conduction time in the heart.

Rheumatic fever is only one of the diseases that may engender these changes in conduction time. For that reason it is necessary to realize that no finding on the electrocardiograph is specific for rheumatic fever. On the other hand, in conjunction with clinical findings the ECG is almost perfectly diagnostic.

It may be that electrolyte changes engender the conduction alteration or it may be that actual inflammatory changes in the fibers themselves have some bearing. This is not known. Specifically, a prolongation of the conduction time means only that there is or has been some type of damage to the myocardium.

The ECG

The normal P-R interval is not more than 0.20 second. In the presence of active myocardial changes it is usually prolonged to 0.24 second or longer, like this:

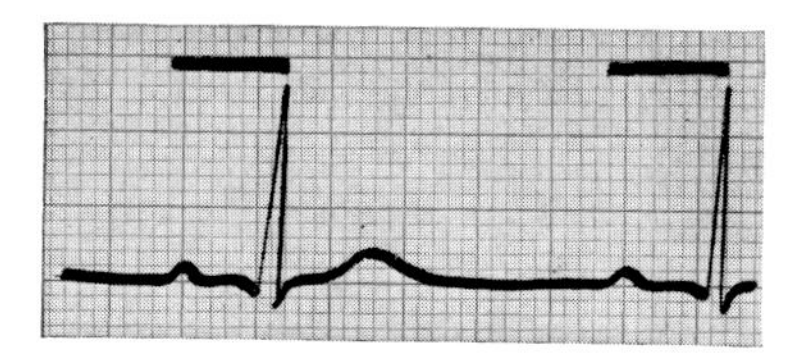

The QRS complexes may be blurred or widened due to slow conductivity, and the Q-T interval is often longer than normal, like this:

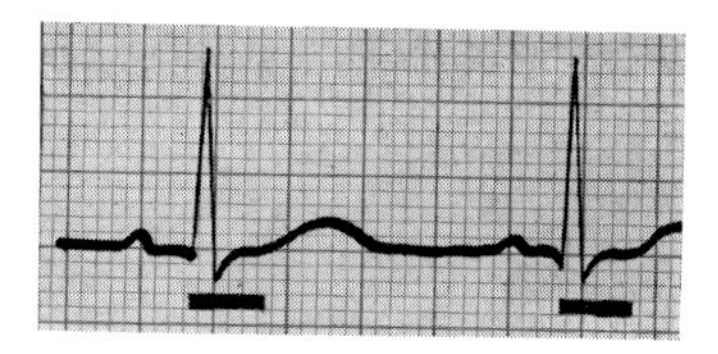

Errors

There are two common mistakes in interpretation. The first is to assume that any prolongation of the conduction time indicates rheumatic fever. This is not true. It indicates some damage to the conductive system of the heart, usually myocardial in origin.

In some cases of cardiac damage the conductivity of fibers is permanently lowered. This happens, not often but occasionally, in rheumatic fever. When this is true a prolonged P-R interval will appear so consistently that it is said to be fixed.

If one does not keep these facts in mind, an occasional bad diagnostic error may be made in the case in which there is a fixed, prolonged P-R interval.

Interpretation

As was previously said, the prolongation of the P-R interval indicates only some sort of damage to the conducting mechanism of the heart. In view of this, any interpretation must be in the light of clinical symptoms and not taken purely from the ECG alone. It is probably true that at least 90 per cent of such prolongations are due to the rheumatic diseases, but by no means all of them.

A-V BLOCK

In some cases the A-V block is probably an extension of the process involved in increase of the P-R interval. Certainly the conducting mechanism may be at first depressed to the point where it functions slowly and is finally stopped completely. As such, one would expect this to occur infrequently in various infectious diseases, which it most certainly does.

More often the advanced degrees of conduction difficulty are caused by arteriosclerotic heart disease, in which the conduction bundle is rendered permanently incompetent or the function permanently depressed. Other conditions may unquestionably be at the root of this difficulty, but by far the greatest number will be found in older individuals with arteriosclerotic changes.

The ECG

Progressively the changes are as follows:

(1) There is a prolongation of the conduction time with an increased P-R interval, like this:

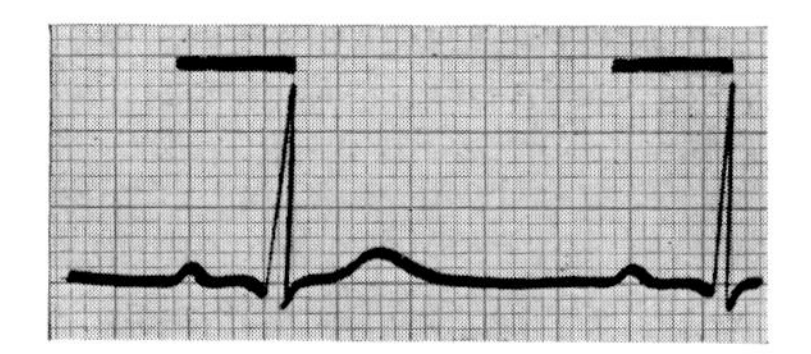

(2) Then there is an occasional dropped beat. Perhaps every six or seven beats the apial impulse will not get through to the ventricle, and the ventricular complex will be missed like this:

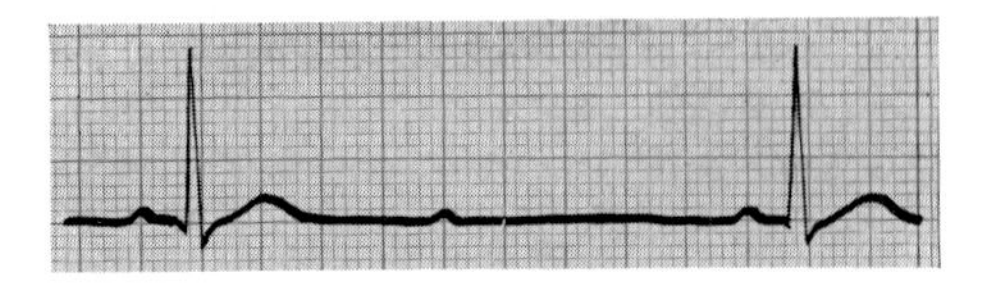

(3) Finally, there is an increasing dissociation until few or none of the auricular beats get through and the ventricles assume their own rhythm, like this:

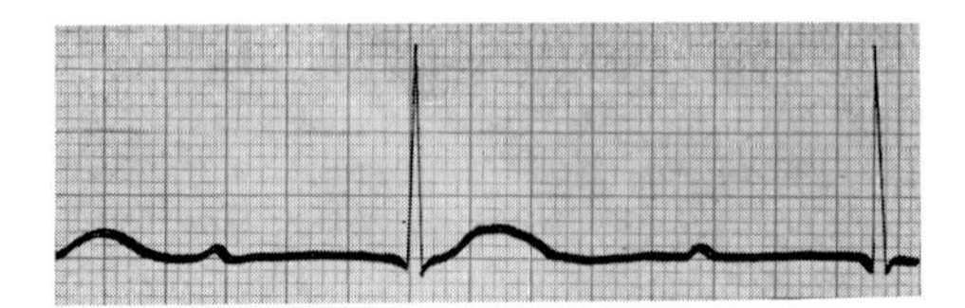

Errors

Probably the most frequent error is to assume some definite diagnostic conclusion from the presence of heart block. Anything that depresses or knocks out the conducting fibers may cause heart block. This would vary from a stab wound to an overdose of digitalis. The finding is indication for a careful and thorough search for the source of the damage—not an indication for diagnostic complacency.

Interpretation

In the older individual arteriosclerotic heart disease is unquestionably responsible for the great majority of heart blocks, and a careful search should be made for evidences of early congestive failure. Historically one should ask about episodes of cardiac pain because minor infarctions are frequently involved.

An extensive application of foxglove is one of the commonest causes and careful inquiry should be made as to whether digitalis is being taken and in what dosage. Occasionally, quinidine may also be a factor.

Rarely, particularly in younger people, it seems possible that there can be a functional depression of conduction. This is not easily explainable, but it seems so well proved that one should keep it in mind.

BUNDLE BRANCH BLOCK

The bundle of His descends the interventricular septum for a short distance and then bifurcates to arborize like this:

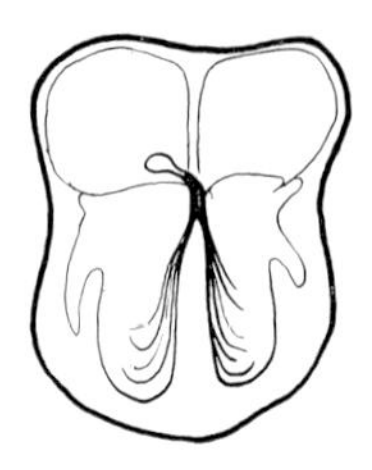

Occasionally an insult may be applied to the conducting fibers in this area:

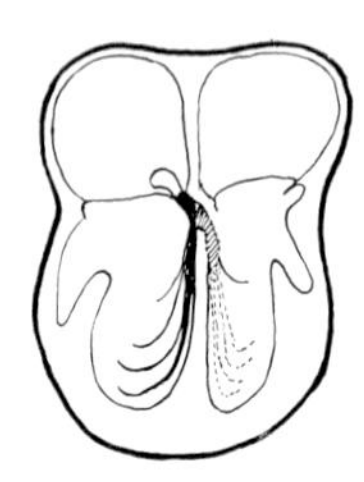

When it happens that only one of the bundles is affected by the pathologic change and conduction to one chamber of the heart is impaired, one notes an irregular ventricular contraction. The chamber with intact conduction supply contracts first and is followed almost immediately by the chamber with an injured Purkinje system.

These insults are most often vascular in origin but rarely may be due to toxic influences in conditions such as uremia or in inflammatory diseases such as rheumatic heart disease and diphtheria.

For practical purposes such lesions are caused by deficient circulation or infarction.

The ECG

The P-R interval is usually prolonged except in the Wolff-Parkinson-White syndrome, in which it is short. This syndrome is rare and will not often be seen by the practitioner.

The QRS complexes are wide, prolonged to greater than 0.12 second, and usually bizarrely notched or slurred. In left bundle branch block the QRS complex is upright in Lead I and the main deflection is downward in Lead III. It looks like this:

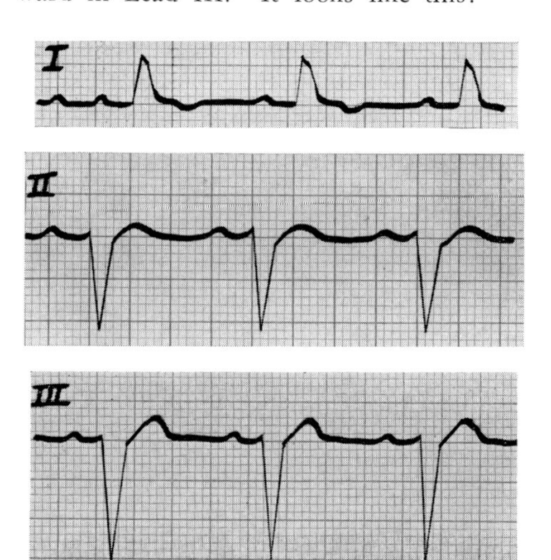

Rarely, in right bundle branch block exactly the opposite may obtain, the main deflection being downward in Lead I and upward in Lead III, like this:

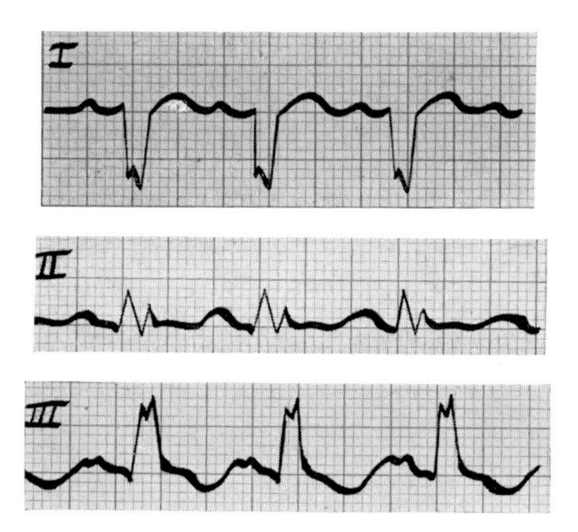

Right bundle branch block is seldom so clearly delineated. More often there is a deep "S" wave in Lead I, although the main complex is upright, and the same applies in Leads II and III. The T wave in Lead III is usually inverted like this:

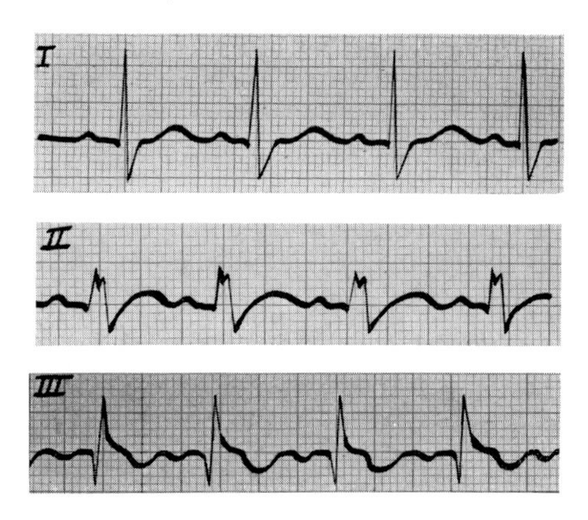

Errors

Errors in the interpretation of bundle branch block are practically unknown.

Interpretation

The presence of bundle branch block means that something is interfering with a portion of the conduction system below its bifurcation. What this something is depends upon clinical interpretation. For practical usage one may assume arteriosclerotic or other circulatory changes, for the practitioner will not see once in three years a case of bundle branch block with any other etiology.

In rare cases in which circulatory changes do not seem to be the cause and in which no toxic factors sufficient to account for the disease are present, the services of an expert cardiologist should be sought.

ARTERIOSCLEROTIC HEART DISEASE

Atherosclerosis of the coronary arteries is unquestionably the most effective killer of productive men today. With the perversity which we medical men bemoan (whether it exists or not), the diagnostic signs of early atherosclerotic change are inconstant and difficult to interpret.

To date no one has elucidated exactly what electrocardiographic changes may be thought entirely characteristic of arteriosclerotic heart disease, nor do we know why those that occur with some regularity are present. From the electrocardiographic standpoint, diagnosis of arteriosclerotic heart disease is purely on an empirical basis, at least in its early stages.

Unfortunately clinical symptoms are not clear-cut either, and the diagnosis is most often made on the basis of history and a shrewd guess on the part of the physician.

The ECG

One of the first changes that occurs is inversion of the T waves in Leads I and II. Inversion of T_3 is more often due to positioning of the heart, and occasionally this change in positioning which produces an inverted T_3 will also invert T_2.

Unfortunately other diseases than atherosclerosis can induce the same changes in T waves. Nonetheless, the ECG may be of some help. These are significant tracings:

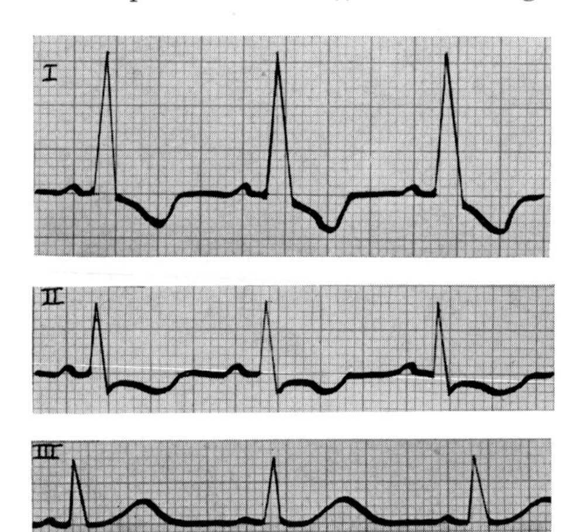

and these are not:

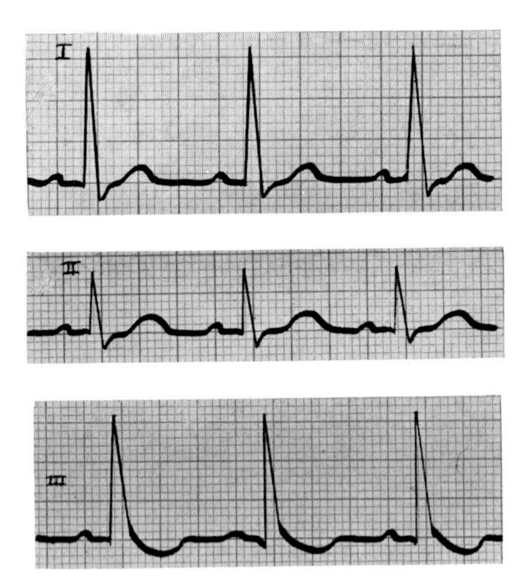

When a significant tracing is found, take three routine precordial leads at the points shown:

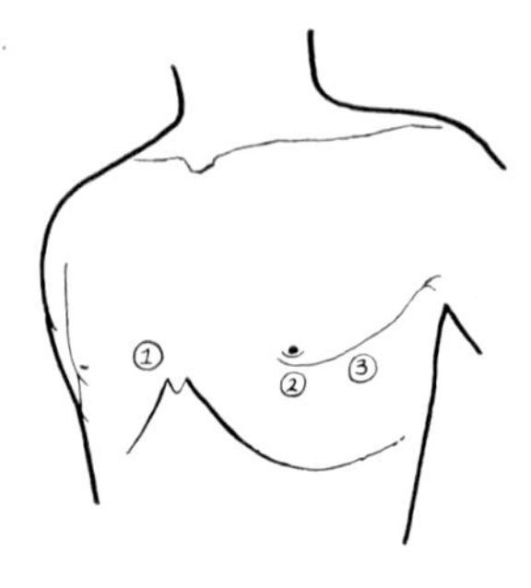

and look for inversion of the T waves. The presence of inversion in these leads is even more significant than that found in the three standard leads.

In marked high blood pressure one sometimes finds an inversion of T and a depression of the S-T segment in the same lead, like this:

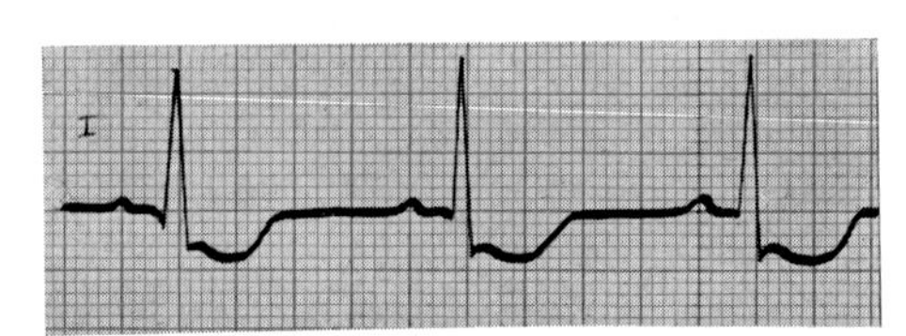

This, again, is not too helpful for it may occur in other conditions.

Errors

In particular, digitalis may mimic all of the changes mentioned above and destroy any significant information to be gained from them. It is an error, also, to read too much into the electrocardiogram in such cases.

Interpretation

It is inevitable that the practitioner in the course of taking electrocardiograms will find some persons with atherosclerosis of the coronary vessels. Perhaps the best advice that can be given is to note the changes for information only and place absolutely no diagnostic faith in them. For the moment, at least, our best diagnosis of early hypertensive changes is based on history and clinical findings, not on the electrocardiogram.

ANGINA PECTORIS

Angina pectoris apparently results from a localized and transient ischemia of the cardiac musculature. It is usually induced by effort and is relieved by rest. The practitioner will seldom get an opportunity to take an electrocardiogram during a spontaneous attack of angina pectoris and the disease is usually so easily identified by historical means that there is probably little excuse deliberately to produce an attack in order to record it on the electrocardiogram. I have always thought it best to avoid the possibility of producing a gentleman's last attack of angina.

Changes characteristic of atherosclerotic heart disease may occur during freedom from anginal attacks but usually the ECG is entirely normal. One concept is important for the practitioner to grasp. A normal ECG simply means that the myocardium and conduction systems are functioning normally at the moment. There is nothing to prevent the patient with a perfectly normal ECG from leaving the office, attempting to climb a flight of stairs, and dropping dead.

Here, again, is a point where patients have undue faith in the findings of the electrocardiogram. Doctors owe it both to themselves and to their patients to have it clearly understood that the electrocardiogram in disease of the coronary arteries is significant only when circulatory changes are obviously present in the tracing or when permanent myocardial changes have been induced. A normal ECG means nothing.

In other words, the best diagnostic instrument I know in disease of the coronary artery is the wise, thoughtful practitioner who has seen many such cases and who will take time to obtain an adequate history and use his stethoscope.

THE CORONARY ATTACK

The heading on this discussion is deliberately generalized for several reasons. Any patient with an acute and clinically obvious myocardial infarction should not be in the practitioner's office for an electrocardiogram. He should either be hospitalized immediately or, if this is impractical, kept at home. Patients with such attacks can often be followed at home if facilities for adequate care are available.

Unquestionably there exists such an entity as coronary spasm, which may cause pain for a duration of several hours or days without developing into a full-blown infarction. This may often be diagnosed in the patient's home, using a portable electrocardiograph, although it is difficult, if not impossible, to distinguish between the full-blown infarction and the severe ischemia.

Apparently electrocardiographic changes related to myocardial infarction stem from changes in conductivity. At first when the blood supply is cut off, the muscle will remain alive for several hours and probably will conduct normally. Particularly is this true if the infarcted area is small. The ECG will be entirely normal.

In massive infarctions, of course, the muscle tissue near the center (i.e., furthest from possible blood supply of the infarcted area) shows almost immediate conduction changes and therefore the expected alteration appears in the electrocardiogram. It is obvious that such patients are experiencing severe coronary attacks and therefore should be hospitalized immediately and neither cared for at home nor under any conditions taken to the practitioner's laboratory for electrocardiograms.

Patients with more minor degrees of infarction with no electrocardiographic changes, or at least minor changes, sometimes are best followed in the home. One should never forget the possibility that the infarcted area may spread and that a case which at first looked minor may soon assume death-dealing proportions.

The patient showing no electrocardiographic changes at first should be carefully followed clinically and repeat electrocardiograms taken every six to twelve hours until the expected changes appear.

After the patient has recovered from the myocardial infarction, electrocardiograms *may* be taken every six months as a measure of cardiac recovery, the interpretations to be made by a regional cardiologist and not by the practitioner.

However, since such tracings rarely show any signs except that there had been an infarction (and this is not always evident) and it is practically impossible to make a definite prediction with even the most elaborate tracings taken six months or more after a typical infarction, I see no reason to take them unless there are specific evidences that disease remains or is about to recur.

The ECG

There are as many patterns characteristic of cardiac infarction as there are places for infarction to occur and all sorts of "bizarrities" may be seen in the electrocardiogram. Fortunately, however, at least 90 per cent of true infarctions occur in areas where a typical Q_1, T_1 or Q_3, T_3 pattern makes diagnosis easy.

In taking the tracings on a patient suspected of infarction, one should take the three standard leads and an apical lead as a minimum. As one becomes more familiar with the problems of interpretation the six chest leads should be added. Most important of all, a single negative tracing taken soon after the onset of pain should not be considered in making the diagnosis. Sometimes electrocardiographic changes are delayed and may not become apparent for some time. In addition, diagnosis is better made by serial changes than by single alterations in any one tracing.

Another point that seems scarcely worth mentioning is that if the patient appears to be seriously ill, one should not delay hospitalization to take an electrocardiogram. Most acute cases of myocardial infarction may be diagnosed clinically and the electrocardiogram becomes a secondary factor which does not warrant delay.

For the sake of convenience in discussing the changes that occur, we will divide this section into discussions of the Q_1, T_1 and the Q_3, T_3 patterns. In anterior infarction it is usual to see the Q_1, T_1.

Often the first changes which may lead one to suspect difficulty are discordantly high T waves which appear in Leads I and II, like this:

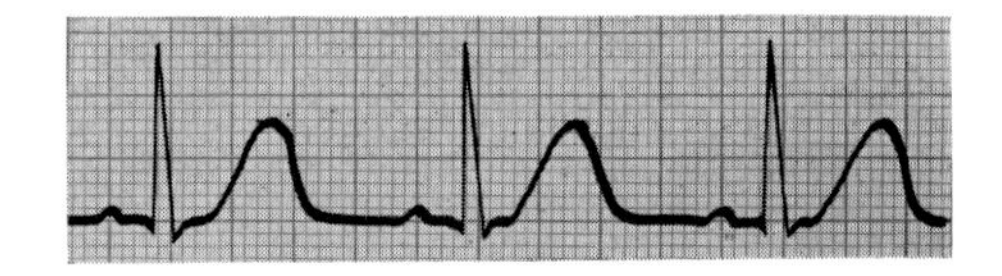

This is not diagnostic of myocardial infarction but frequently along with clinical signs may be taken to point in that direction. They usually occur within an hour or two after onset of pain, but may be delayed as much as six to eight hours.

The next typical finding is an elevation of the S-T segment, that is, the high take-off so commonly referred to. It occurs in Lead I and sometimes in Lead II and looks like this:

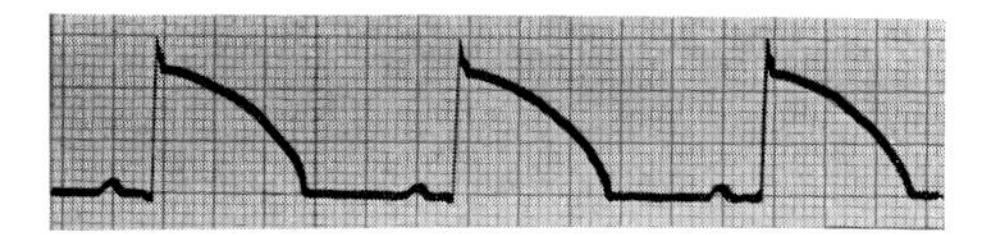

Notice the curvature or arc shape of this elevated segment which is not common in any electrocardiographic tracing and which is striking in early myocardial infarction. This change apparently depends upon a current of injury set up in the devitalized muscle and, of course, is not present until the muscle is devitalized. This may range from one to two hours after onset of pain to as much as twenty-four hours later. It is for reasons like this, of course, that serial tracings are of the utmost value.

The next change that usually occurs is a flattening or biphasic change in the T wave. This is a typical flattened T wave in Lead I:

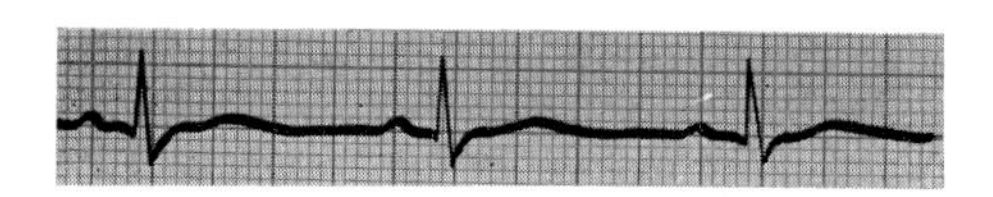

and this is typical biphasic in the same lead:

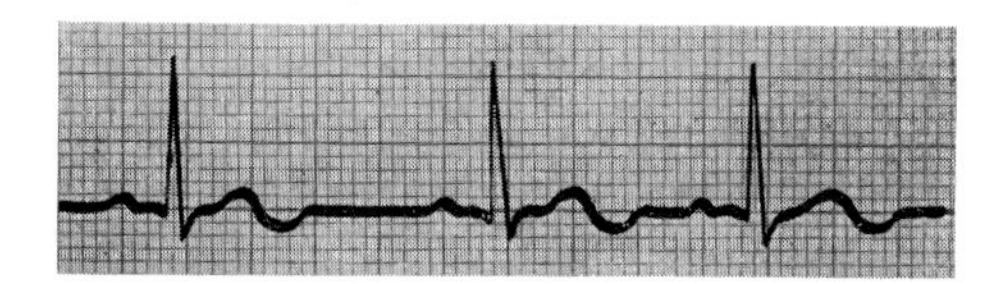

This change may occur as much as twenty-four hours after the original infarction and has been known not to appear for several days. The T wave ultimately becomes inverted like this:

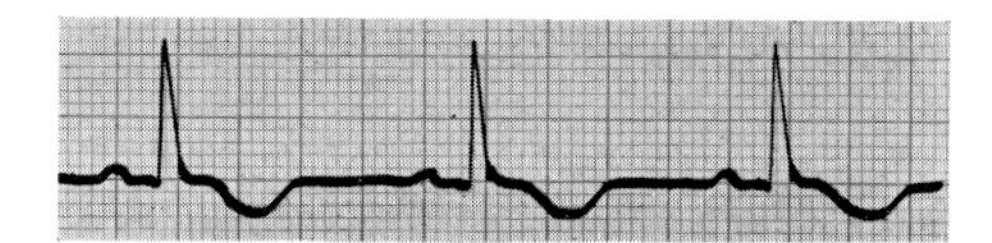

Usually before this inversion of the T wave there appears a prominent Q wave in Lead I, like this:

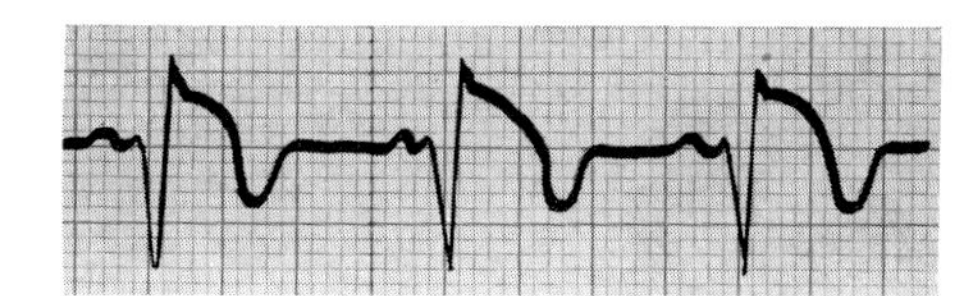

By the time that Q_1,T_1 changes are quite apparent—that is, by the time a prominent Q wave is present and the T wave is inverted in Lead I—the S-T segment which was at first elevated like this:

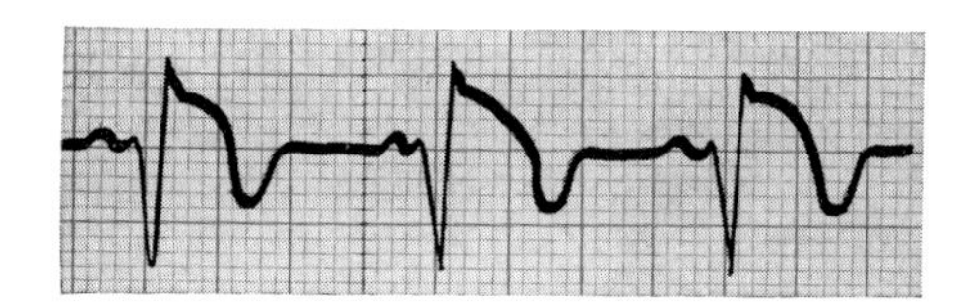

usually approaches the isoelectric line so that the tracing after a day or two looks like this:

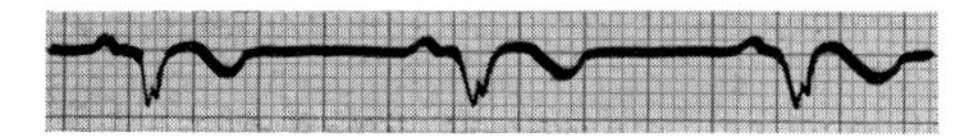

Over a period of weeks the S-T segment reaches absolute normal and the Q wave usually disappears to some degree, but months may elapse before the T wave reassumes normal configuration.

In Lead IV there is usually a great elevation of the S-T segment, beginning with an upward convex shape like this:

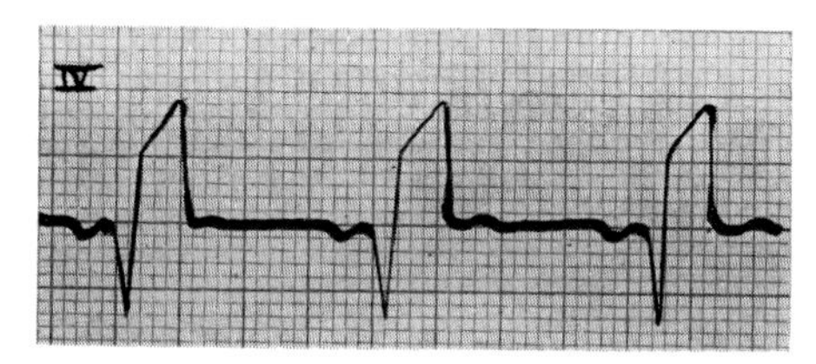

"Bizarrities" in Lead IV often may appear and become somewhat diagnostic before the typical changes in Lead I and Lead II occur.

In the Q_3,T_3 pattern the sequence of events is largely reversed, the principal deviation of the R-T segment appearing in Lead III and the typical Q and T waves appearing in Lead III and sometimes in Lead II, like this:

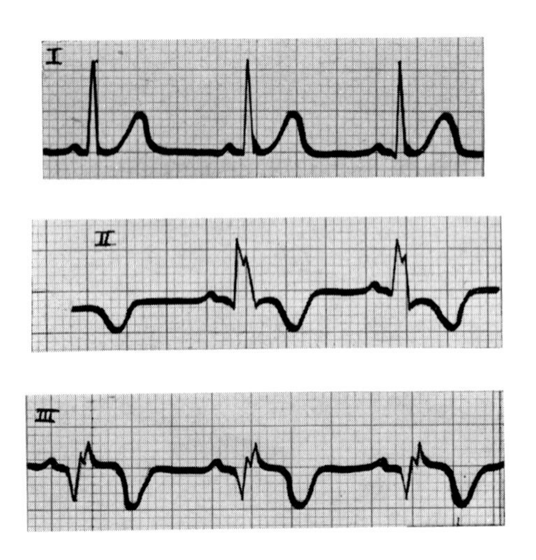

This is a typical posterior infarction in several stages, illustrating the almost normal tracing seen on the first day and the sequence of changes during two and one-half weeks:

First Day

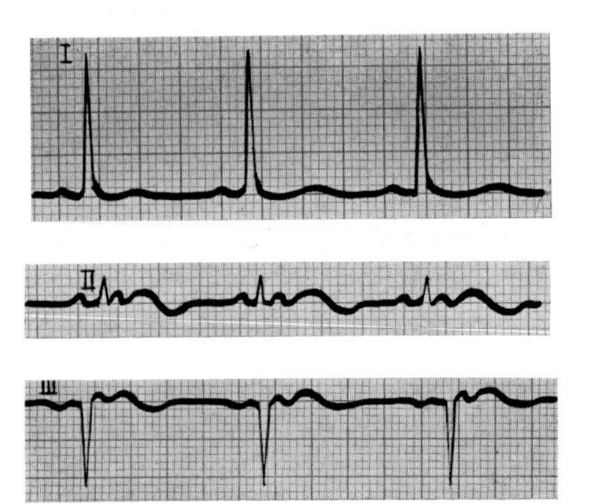

Third Day

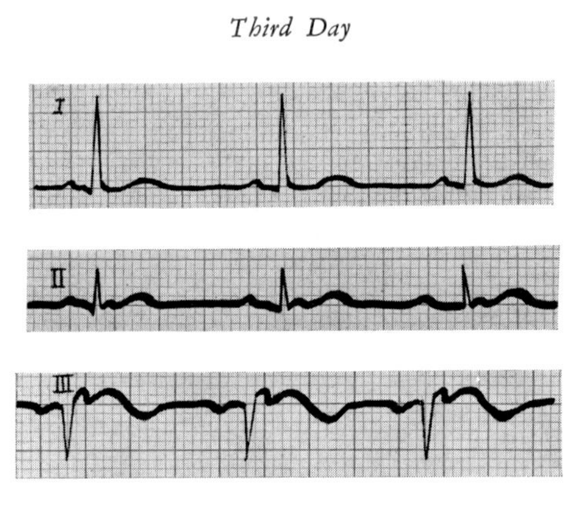

Tenth Day

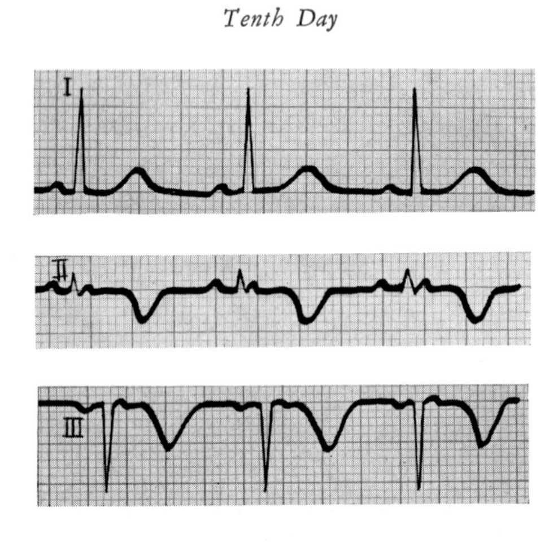

Seventeeth Day

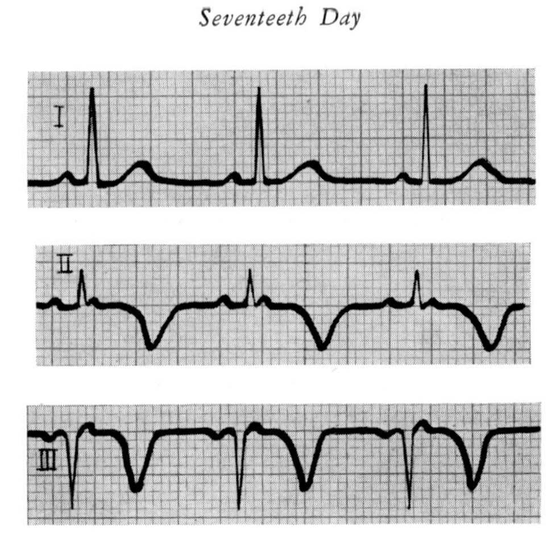

Errors

Probably the principal error is to assume that no infarction is present when one gets an essentially negative tracing on the first try. It cannot be repeated too often that serial electrocardiograms are the means by which coronary infarction is diagnosed. Often a single electrocardiogram taken at a propitious time will give one most of the information needed, but a single negative electrocardiogram is never of significance.

Occasionally one sees a heart that just literally goes to pieces with multiple infarctions so that no clear-cut pattern is observable but it is obvious that there are major conduction changes. Such massive infarction obviously means immediate hospitalization and desperation measures, even though the electrocardiographic changes are not typical of any particular pattern.

Interpretation

Over a period of time the electrocardiogram will give an accurate picture of the amount of damage that has been done to the myocardium. During the early hours of an infarction it is not reliable. The process of infarction itself is a dynamic changing entity and a spot check, such as the ECG, may be misleading. After several days to a week the process has usually reached its maximum in tissue destruction. One may then examine serial electrocardiograms with some confidence for signs of impairment from the infarction.

In other words, one major danger in interpretation is to attempt to read too much into a single tracing.

AXIS DEVIATION

Probably the most common electrocardiographic finding seen by the practitioner is deviation in the electrical axis of the heart. In most cases such deviation indicates preponderance of the corresponding ventricle, that is, left axis deviation means left ventricular dilatation and right axis deviation means dilatation of the right heart.

These findings are not absolutely correlated. There are a few cases of left axis deviation in which the left heart is not enlarged, but these are distinctly the exception rather than the rule.

Actually, clinical diagnosis by means of a carefully taken history and a competent physical examination is just as good and sometimes a better means of distinguishing the enlarged heart as electrocardiography. For that reason we will only mention the typical electrocardiographic patterns. Once again, it is best to rely on the stethoscope and the palpating finger rather than the ECG.

In left axis deviation the QRS complex is upright in Lead I and taller than the QRS in Lead II. QRS is deeply inverted in Lead III. T_3 and sometimes P_3 may be inverted. Following are typical tracings:

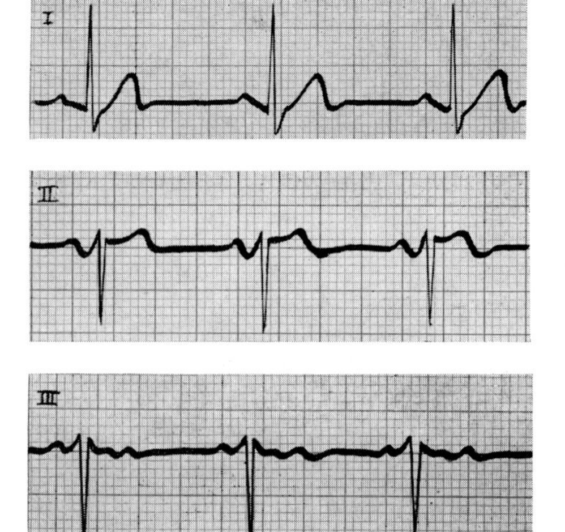

Right axis deviation shows an upright QRS in Lead III, taller than the QRS in Lead II. QRS in Lead I is deeply inverted.

T_1 and P_1 sometimes are flat or inverted. Following are such tracings:

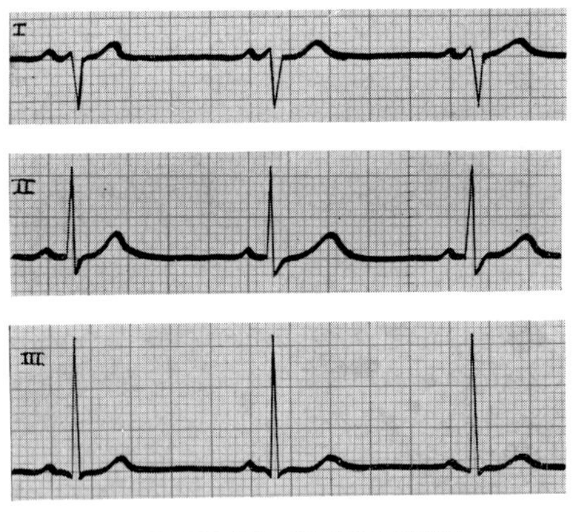

GENERAL COMMENT

Of necessity, this chapter has been a brief summary of the information to be gained in the office from an electrocardiogram. If the practitioner will use his machine conservatively and cautiously and subject any questionable patient to examination and electrocardiography by an expert cardiologist, he will find himself an exceedingly competent minor cardiologist in a few years, capable of handling at least 90 per cent of the patients who consult him.

Again, although it transgresses common custom, I do not think much of the idea of sending a tracing to a cardiologist along with a casual note requesting a diagnosis. This places the cardiologist at a tremendous disadvantage. I would suggest that the practitioner do as much cardiology as he feels himself competent to handle and then send all questionable cases—both patient and electrocardiogram—to a regional cardiologist for further check.

Section Two

CHAPTER EIGHTEEN

Office X-ray

INTRODUCTION

The problem for the practitioner is to obtain as much practical information as possible with his x-ray machine without impinging upon detailed roentgenologic techniques and interpretations which are best left in the hands of the trained specialist. It is not always easy to say just exactly what the practitioner should and should not do.

In this section I have been somewhat arbitrary in selecting procedures theoretically within the range of the average physician. In some places it is herein indicated that the practitioner should go a great deal further than the average roentgenologist thinks he should; in others, distinct over-conservatism will be apparent. These limitations were based not only on my own personal ideas, but also on the careful evaluation of the practices of many other physicians.

Actual physical factors and techniques, such as peak kilovoltage and milliamperage settings and time of exposure, are not mentioned. Each machine is usually accompanied by a chart of definite recommendations by its maker and this, along with alterations found necessary through the practitioner's experience, is usually ample.

The x-ray, like the laboratory, should not be held rigidly to certain preconceived positions and techniques. Its purpose is to offer information, not to accomplish routine tasks. Sometimes an unusual position or an unusual view will give far more information than the standard techniques and most assuredly should be used. Therefore always keep in mind, the x-ray is a tool, not a routine clinical department.

CHAPTER NINETEEN

The Skull

Detailed interpretation of skull films is one of the most technical and difficult problems faced by the roentgenologist. The practitioner should confine himself to certain simple interpretations and leave the more complex surveys of intracranial matter to the trained specialist. There are certain normal markings which must be recognized.

The normal suture lines are as shown:

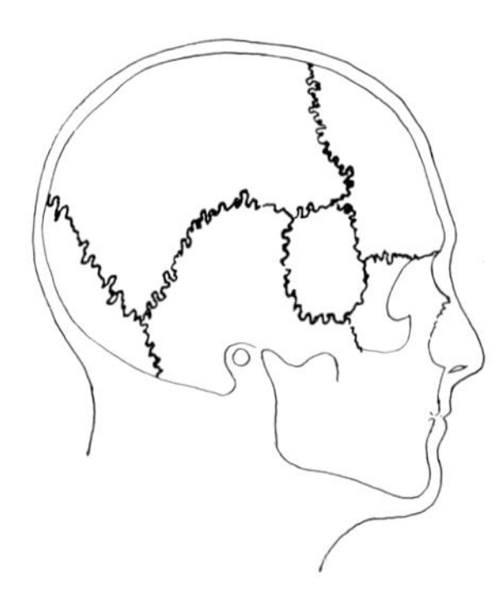

Sutures in the newborn infant, of course, are widespread and look like this:

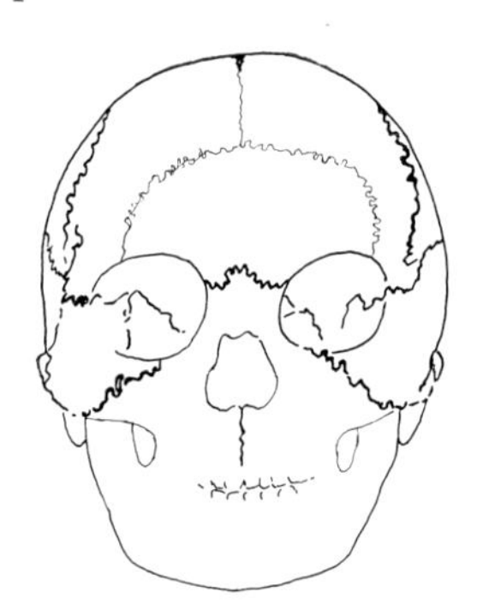

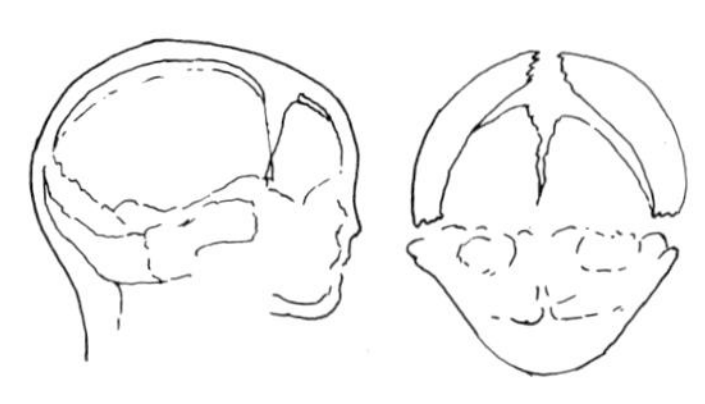

In the adult the suture in the external table of the skull differs considerably from that in the internal. The external is more serrated, like this:

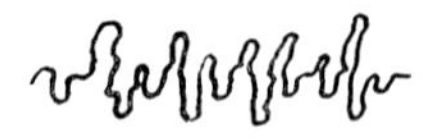

and the internal more nearly straight, like this:

A typical projection of such a suture in the roentgenograph looks like this:

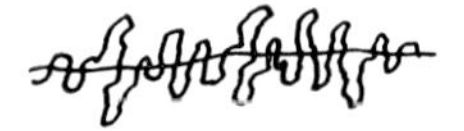

Occasionally the suture lines separate so that a small plate of bone is included between the separation. These small isolated bones are called Wormian bones and are most often found here:

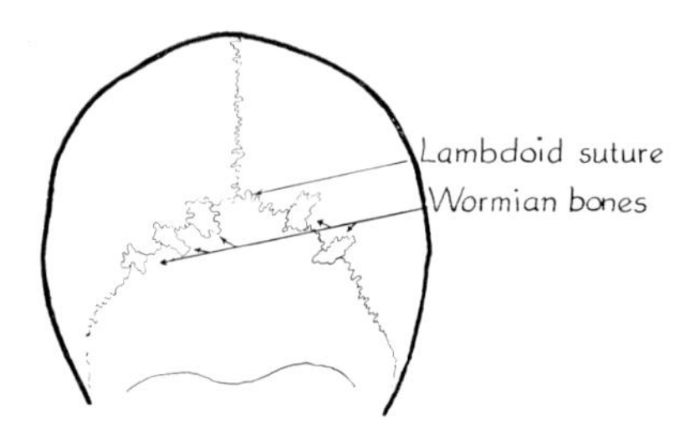

Another series of normal markings are the arterial grooves. They are channels worn by the pulsating arteries and may show some thickening of bone at the edge of the groove, like this:

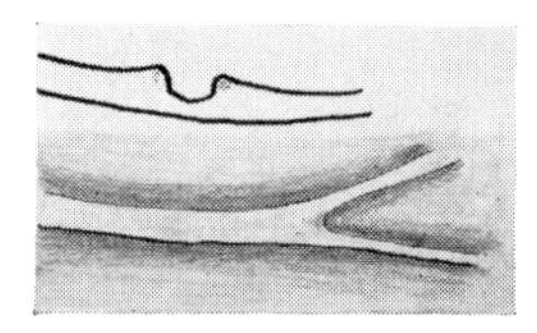

They move in more or less wide-sweeping curves and typically show a gradually diminishing size from below upward. The most readily identified one is the groove of the middle meningeal vessels which usually occupy this position:

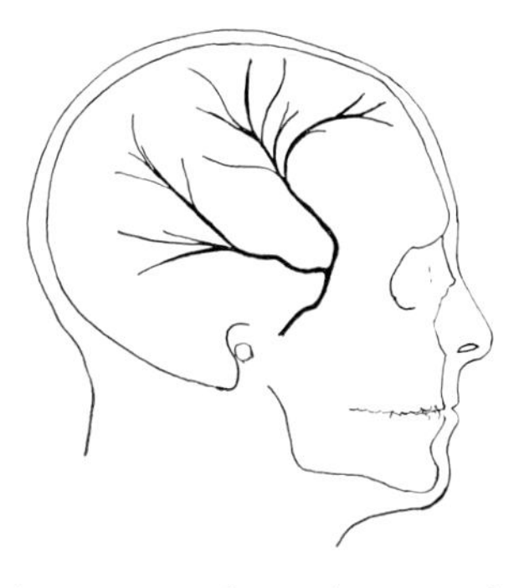

Diploic venous channels are often seen in older subjects but are seldom made out in children. They are most often seen roentgenographically in the parietal area:

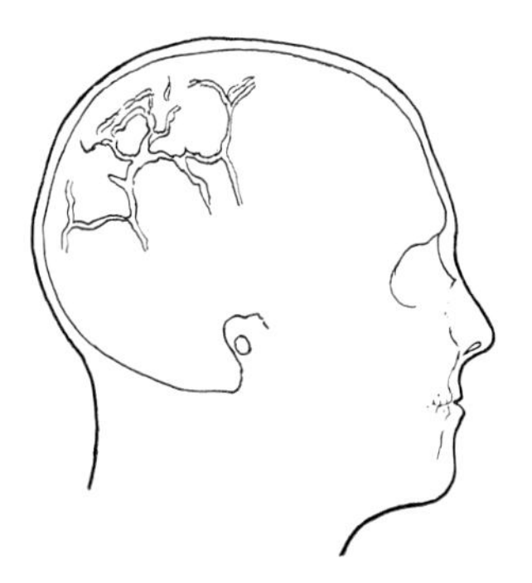

Notice that these vessels show no distinct course but branch and entwine indiscriminately, often forming patterns of almost stellate configuration. Notice, too, that the outline is irregular and fuzzy in appearance and that changes in size in the veins, almost from millimeter to millimeter, give these channels a beaded appearance. Differentiation of these channels from typical skull fracture will be mentioned later.

The skull is subject to so many other normal variations that one point stands out in considering it roentgenographically. Under no circumstances should the physician ever make a diagnosis or predicate treatment on findings that are not clear-cut. If there is doubt, re-x-ray, and if there is still doubt, base treatment on clinical findings until a skull survey can be made by an expert radiologist.

SKULL FRACTURE

A skull fracture is probably a great deal more common than many physicians think. This lesion is extremely common in children, and many small linear fractures are missed because they are not delineated clearly enough by the usual roentgenographic technique.

In adults this is probably particularly true of minor basilar fractures. With present roentgenographic techniques it is difficult and sometimes almost impossible to demonstrate a small linear fracture in the basilar area, and post-mortem reports have been published which show that in as high as 1 per cent of the cases the subjects had sustained such fractures without knowledge of it at some time during life.

The patient with a skull fracture and serious underlying cerebral damage has no business in the doctor's office or, for that matter, in x-ray in the hospital. It is not this seriously injured group of patients that we will consider here, but rather the man who experiences a blow on the head and does not appear to be acutely injured.

For practical consideration, skull fractures may be divided into four classes:

1. By far the most frequent are fractures of the vault. Many of these are missed completely. Such fractures have *absolutely no significance* in themselves other than the possible damage to underlying vessels and brain tissue. They are highly innocuous from the standpoint of the bony damage itself. A patient with a suspected head injury should be examined clinically for cerebral damage. If there are clinical signs the patient should be followed whether or not he has a "negative" x-ray.

2. Fractures of the anterior fossa, on the other hand, have certain dangerous implications which may continue to be a threat for years. If the fracture line runs into one of the sinuses or into the cavity of the nose, which it often does, a connection is established between the outside of the body and the dural contents. In this area the dura is attached firmly to the underlying bone and does not readily initiate repair of any tear. For this reason a rip in the dura in the anterior fossa may remain open for years and cases have been reported in which mennigitis occurred from an obvious dural tear as long as fifteen years after the original injury. This lapse in healing (or at least lack of adequate healing) in the dura presents a real threat to the patient with an anterior fracture, and at times surgical repair must be undertaken to protect the patient.

The floor and portions of the anterior wall of this fossa are irregular. The bone may vary this much in thickness:

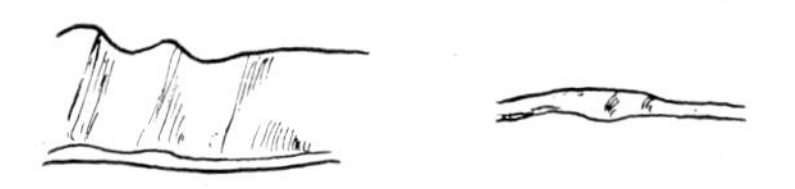

A fracture line approaching one of the thick areas while the fracture is occurring seeks the area of least resistance. It may approach the thick area like this:

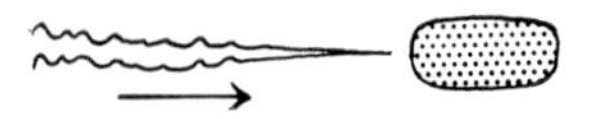

Notice the separation of the fracture line. This continues until the fracture actually isolates the thickened area of the bone like this:

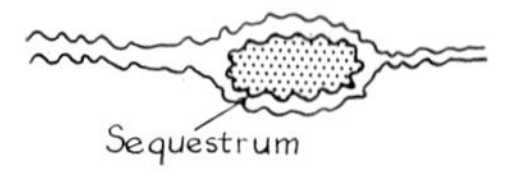

If the blood supply to the thickened area of the bone is cut off, and it often is, the bone actually becomes a sequestrum and may be absorbed. If this is in the orbital roof, for instance, it is not so serious, but suppose it were to overlie an ethmoid cell. The final result would be this:

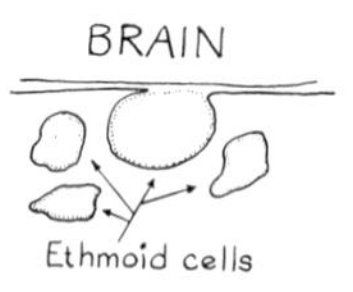

with only the thinnest membrane separating the cranial content from the infected or potentially infected ethmoid area. Such an injury places the patient in the pleasant position of sitting on a powder keg striking matches.

3. Lateral fractures in the area of the middle cranial fossa are sometimes seen in minor injuries and can be clearly discerned on the average x-ray film, but fractures into the structures of the base of the middle fossa are usually such serious injuries that they are seen only in the hospital.

4. Fractures of the posterior fossa seem to be divided into two sharply defined categories. They may be among the most serious and fatal head injuries seen and, of course, will not be office problems. Also, trivial cracks may occur without much in

the way of active symptomatology. Unfortunately, this "trivial-crack" type of fracture is difficult if not impossible to detect by x-ray.

Skull fractures in children usually heal with some rapidity. There is often no appreciable change shown on the x-ray film six to eight months after the fracture. Adults, on the other hand, show great prolongation of healing time, three or four years sometimes elapsing before firm union from the x-ray standpoint has occurred. Sometimes the evidence of fracture persists throughout life. Before you venture a positive interpretation be sure to ask the patient about previous cranial trauma. Evidence of the healing processes usually, *but not always,* can be seen in the films.

One other point is of great importance in discussing these skull injuries—a severe blow that may result principally in separation of the suture lines. Usually these suture lines are not absolutely firm until approximately the age of 35. In young adults one occasionally sees trauma resulting only in the pulling apart of the skull at one of its lines of suture. This should be kept in mind and considered, because it will occur in an occasional case and give positive neurologic findings.

Technique

We generally use four or five positions.

The first is the Caldwell position, taken like this:

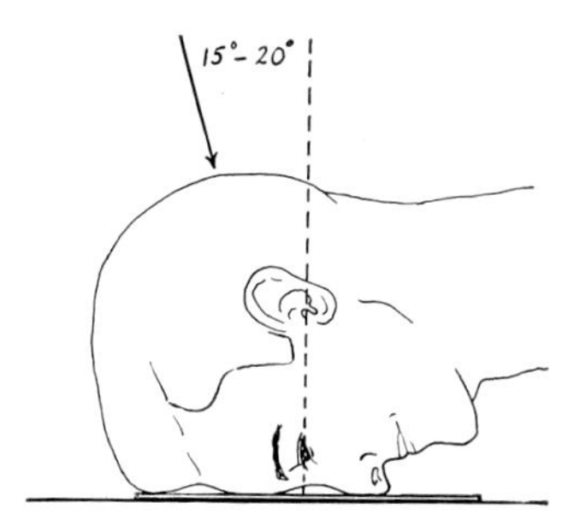

Following is a drawing, showing the important structures to be seen in this position.

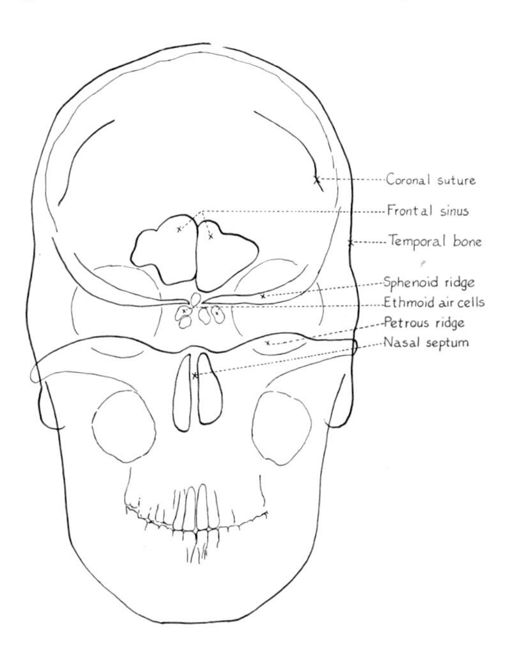

In these sketches we have deliberately omitted all unnecessary lines. Where there is some question about recognizing a structure or where certain relationships need to be shown, we have included less important structures. After looking at these drawings, compare the drawing with a typical film and identify on the film each of the major structures shown in the drawing.

Next is the Towne position, which gives an excellent demonstration of the occipital bone and the petrous ridges. It is taken like this:

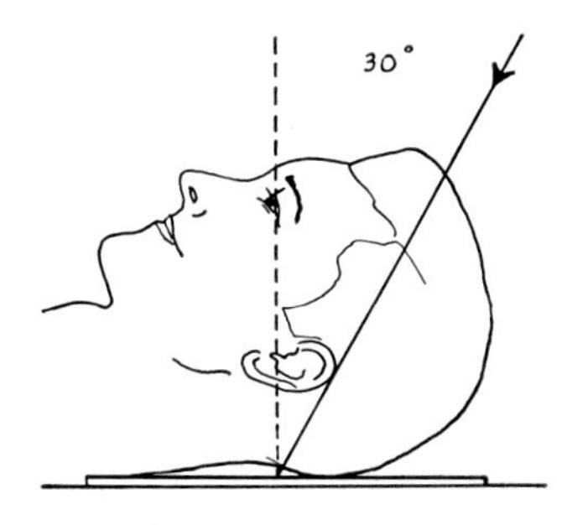

Following are the important structures to be delineated:

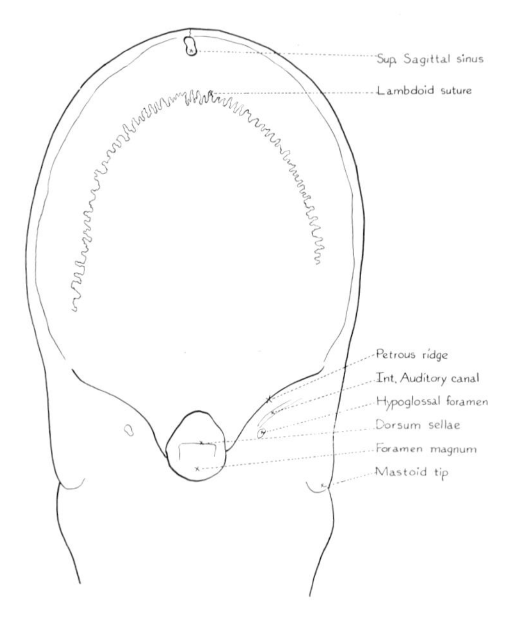

Take two straight lateral films, one with the right side nearest the film and the second with the left side near the film. It is extremely important that two lateral films be taken, for details of the side opposite the film are not clearly delineated. Position the patient like this:

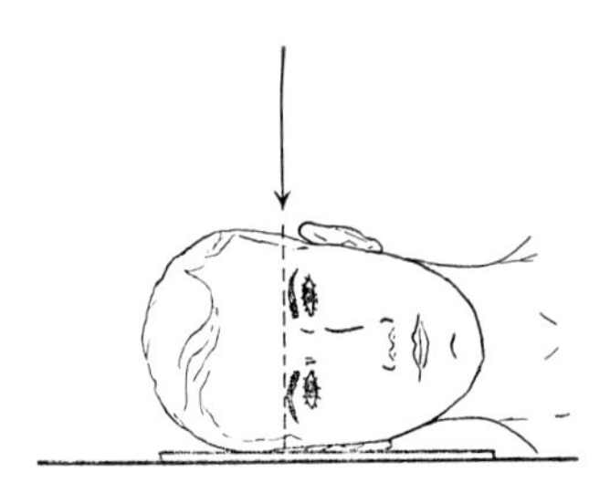

Have the x-rays enter the skull above the ear.

Surprisingly, one of the commonest errors is failure to mark the film in such a way that one knows which side was nearest the cassette. We put a coin on the lateral film with the right side down.

Following are the important details of the resultant film:

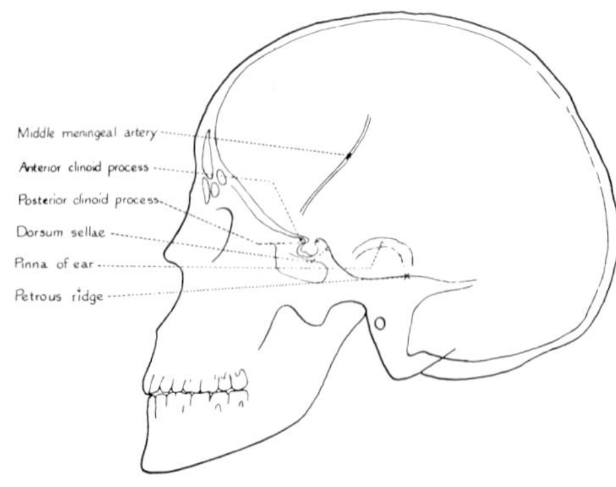

Occasionally the straight posteroanterior film will be of some service. Place the patient in this position:

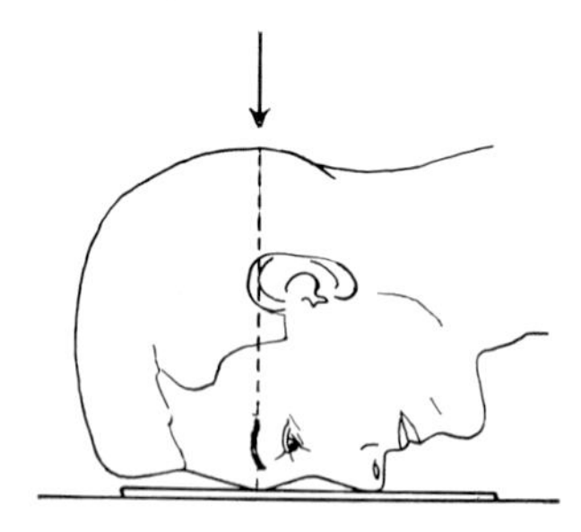

Following are the important structures to be found in the resultant film:

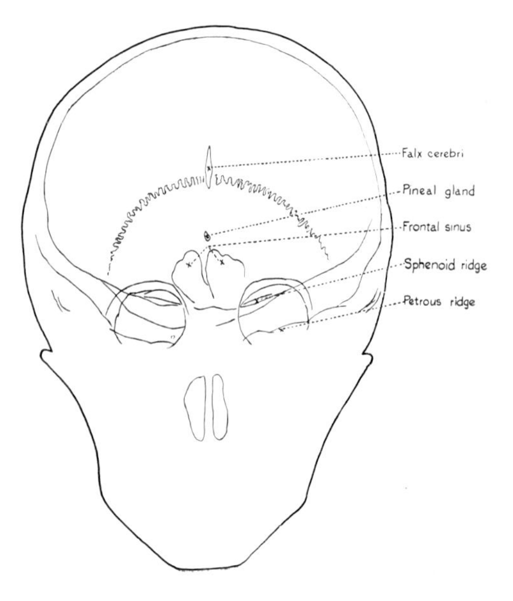

One important point in technique cannot be standardized. If there is a question about the depression of a bony fragment following fracture, the tangential view should always be taken. For example, if this shows up on the lateral film:

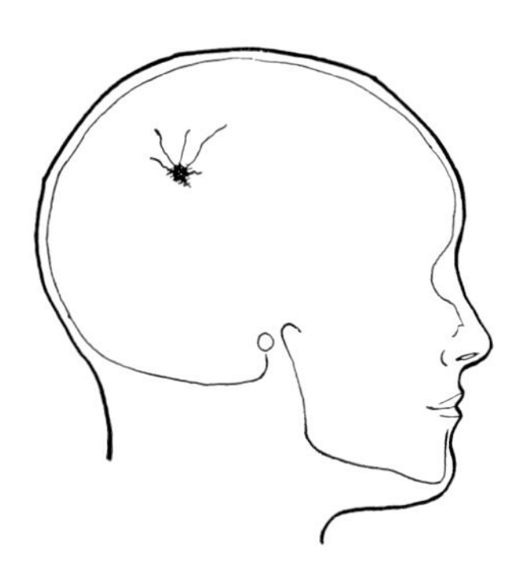

and this on anteroposterior film:

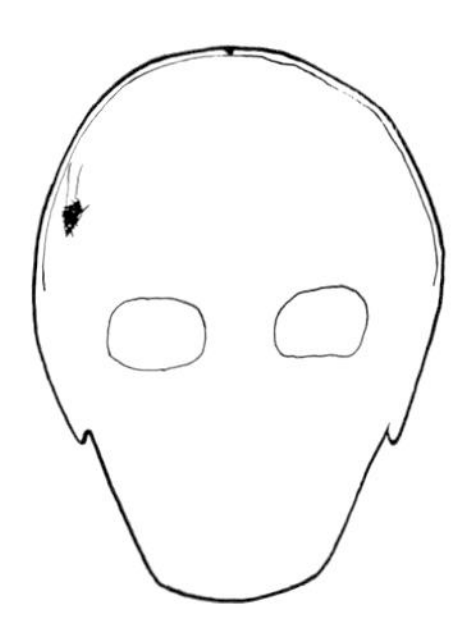

one has every indication that a depressed skull fracture exists, but in order to get a good delineation of it, take a view like this:

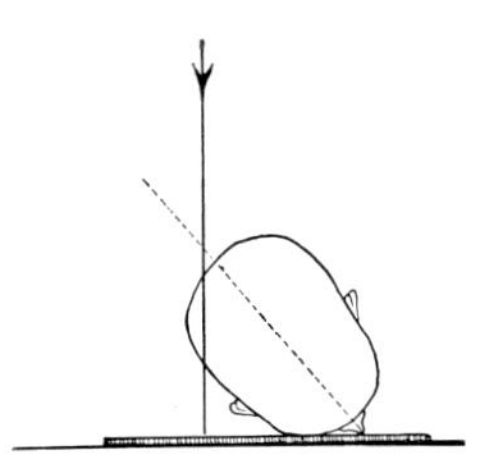

Interpretation

Fortunately for us practitioners at least 75 and probably 85 per cent of the minor fractures we see involve the vault without extending to structures in the base of either of the three fossae. Fractures of the vault occur approximately 25 per cent in the anterior third, 25 per cent in the posterior third, and 50 per cent in the middle third.

In examining films the only problem that exists is the linear skull fracture. Stellate fractures, depressed fractures, and various other forms are so apparent that there can be no question as to their identification. The linear fracture, on the other hand, may look exactly like a vascular or diploic channel or may so closely approximate a suture line that it is difficult to tell the difference. Certain findings are characteristic.

The fracture tends to change direction by sharp angles, while vascular and suture markings usually show broad curves. Such is perhaps the most important single characteristic of fracture.

As an example, this is a vascular marking:

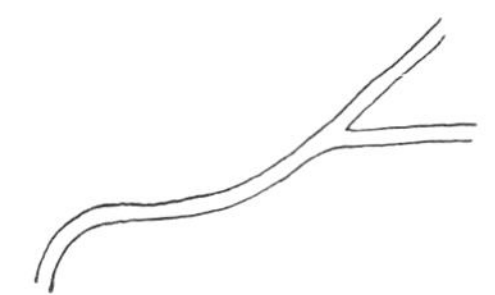

and this is a fracture:

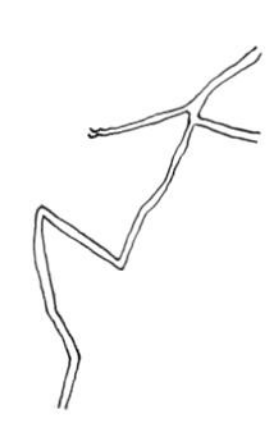

The edges of a fracture are clear-cut and sharply defined. This usually prevents confusion with diploic channels which are fuzzy and beaded. This is a diploic channel:

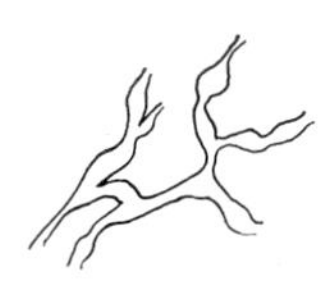

and this is a fracture:

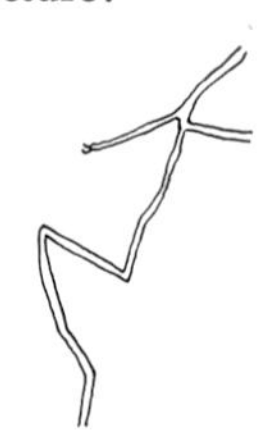

A fracture may show differing courses in the inner and outer table, like this:

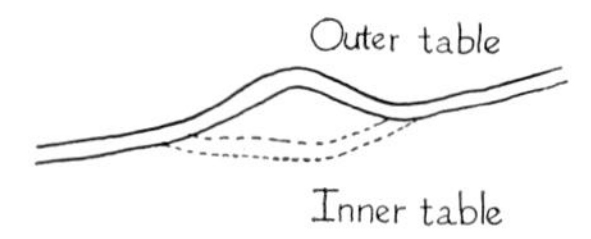

If after careful examination, using the anatomic knowledge at your command and the information regarding the characteristics of the fractures herein delineated, you still cannot be sure whether or not a small linear skull fracture exists, the matter is probably an insignificant one. Some of these fractures puzzle even the most expert radiologists, and when clinical signs are nil or nearly so and x-ray signs inconclusive, the interpretation is probably of more academic importance than clinical importance.

Errors

We previously mentioned some of the common findings that may be confused with fracture of the skull. There are two or three other points of confusion that should be kept in mind by the practitioner.

Instead of the bone actually breaking, sutures may be jerked apart, as shown here:

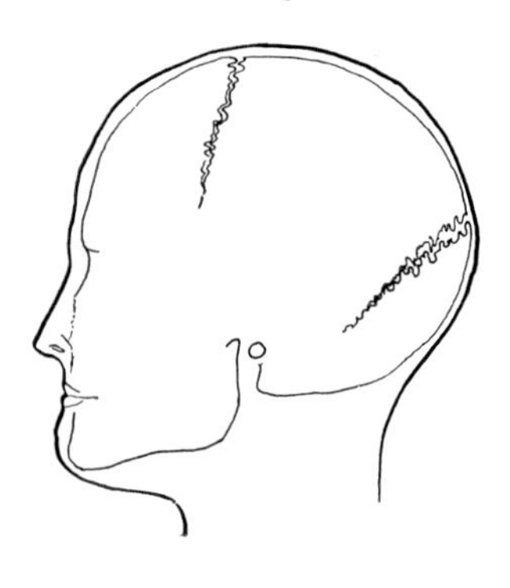

When this happens it becomes a matter of judgment. Occasionally some information may be gained by comparing the two suture lines on opposite sides. A slight difference in width can and does occur normally, but differences of more than 2 or 3 mm. probably represent the result of trauma.

The most common error is to assume that a negative x-ray film proves the absence of fracture. Since many minor and a few major skull fractures go undetected even though x-ray films have been taken and examined by competent men, one should never make the assumption. The care of a head injury should and must be determined by the clinical findings and not upon the basis of roentgenographs. X-rays can and do help but are not the final arbiter.

For example, it is possible that there is a tear in the meningeal artery although there are no findings of a fracture in the area, and it is equally possible that a fracture line crosses the meningeal channel without disrupting the continuity of the artery and its accompanying veins. If a fracture line seems to cross the channel, one is then, of course, suspicious that the vessels may have been torn, but the determination is made clinically, not on the basis of x-ray findings.

A fracture into a sinus is a potentially serious injury since the dura may remain open. On the other hand, a significant number of these heal without clinical aftermath. Such an injury, incidentally, is a matter for the most carefully reasoned and expert clinical judgment. Even though the injury may appear trivial, the opinion of a trained neurosurgeon is valuable in such a case.

INCREASED INTRACRANIAL PRESSURE

The pathologic entities that may cause increased intracranial pressure are legion. Tumors of all kinds, obstructions to the outflow of the cerebral spinal fluid, vascular insults, scarring resulting from direct trauma or infection, and numerous other conditions may be responsible.

Detailed diagnostic aid may be given by an adequate roentgen-ray survey, but the average practitioner has no part in this. Beyond knowing and being able to demonstrate on a proper film the signs of increased intracranial pressure, the physician has no responsibility. To attempt further diagnostic procedures is to court disaster. Like all the rules, however, this may not apply in isolated areas where the services of a trained roentgenologist are not available, but it is certainly true in most localities in the United States.

The important structure to examine in checking for increased intracranial pressure is the sella turcica. The normal sella turcica looks like this:

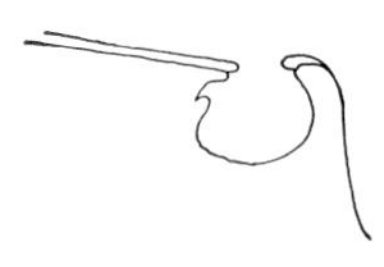

There are two variations that rarely occur in the normal structure but which should be appreciated when present. Occasionally the petro-clinoid ligaments will become calcified, even in young persons, and present a shadow like this:

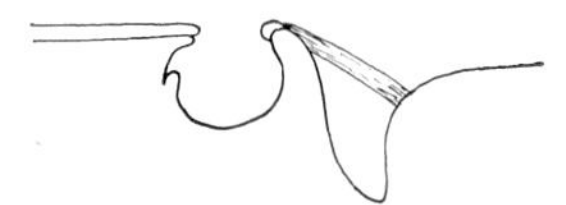

It does not represent abnormality. Occasionally there will be some calcification between the anterior and posterior clinoid processes so that the sella turcica is said to be bridged. The clinoid processes look like this:

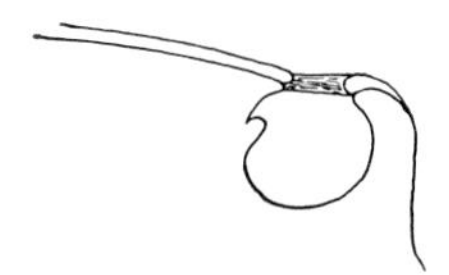

These normal variations are not often seen.

One should realize that it takes a prolonged increase in the intracranial pressure to make changes in the sella turcica or in other structures appreciable roentgenographically. Sudden, acute rises in intracranial pressure are not diagnosable by routine x-ray procedures. After three to six months changes become apparent and diagnostic.

Technique

The straight lateral film taken like this:

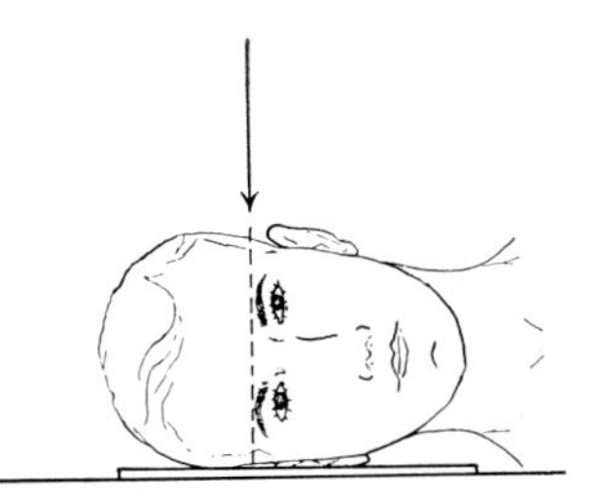

is entirely adequate for demonstration of sellar changes.

Interpretation

Persistent increase in intracranial pressure causes thinning and ultimate destruction of the posterior clinoid processes. This is a normal sella turcica:

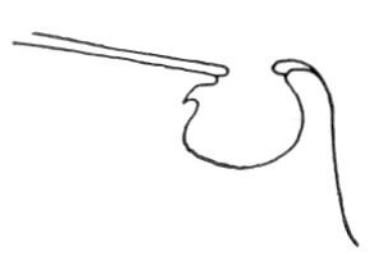

This is one with thinning of the posterior clinoid process:

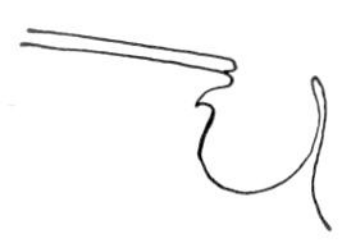

and this is one with destruction of the posterior clinoid processes and a portion of the dorsum sella:

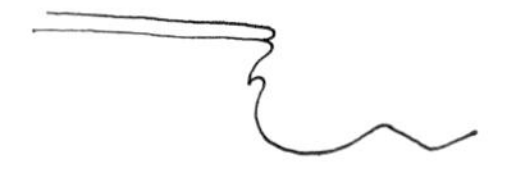

Along with this process the sella turcica may enlarge and become somewhat flattened, although this is by no means always the case. The important point for observation is the destruction of the posterior clinoid processes.

After long-continued, heightened intracranial pressure, the convolutions of the brain may mark the inner table of the skull so that it has the typical "beaten-silver" appearance. Changes in the clinoid processes, however, usually antedate this and it becomes more of academic interest than of diagnostic value.

If there are asymmetrical changes in the sella turcica or if the anterior processes are involved, it is best to submit the film to an expert radiologist for interpretation.

Errors

Minute changes in the posterior clinoid process may occur in normal persons; therefore, do not attempt to read too much into one of these films. Obvious changes in the clinoid processes are usually accompanied by equally obvious signs, and the x-ray film simply tends to confirm an impression already held from clinical examination. If the clinical findings are distinctly at variance with the x-ray film, carefully recheck the clinical signs. If there is still variance, submit the film to a roentgenologist.

Discussion

The x-ray is a valuable adjunct but not a substitute for clinical acumen. Those who are familiar with this examination usually tend to overuse it and it is sometimes employed to replace careful clinical evaluation.

OSTEOMYELITIS

Infections of the skull are not common. In the average practice one sees such a case perhaps once every two or three years.

Local lesions of the scalp rarely spread to involve the bone beneath. Occasionally there is extension from an acutely infected sinus and occasionally the disease is of hematogenous origin.

Clinical symptoms are usually those of an acute inflammatory process, and the local findings are exactly those which would be expected in such a case.

Technique

Straight lateral projections and a projection through the skull, with the involved area nearest the film, are usually all that are needed.

Repeated examinations are both confirmatory from a diagnostic standpoint and an excellent guide to treatment.

Interpretation

As with osteomyelitis elsewhere, during the acute stage of the infection there are usually few if any visible changes to be seen in the x-ray films. Obvious diagnostic findings seldom appear until ten to twenty days after the onset of symptoms.

The first finding is one patch or several patches of obvious thinning, the edges being fuzzy and indistinct, and the thinned-out areas of a heterogeneous density, like this:

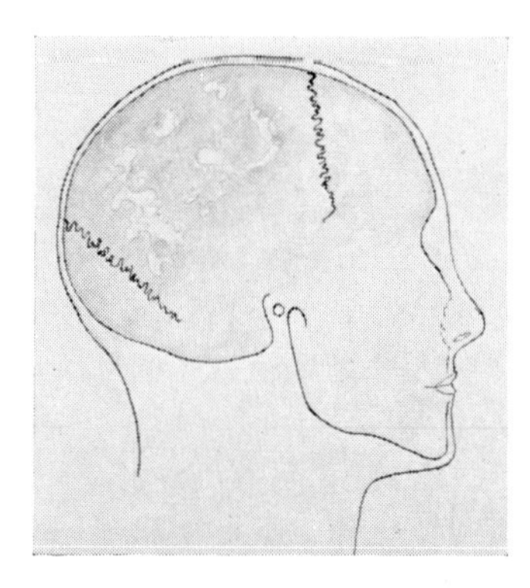

As the disease progresses there may be spread, with increasing bone destruction in the original areas. An important diagnostic point is that osteomyelitis destroys the fine trabeculations of the bone but does not quickly destroy the coarser, bony septa. A tumor, on the other hand, destroys everything within its path without regard to size. Examination of the film with a hand lens will best show this.

With further progression sequestra may form. Increasingly dense spicules are shown at the edge of the destroyed areas. This thickening and sclerosis serves in the x-ray film to "set off" the areas of destruction. It looks like this:

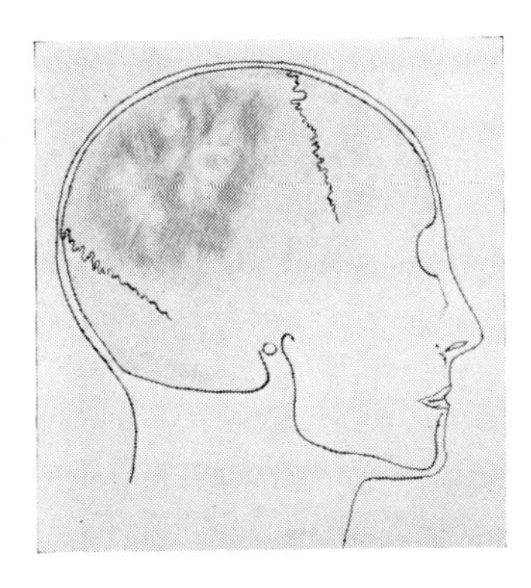

In the recovery period there is a gradual filling in of some destroyed areas with dense bone, but such areas seldom if ever assume an entirely normal appearance again.

When considering this disease one should read the more complete section on osteomyelitis on page 313.

Errors

The most frequent error is to take an x-ray film during the early changes in the process and, because it is negative, to assume that no infection is present. It cannot be repeated too often that from ten to twenty days are needed before any changes on the x-ray film become apparent. With our modern antibiotics many cases of osteomyelitis are cleared up completely before they become apparent by x-ray.

The second error is to confuse acute osteomyelitis of the skull with invasion by a malignant tumor. The obvious clinical presence of a pyogenic infection is some help in the differentiation and the typical radiologic features of osteomyelitis usually serve to make the differentiation without difficulty.

THE MASTOIDS

With modern antibiotics in such common use, mastoid disease is extremely rare and operation or the necessity of radiologic examination is practically unknown in practice.

However, within the past few years an interesting concept has come to our attention that may be of the utmost service to us in another disease. Diamant has stated categorically that the relative pneumatization of the mastoids is directly related to the presence of otitis media. In our limited experience his contention is entirely correct.

The infantile type of mastoid, with few air cells, is much less likely to support an acute otitis media and much more likely to support a chronic otitis media. The adult, or fully pneumatized, type practically never supports a chronic otitis media, although the acute disease is rather common. This finding actually has some prognostic value in practice. It is also of great value in judging the extent of treatment.

Technique

The degree of pneumatization in mastoids is best seen in the posteroanterior oblique projections which are taken like this:

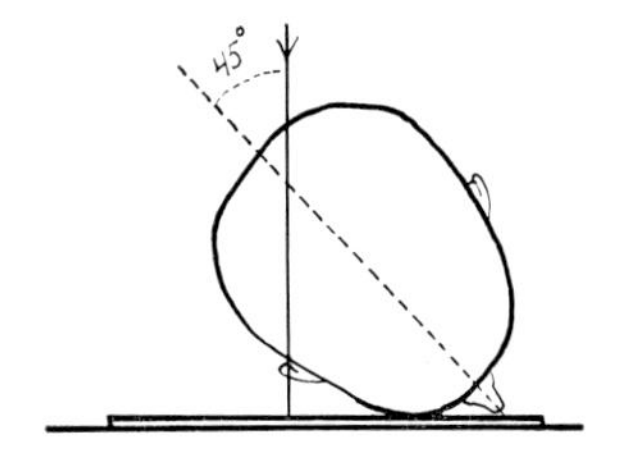

Interpretation

The infantile type of mastoid, poorly pneumatized, looks like this:

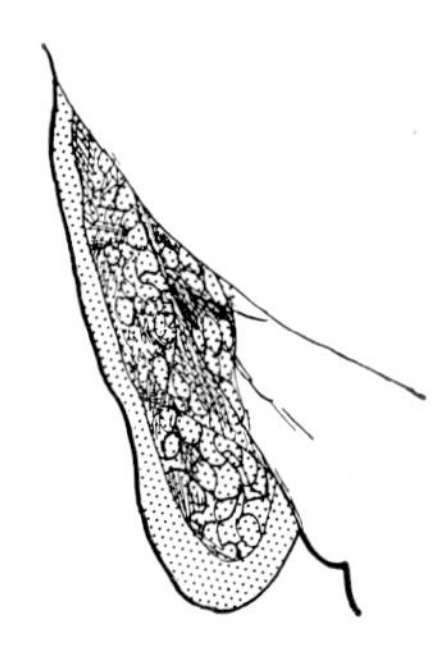

The adequate, fully aerated mastoid looks like this:

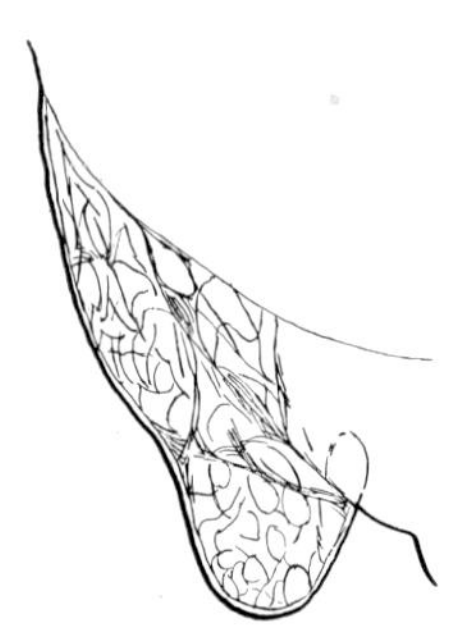

The infantile type is likely to support chronic infection, which is practically never seen in the adult type.

Errors

Errors in either technique or interpretation are rare, for the procedure is simple and interpretation clear-cut.

There are, of course, degrees of differences between the fully pneumatized and the infantile mastoid, but we have not seen a case in which we could not make at least a reasonable effort at classification. This is another case in which experienced judgment will outweigh mathematical analysis.

Discussion

Immediately upon reading this discussion of mastoids the question will arise that we have been talking about middle-ear infections and taking pictures of mastoids. Actually, they are, essentially, synonymous. The mastoid is connected directly to the middle ear, as you know, and probably no case of otitis media occurs without some involvement of mastoid cells. Why the poorly aerated mastoid should support chronic infection, whereas the well-aerated one does not, is still in the field of conjecture. The fact remains that this has been demonstrated conclusively to be the case.

CHAPTER TWENTY

The Sinuses

Radiography of the paranasal sinuses is a difficult task, but it can be done satisfactorily with average equipment if the physician will be meticulous in technique and cautious in interpretation. There are so many bony structures in the skull that cast shadows upon the film that positioning assumes paramount importance. A high degree of exactitude is necessary for every exposure.

Interpretation of film is beset with limitations, but if one recognizes these limitations and does not attempt to exceed them, there is every possibility of highly successful work.

Technique

In ordinary office practice there are three positions for sinus radiography: the Caldwell position and the Waters position in both recumbent and erect stance.

Technical factors will vary with the machine used; therefore, it is best to follow the instructions which accompany the machine rather than to try to list a general set of factors which will encompass all machines.

For the Caldwell position, place the cassette on top of the x-ray table, with the patient lying face down so that the nose and forehead touch the surface of the cassette. Then slant the x-ray tube from 15 to 20 degrees caudalward and extend the cone until it touches or nearly touches the patient's head. This is the proper positioning for the projection:

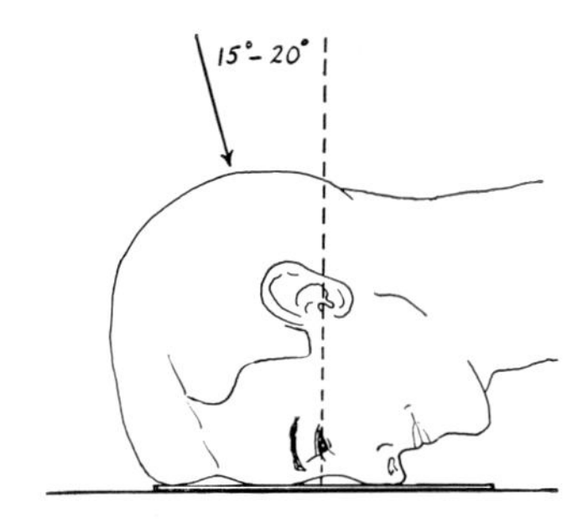

The resultant x-ray will give relatively clear delineation of the ethmoid sinuses, a clear picture of the frontal sinuses, but the petrous ridges may obscure the maxillary sinuses. A typical x-ray film shows these essential points:

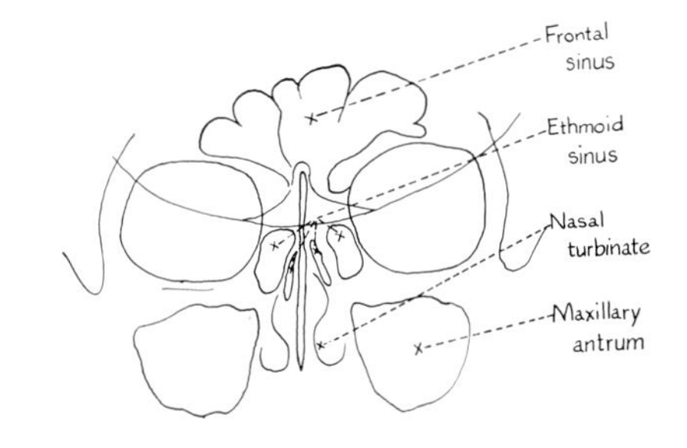

For the Waters projection, place the patient in the prone position so that the chin touches the cassette and the nose is 2 to 3

cm. above it. The axis of the x-rays is vertical, like this:

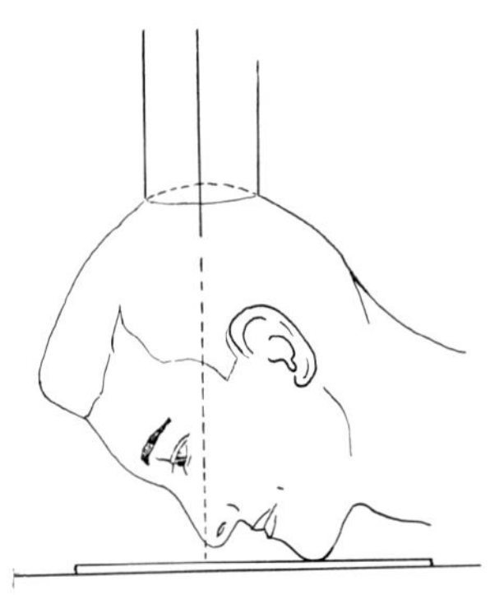

The mouth may be opened widely, which will usually allow adequate visualization of the sphenoidal sinuses. Frontal and ethmoid sinuses are inadequately visualized but the maxillary antra are clearly shown.

If there is a question of fluid in the maxillary sinuses, repeat the position with the patient erect and the axis of the x-rays horizontal. A fluid level will be shown in this picture when it cannot be seen in the film taken with the patient reclining. The proper position for a standing Waters projection is this:

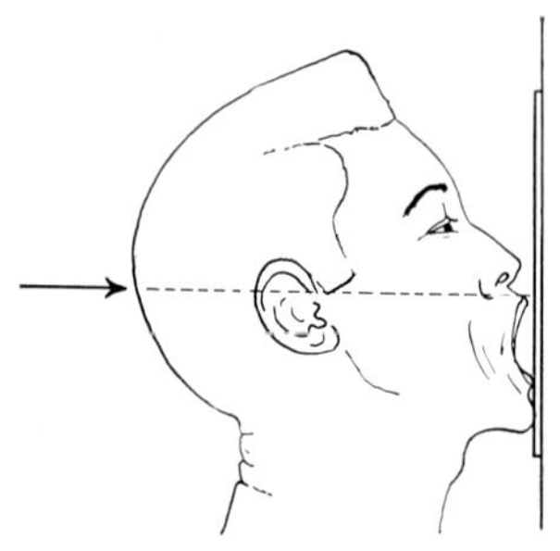

If the film is to be satisfactory, the technician must be particularly alert in seeing that the position is exact. It is most important that there be no rotatory movement of the head. The principal beam of the x-ray must go through the sagittal plane without any rotation around the center axis of the body. If rotation occurs, a portion of the sinus wall may be obscured, and many factors in interpretation concern these walls.

Technical factors having to do with penetration of the rays and printing of the pictures must be precise if one is to achieve films that can be used to obtain maximum information. The lining membranes must be clearly delineated and this sometimes means a "softer" beam.

Interpretation

The normal sinuses vary greatly in size and shape and may vary from one side to the other. The bony margins are sharp and clear-cut, with bone of normal density, as compared with other bony projections in the immediate area. Unless these bony margins are paper thin and consist largely of two opposing surfaces of cortical bone, evidence of a typical medullary structure between the cortices may be seen.

The mucous membrane in a normal sinus can seldom be seen. Rarely the normal mucosa may be appreciable as a line of 1 mm. thickness or less outlining the bony cavity. This is the exception rather than the rule.

Normally bony details of other portions of the skull that are projected through the sinuses show sharp delineation with clear-cut edges and occasionally with noticeable medullary structure. This visualization of other structures projected through the sinuses is one of the most important parts of radiologic diagnosis. One should observe normal films until certain of the usual appearance of these structures.

The relative opacity of the sinuses depends upon the thickness of their bony walls which may vary within wide limits, both between individuals and between contralateral sinuses.

Normally the maxillary antra are more transparent to the x-rays than the orbit and the frontal sinuses slightly less transparent than the orbit. This is a good fact to remember in basic interpretation of films.

Before examining the finished films for evidence of pathology, check them to see that proper projection of the questionable sinuses is present. Be sure to notice any rotation from the sagittal plane, having new films taken if rotation is present.

First, look at the structures projected through the sinuses and notice whether they are clear and sharply defined. This sketch shows an exaggerated idea of the difference between clearly projected structures and those which might be called "fuzzy":

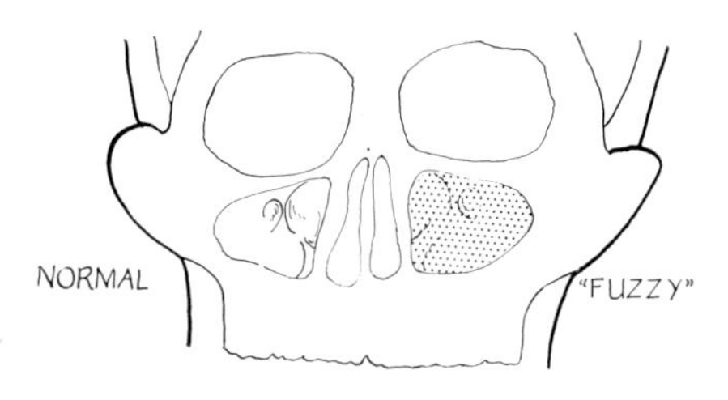

When this fuzziness occurs it is usually evidence of swollen mucous membrane or fluid in the sinus, which distorts the image of structures behind the sinus itself.

Next, examine the mucous membrane inside the bony borders of the sinuses. Notice any thickening which is present. If the membrane can be clearly delineated and is more than 1 mm. thick, you may assume that there is *or has been* some pathology. Notice the contour of the membrane and whether it parallels the sinus wall or bulges into the sinus cavity. Make a note of the relative thickness of the membrane as compared with the more transparent central area in the sinus.

Finally, examine the bony walls of the sinus and notice whether they are sharp and clearly defined, with structures clearly apparent, or whether they show extraordinarily heavy deposits of calcium in the cortices or possible lightening of the bony outlines of the structure.

Should there be what seems to be a fluid level in the maxillary sinuses, have the patient return to the x-ray room and tilt his head approximately 15 degrees off the vertical. Have the patient hold this position for at least three minutes and then x-ray in the Waters position modified by the continuing tilt of the head. If there is truly a fluid level, its surface will remain horizontal. Now re-examine the film of the Waters projection taken with the patient lying face down. The fluid level should not have been apparent in this picture.

In acute infectious sinusitis, the principal change noted is that the involved sinus becomes more opaque than normal and the structures projected through it are not clearly outlined. The bony walls of the sinus are not affected unless there has been previous chronic sinusitis. This point is better determined historically than by radiologic technique.

In the earliest stages the mucous membrane is often not seen. As the infection progresses, particularly if there are strong bodily defenses, there may be a slight clearing near the center of the sinus and the membrane may be observed as a line paralleling the bony walls. It is usually 2 to 4 mm. thick, like this:

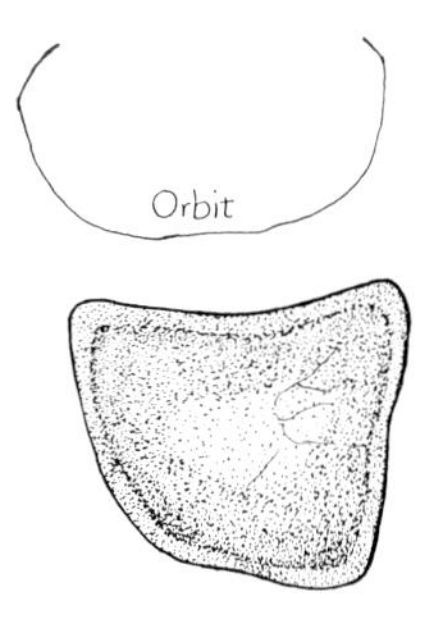

Should the infection become increasingly severe, the whole sinus may assume a homogeneous cloudy density, making it difficult to determine where the sinus ends and the bony wall begins. This can happen in a period of less than twenty-four hours, but more often it takes at least forty-eight hours. With our present methods of therapy this is not the usual course, and these findings are becoming increasingly rare.

In chronic disease there is usually obvious thickening of the mucous membrane, which parallels the sinus walls and may extend as much as 5 mm. into the cavity. Bony changes are frequent. The first and most rarely seen bony change is rarefication. This occurs following an acute infection that has changed recently to chronic disease. The bony walls are not sharply outlined and there are patches of lessened density alternating with normal bone, like this:

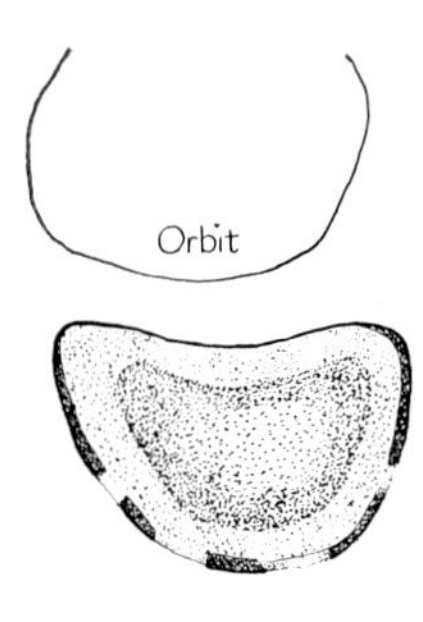

The more common changes seen in chronic sinusitis are thickening of the lining membrane and a sclerosing osteitis of the bony wall. The heavy deposit of calcium appears to outline the cavity with a dense wall. Such a picture gives no clue as to whether there is an existing infection or whether the infection may have occurred previously and is no longer active.

If the case be acute, allergic disease of the sinuses shows clouding, which is typical of that seen in infectious disease. It is seldom quite so intense. In such an acute case the history and a nasal smear are far more valuable in making the diagnosis than are roentgen studies. As the clouding starts to resolve one may begin to see the affected mucous membrane outlined against a translucent area in the center of the sinus. It is thickened and tends to bulge into the cavity of the sinus, exhibiting a convex surface like this:

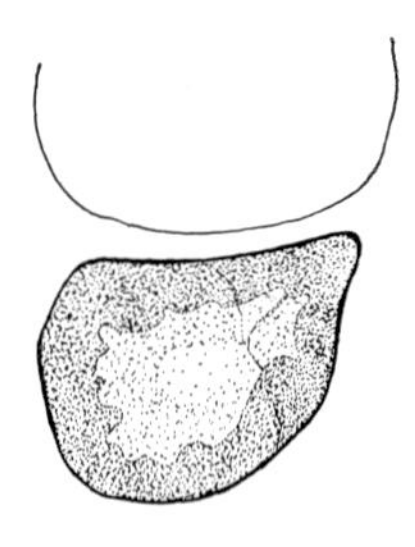

The bony changes of osteoporosis which has been followed over a period of months by sclerosis are not nearly so marked in allergic disease. They are persent, however, to some slight extent and may serve to confuse the picture.

Polyps are frequently seen in the sinuses, particularly in the frontal and maxillary cavities. They look like projections from the mucous membrane into the cavity but seldom have the typical tear-drop shape. To me they look like the shadow of a thumb protruding into the sinus. Occasionally they may show some narrowing of the base of the shadow, but this is not common. These shadows are seldom seen in the sinuses without accompanying intranasal changes indicating allergy. Intranasal polyps usually are found with sinus polyps. Clinical findings must be correlated with the x-ray findings if proper interpretation is to be made.

Errors

Errors in technique made when the films are taken have been previously discussed. They are relatively frequent but can be corrected by meticulous attention to detail. Errors in interpretation, on the other hand, are legion and the physician must guard against them to avoid an occasional inaccurate diagnosis.

The practitioner must remember that sinus radiology will give an indication of the processes going on, but this indication may be grossly inaccurate unless carefully correlated with clinical findings.

The patient should be examined thoroughly, using acceptable clinical techniques. A complete history should be taken and the findings of the physical examination correlated with this history before x-ray is employed. It is only in conjunction with a complete history and physical examination that the x-ray may be used to secure adequate information.

In the discussion on interpretation, I have perhaps indicated that one could be sure of the diagnosis, as between allergic and infectious disease, simply by examining films. This of course, is not true. It is true that there are many cases in which the differentiation can be made by glancing at the film. Unfortunately, though, in the majority of cases x-ray evidence is only contributory and then only to a minor degree.

A frequent source of error is to attempt to compare sinuses. Previous disease in one sinus, unequal development, chronic hypertrophy of the mucosa on one side, and even a foreign body may all enter to confuse the picture. Each sinus should be examined as a unit *without* comparison with the sinus on the opposite side.

As an example, one may look at films of the maxillary antra and notice a thickened mucous membrane on one side. Attention will be drawn to that side and careful examination will show changes in the bony walls which would be expected with chronic sinus disease. After a ten-minute examination we may decide that we are dealing with a chronic sinusitis of the right maxillary antrum. Unless we look closely at the *left* antrum the slight haziness of structures behind it will not be noticed. Comparison, if made will show the right antrum to have both bony and membranous changes not present on the left. Our diagnosis may be chronic disease of the right antrum, but the patient will have acute disease of the left antrum. Such mistakes are intolerable but are made frequently when one attempts to compare sinuses.

Another error that is all too frequent is to diagnose chronic disease when, actually, acute disease is present. An acute infection as an exacerbation of chronic disease may be undetectable by means of x-ray.

Interpretation of sinus disease in children is hazardous because of the extreme variations which children's sinuses show. If one x-rays a child for possible sinusitis the x-ray film should receive the most careful interpretation and painstaking correlation with the clinical findings.

Following are sketches of typical sinus disease with short expository paragraphs to describe the findings in each case:

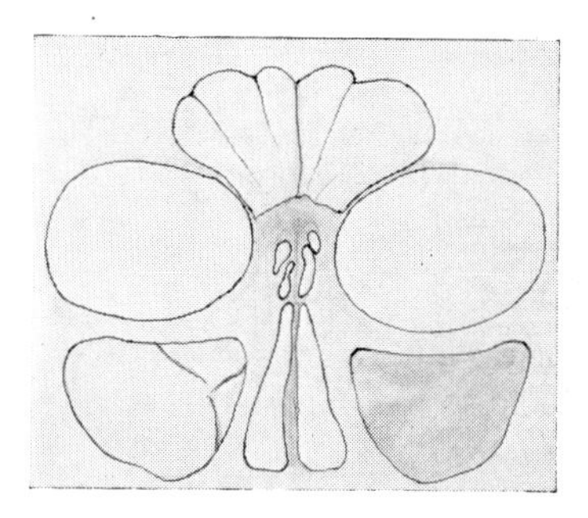

A case of acute suppuration of the left antrum. There is no involvement of the frontal or ethmoid sinuses or right antrum, nor are there signs of previous sinus disease.

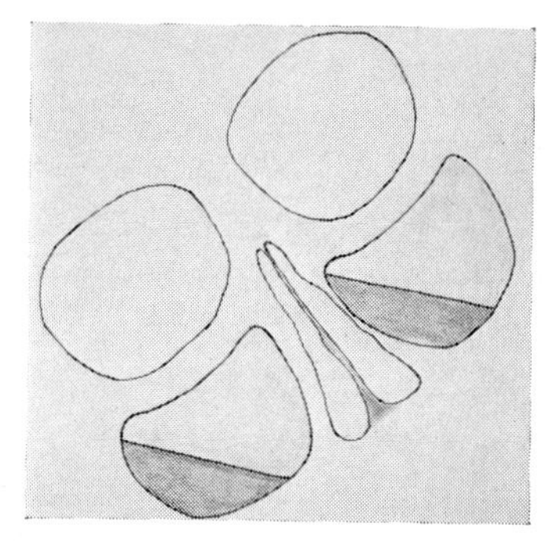

An empyema of the maxillary sinuses. There is no involvement of the bony walls, which would indicate that the infection is of relatively recent origin. Even so, empyema does not occur in a day or two. The implication would be that this patient has not had chronic sinus trouble but has recently had an acute episode and future difficulty is likely.

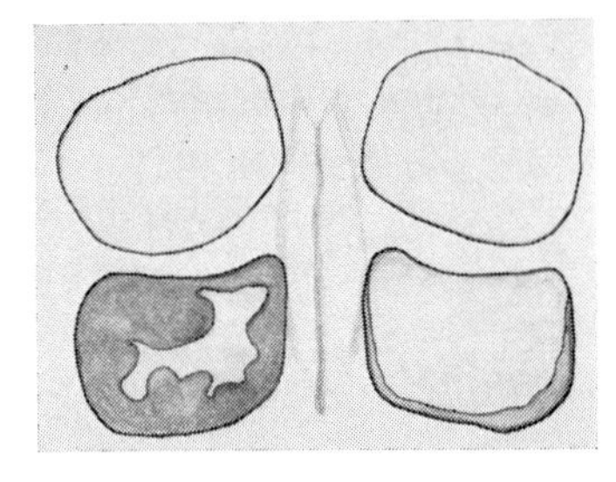

Allergic sinusitis involving the right antrum. Seldom do we see a "textbook" case like this, but it is well to know that they do occur. This was sketched from an actual film.

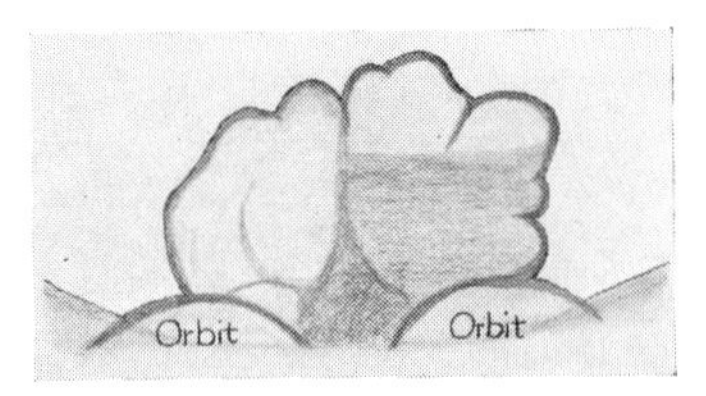

A fluid level in a frontal sinus. It has resulted from an acute episode superimposed upon chronic disease.

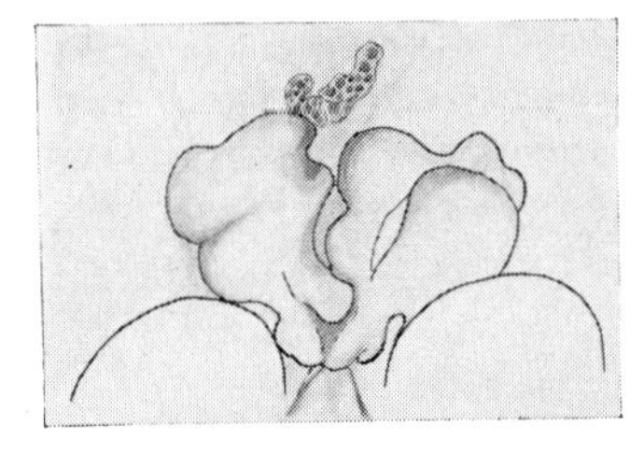

Sinusitis and osteomyelitis. Not as serious as it looks, but a disease with a great tendency to chronicity.

Discussion

Radiography of the paranasal sinuses is sometimes taken rather lightly by the practitioner. Just to "shoot a picture of the head" aerated is not a good means of detecting sinus disease. I would recommend careful x-ray technique and ultraconservative interpretative procedures until the physician becomes well experienced.

A recommended method is to send all films to a qualified radiologist for check interpretation until one is sure of one's own ability to read them properly. There exists no reason why any practitioner who is willing to study and to be checked cannot do basic sinus radiology.

Perhaps the worst factor is the tendency to become overdependent upon radiographs. Sinus disease is still best diagnosed by accurate history taking and physical findings. The x-ray finds its principal usefulness in picking up evidence of chronic sinus disease. One must remember that findings typical of chronic disease do not mean that the chronic disease is active. Activity still must be determined by clinical means.

Hypertrophied lymphoid tissue in the posterior nasopharynx, when it becomes infected, is unquestionably the cause of much postnasal drainage. This is particularly true in the younger person for, there has not been the atrophy of lymphoid tissue which occurs with age.

There exists also a tendency to ascribe many headaches, which are purely of tension origin, to sinus difficulty. Here again the physician can be placed in a somewhat compromising position. A great many people have some slight roentgen evidence of chronic sinus involvement.

The practitioner who does not question and examine his patients carefully and who uses x-ray injudiciously and to excess may find himself diagnosing practically every tension headache he sees as chronic sinusitis because of trivial x-ray findings. This must be rigorously guarded against.

Unless there is relatively positive evidence of involvement of the paranasal sinuses upon routine history taking and physical examination, then it would seem wise to exclude the x-ray.

There are certain rare and complicated diseases of the sinuses, such as malignancies and mucoceles, which do not often lie within the diagnostic purview of the average practitioners. Without regard to how much experience the physician has had in examining sinus films, I would advise that any picture not falling within a known and indisputable pattern be sent immediately to a qualified radiologist for interpretation. Even such a referral leaves something to be desired, for accurate radiology depends upon consultation between the clinician and radiologist for final factual interpretation. It has been my practice, in a questionable case, to seek two-way consultation between the radiologist and otolaryngologist, requesting that they submit a report on the case only after having conferred together.

CHAPTER TWENTY-ONE

The Facial Bones

The facial bones are subject to all the diseases of the bone which will be mentioned later. Here, we are mainly interested in the common techniques for demonstration of traumatic injury. Since these techniques are somewhat specialized, they are given separate consideration. First of all, we will consider the radiologic positioning involved, and, second, discuss briefly some points about demonstrating the injury on the finished film.

As is so often the case, an adequate history and a searching examination may be more accurate than x-ray in pinpointing the injury. It is a distinct mistake—and one often committed—to x-ray before adequate history and examination are completed.

THE MANDIBLE

The common sites for fractures of the mandible are these:

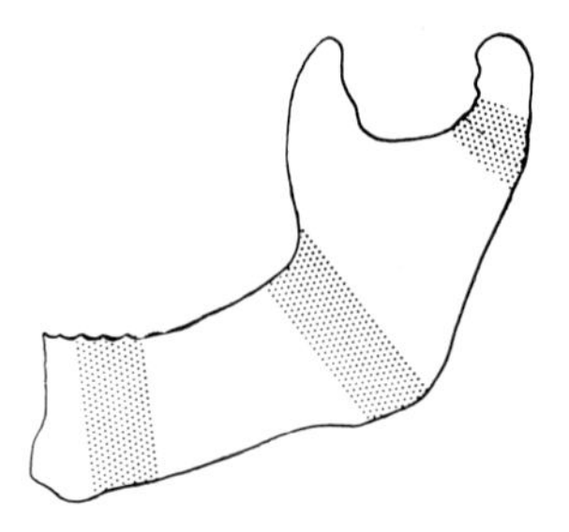

In about 60 per cent of cases there are two fractures rather than one.

The most difficult injury to demonstrate is fracture at the neck of the condyle:

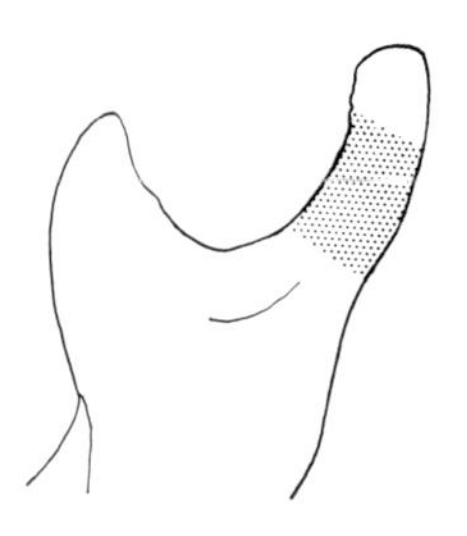

In injury to the mandible, take three views as follows:

A straight posteroanterior view in a position like this:

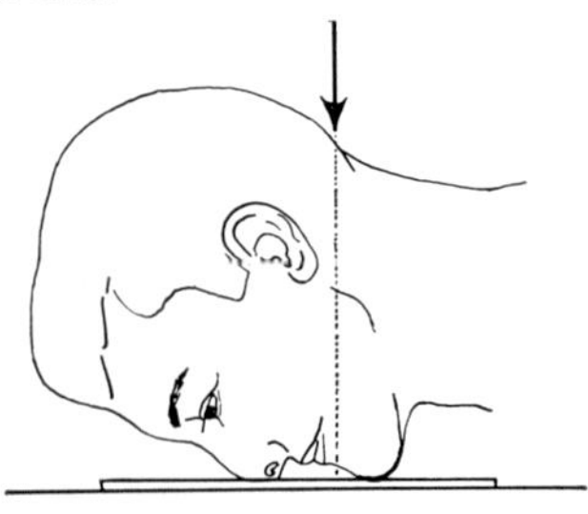

Two oblique views which should be positioned like this:

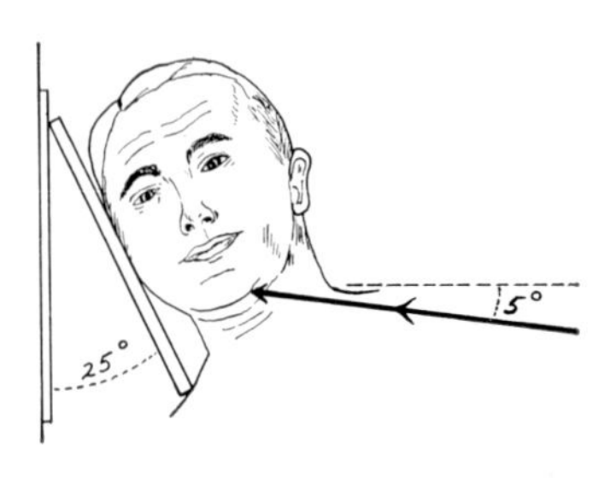

The important areas to be searched for in the films are these:

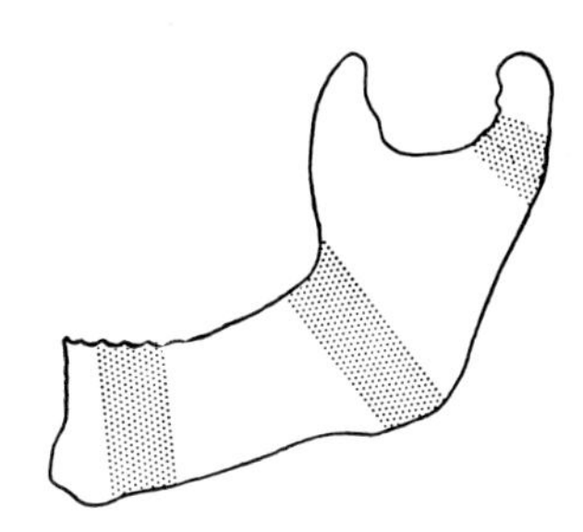

THE ZYGOMA

When one suspects fracture of the zygoma, an x-ray should be taken in the submento-vertical position like this:

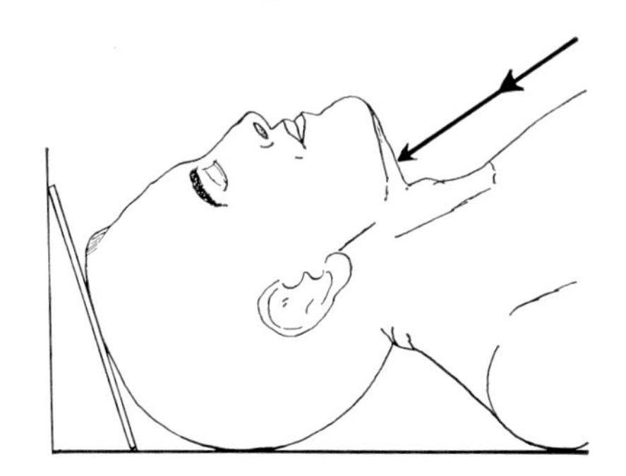

The resultant film will clearly delineate the zygomatic arches like this:

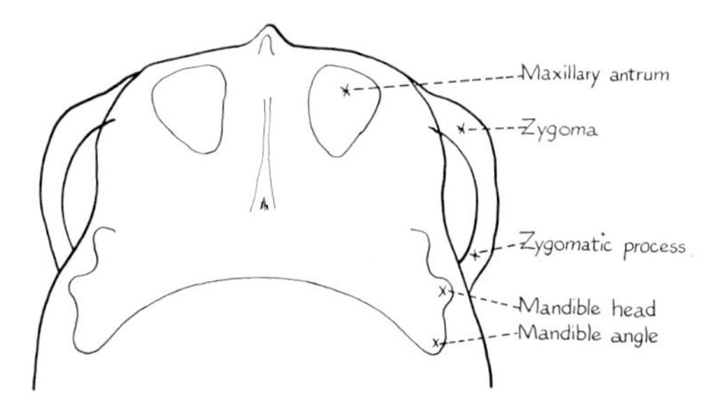

THE MAXILLA

Most maxillary fractures occur in the vicinity of the orbit and are well delineated on plain posteroanterior view. Rarely they may be difficult to see, but there is one small point that is an excellent tip-off in diagnosis. Look at the junction between the frontal and malar bones at the edge of the orbit:

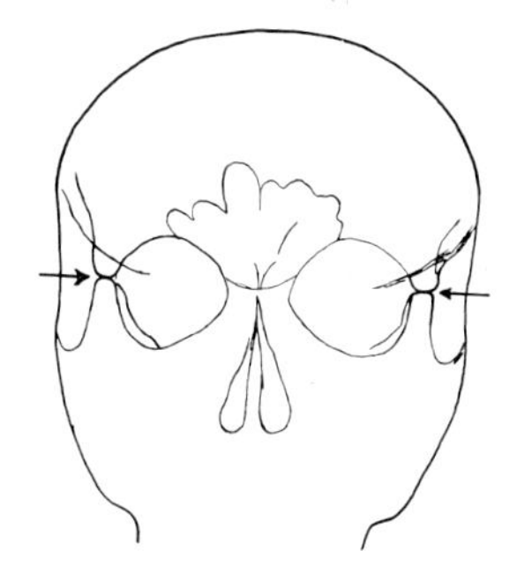

If this junction is pulled apart you may assume there is a fracture of the facial bones and proceed to delineate it more carefully.

THE NOSE

X-raying for fractures of the nose seems to me a senseless procedure. These fractures are easily diagnosed by clinical means.

Discussion

There is little to say about the problem of facial fractures. Careful utilization of standard x-ray techniques and an occasional bit of improvization will serve to demonstrate any of these fractures with entire adequacy.

CHAPTER TWENTY-TWO

The Ribs, and Cervical and Dorsal Spine

THE RIBS

We can dispose of the problem of ribs rather quickly.

Patients with severe fractures with displacement of fragments should be sent without delay to the hospital, where the x-ray films should be made. The rib fracture without displacement is a roentgenologist's terror because innumerable views may have to be taken in order to give an adequate demonstration of the fracture line.

In the case of simple rib fractures, since clinical methods for diagnosis are so accurate it seems unnecessary to x-ray, taking eight or ten plates to locate a fracture known to be present.

THE CERVICAL VERTEBRAE

Severe injuries of the cervical spine are not examined in the office x-ray department. The main interest centers around the minor injuries to which the cervical vertebrae are subject and toward demonstrating the arthritic changes which occasionally occur.

Severe fractures of the cervical vertebrae usually produce some injury to the cord and are accompanied by major neurologic changes. Compression fractures without cord damage are, however, relatively common and may often be demonstrated in the physician's x-ray department.

Surveys have shown that some 10 to 15 per cent of injuries to the spine involve the cervical vertebrae. Of these the great majority are compression fractures produced by sudden sharp flexion of the head and neck. Much more rare are fracture dislocations, with riding forward of one vertebral body upon the other, and possible damage to the articular facets.

These are sketches of a normal cervical vertebra from the anterior and the lateral aspects:

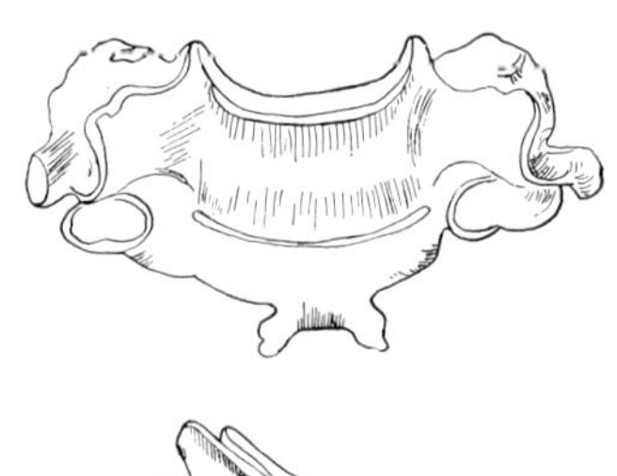

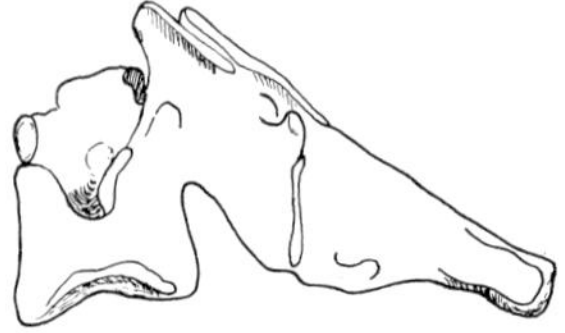

In the ordinary anteroposterior x-ray the vertebral bodies are clearly shown but the lateral bodies are obscured, like this:

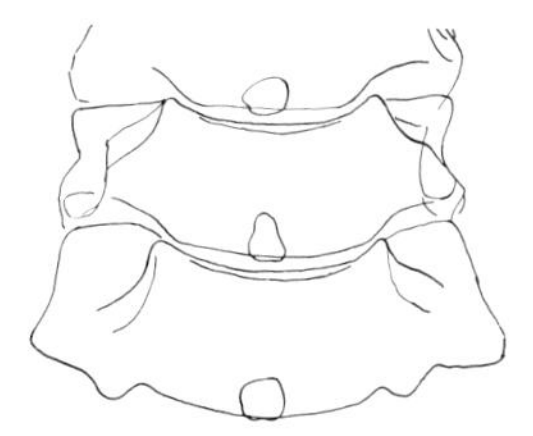

The lateral x-ray, on the other hand, not only shows the vertebral bodies themselves, but also delineates the articular processes with some clarity, like this:

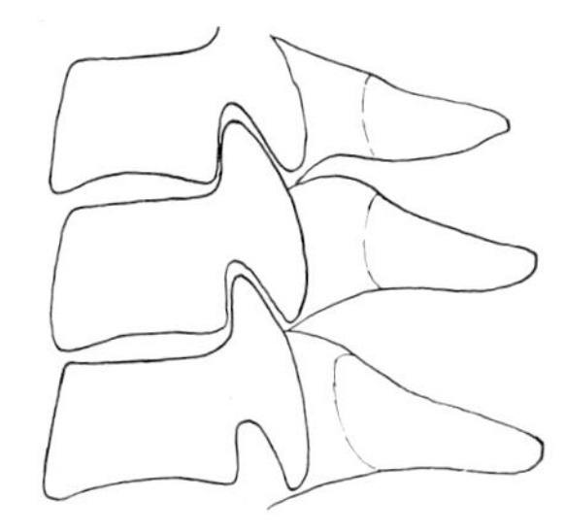

Osteoarthritis of the cervical spine is a common lesion in older persons. The process begins as a degeneration of a joint cartilage, with slight narrowing of the joint spaces. The cartilagenous damage seems most pronounced near the edges of the vertebral bodies in this area:

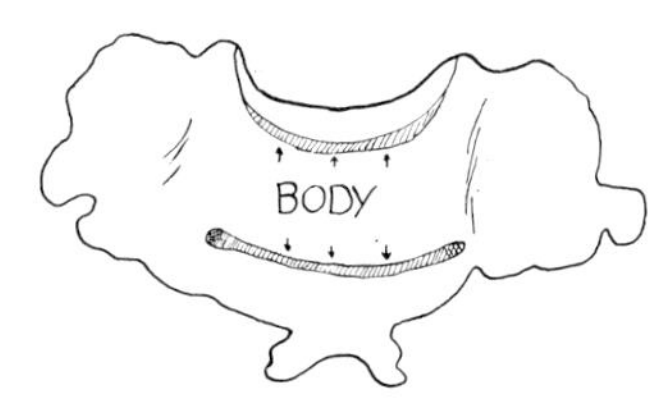

The cartilage is replaced with spicules of new bone which cause spurring. In areas where the cartilage is seriously worn there is great thickening and sclerosis of the bone itself. An affected vertebral body looks like this:

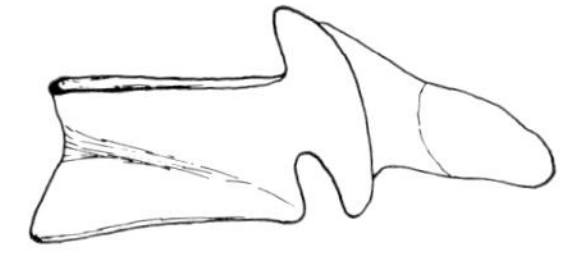

The normal cervical vertebrae are regular in character and aligned as shown in this sketch:

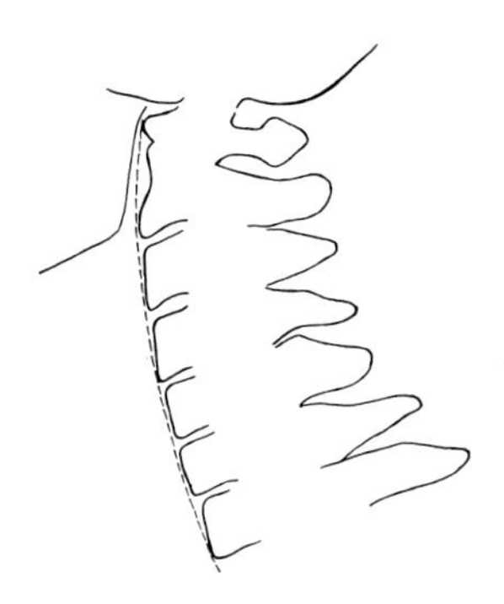

The outstanding exception and the major trap for the unwary is C_5 or C_6 which may appear somewhat narrowed anteriorly, like this:

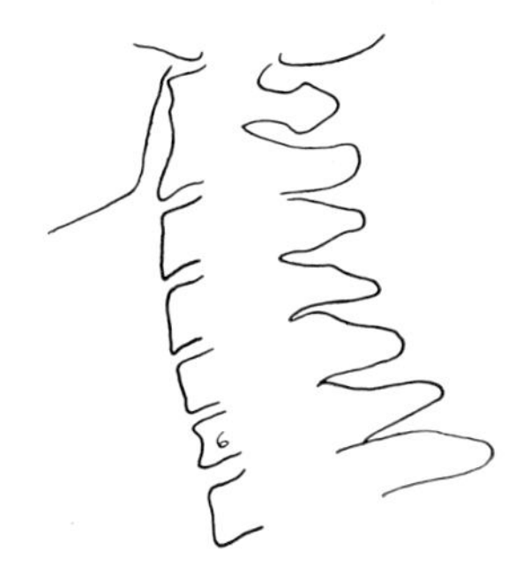

This is not abnormal.

In children all the cervical vertebrae may show this anterior narrowing, as seen in this typical lateral view of a cervical spine of a child:

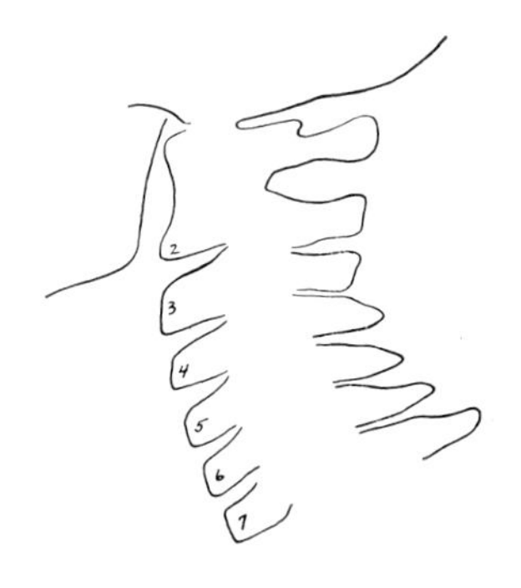

Technique

In ordinary cases two views are all that are necessary.

Take the anteroposterior view in this position:

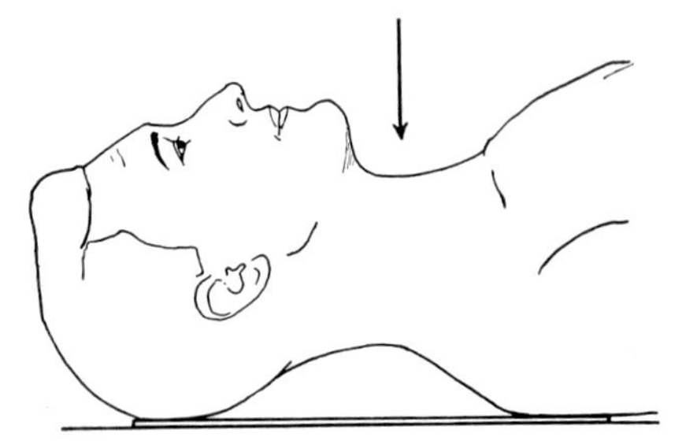

The resultant x-ray film will show the following important structures:

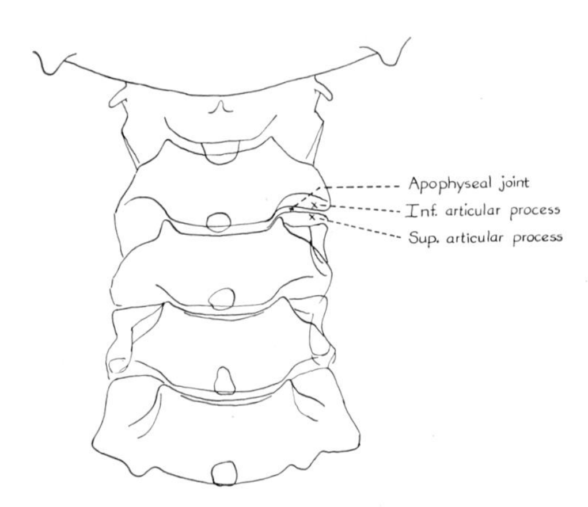

Notice that the auricular processes are not well delineated in this view.

Take the straight lateral view with a six-foot distance between target and film, which will give excellent detail and show clearly the articular and spinous processes. Have the patient grasp the edges of the stool on which he is sitting and bend over so that his shoulders are down as far as possible. Some sort of block should be placed between the patient's head and the casette to minimize head motion. Balsa wood, which can be purchased at any model airplane shop, is good material for this.

The resultant x-ray film will look like this:

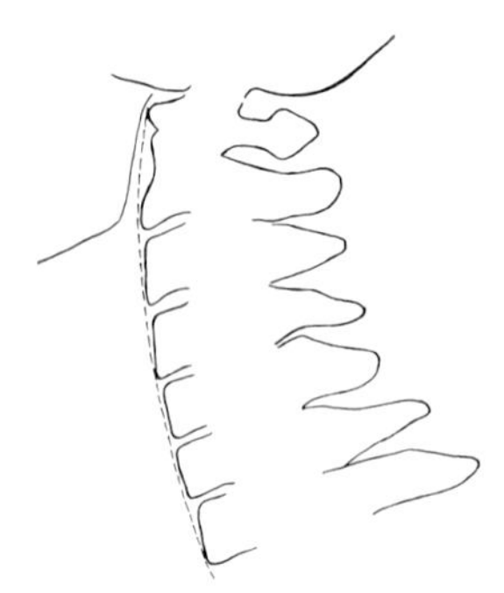

Interpretation

Most fractures of sufficient mildness to be seen in the office practice of medicine are minor compression fractures which look like this:

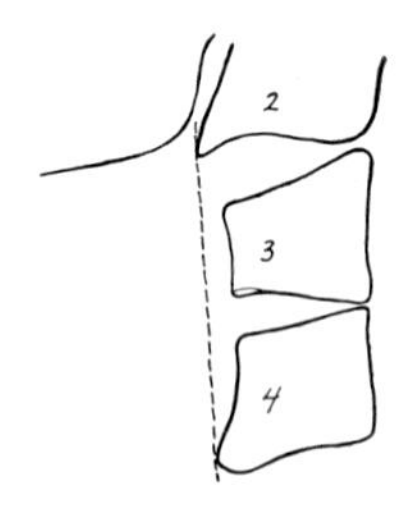

There is no difficulty in locating these fractures unless one forgets the normal foreshortening of the anterior portion of C_5. Occasionally C_6 partakes slightly in this normal change.

A line drawn along the anterior surfaces of a vertebra should flow in a smooth curve without any vertebrae being more than 1/8 inch out of line with the curve. In checking the alignment of the vertebrae with the skull, Chamberlain's line is valuable. It is a straight line drawn from the hard palate to the lowest part of the inner table of the occipital bone and ordinarily it will fall just above the odontoid process. If the odontoid process falls above the line, one should think of crushing or basilar impression.

Next draw a curved line connecting the anterior margins of the spinous processes as here:

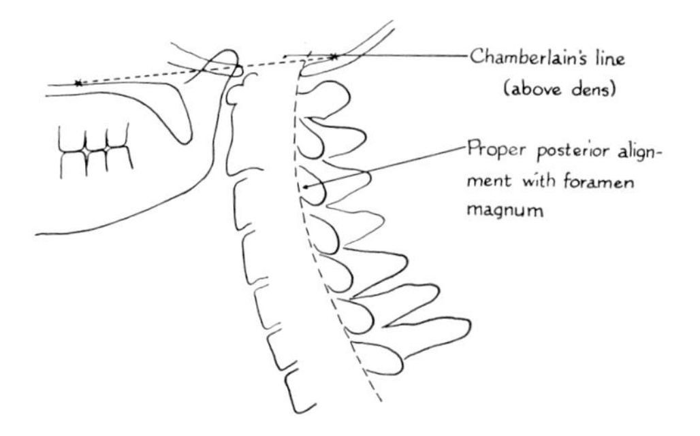

Notice in the normal film that it forms a curve which meets the posterior margin of the foramen magnum.

The changes noted in arthritis have already been mentioned, but one interpretative problem constantly appears. These changes are seen sufficiently often in old people without symptoms—at least with no more than moderate annoyance—that one must be extremely careful before implicating them as a cause of discomfort.

One of the most frequent pathologies that we practitioners see is the aching of neck muscles due to prolonged tension. The fact that the cervical vertebrae show changes typical of arthritis does not mean a thing so far as causation of symptoms is concerned.

Here is a sketch from an x-ray film of a typical case:

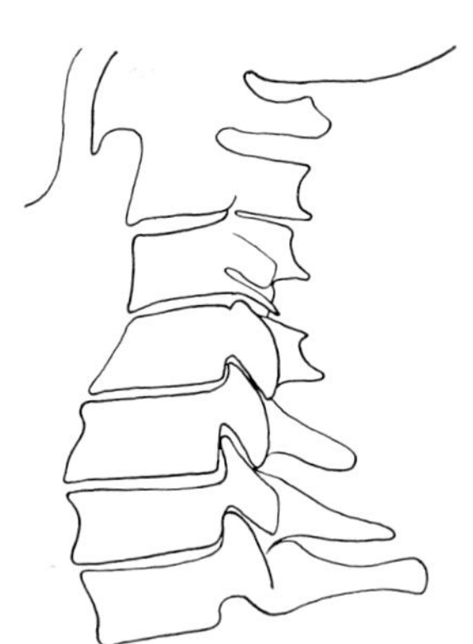

Careful clinical evaluation brought out the fact that this woman had typical headaches and that the aching soreness in her neck, which progressed even far enough to limit motion, was almost invariably associated with a tension headache or occurred immediately following one. She was not informed of the changes in her cervical spine and steps were taken to relieve her headaches. When this was accomplished, no further symptoms were present during the two and one half years we continued our follow-up study.

Errors

Errors in roentgenographic technique are not common. The procedure is so simple that there is no reason for poor films.

If careful clinical examination, as well as x-ray, is done, few fractures will be missed. As a matter of fact, the tendency, lies just the other way. We all have seen cases where the old C_5 trap either caught us or came close to doing so. If a fracture is suspected a most meticulous examination of the supposedly involved vertebrae should be made, using a hand lens to delineate, so far as possible, the bony trabeculae and to look for evidence of crushing. Usually a careful check will result in an accurate diagnosis.

Errors in interpretation of arthritic changes have already been discussed. The changes themselves are usually self-apparent and are not questionable.

When there is question about this point, oblique views of the neck should be taken as shown in this cross section:

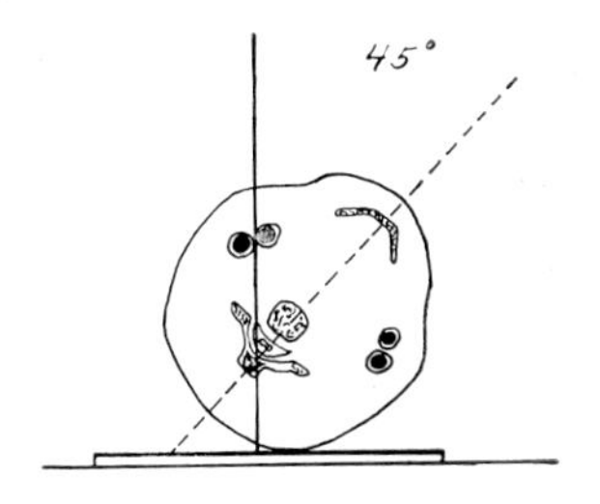

and sent to the nearest roentgenologist for detailed interpretation.

THE THORACIC VERTEBRAE

The thoracic vertebrae are subject to a number of diseases of the bone, which will be discussed on page 311, and are not infrequently the subjects of traumatic injury. Here, our main discussion will center around the fractured vertebral body.

Normally each thoracic vertebra slightly exceeds in size in all dimensions the thoracic vertebra immediately above it. The bodies are slightly foreshortened anteriorly so that a line drawn along the anterior portion of the body is perhaps 1/16 inch shorter than a line drawn along the posterior surface of the body.

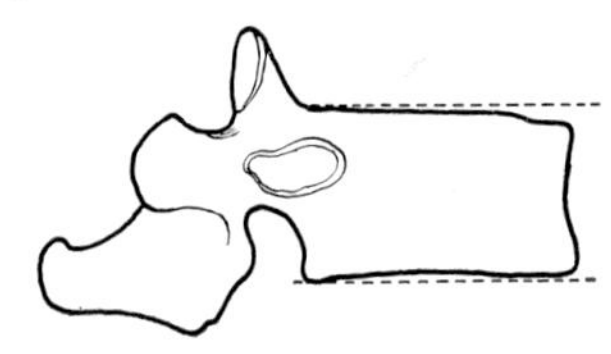

Technique

Take the anteroposterior view in this position:

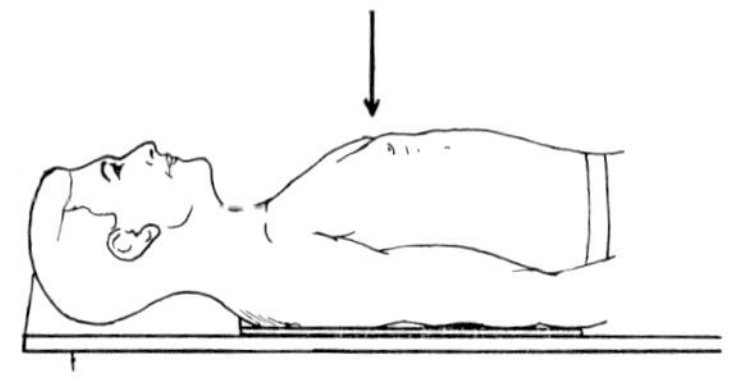

and the lateral view like this:

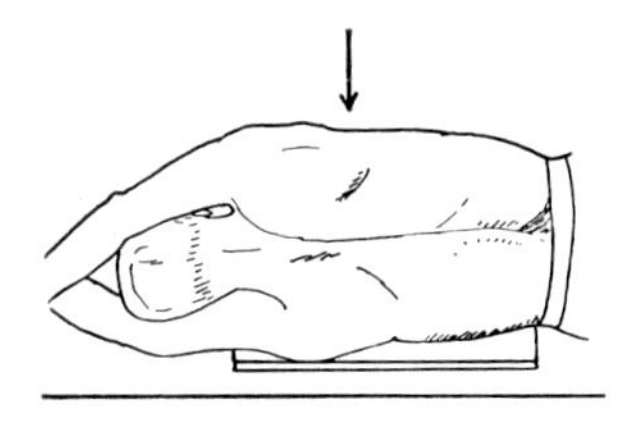

Interpretation

A typical fracture crushes the vertebra and causes resultant wedging like this:

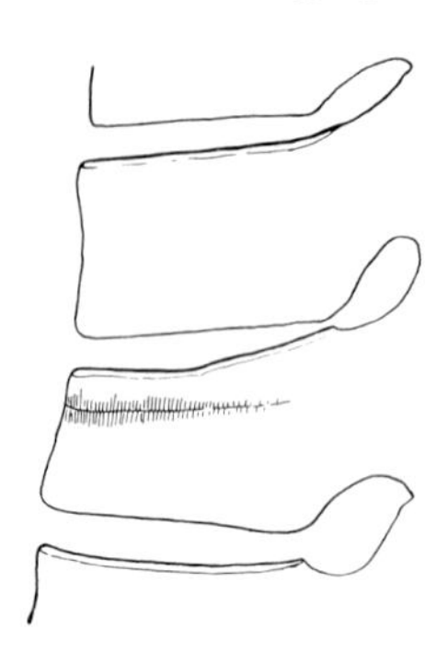

Sometimes it is important to distinguish between recent and old injuries. Surprisingly enough, some persons actually sustain a crush fracture of a vertebra and continue about their business, complaining bitterly of pain in the back but refusing to see a physician. Such persons may show up twenty years later, complaining of back pain and still showing roentgenologic signs of vertebral crushing.

A new fracture shows crushing and distortion of the internal architecture of the bone. As the fracture heals, the deformity may not be corrected but the internal architecture will become normal. Careful examination with the hand lens will serve to clarify this point.

Errors

Ordinarily there are no interpretative errors. The most common error is failure to x-ray. When a careful clinical examination indicates that pathology is not simple and clear-cut, an x-ray is always indicated. Incidentally, there are excellent clinical signs of a crush fracture to a vertebral body and I would suggest you consult a good textbook for this information.

CHAPTER TWENTY-THREE

The Lungs and Pleura

Radiography of the chest is one of the most important contributions of the office x-ray. Information of great value is furnished to the practitioner and he is also given an opportunity to make a complete fool of himself more often than in any other radiologic field except perhaps that of the gastrointestinal system.

Begin by realizing that the field is a highly technical one. If there is any question about interpreting a film it should be sent to a qualified roentgenologist along with a brief clinical history. It is wise for the physician just out of training to submit all chest films for check to a man qualified in x-ray interpretation. If this is done over a period of several years, the practitioner will certainly become an adequate interpreter of chest films.

Another good thing to do is to review in great detail both the gross and radiologic anatomy of the chest and its content. The material presented here is very much preliminary in nature. One of the standard anatomy books, such as Gray, Cunningham, or Morris, is the best for a thorough review. Meschan's *Normal Radiographic Anatomy** is good for reviewing radiologic appearance.

If you are like I am, you will find these things difficult to learn and easy to forget, even in daily use.

NORMAL ANATOMY

The normal interlobar fissures of the lung are located here:

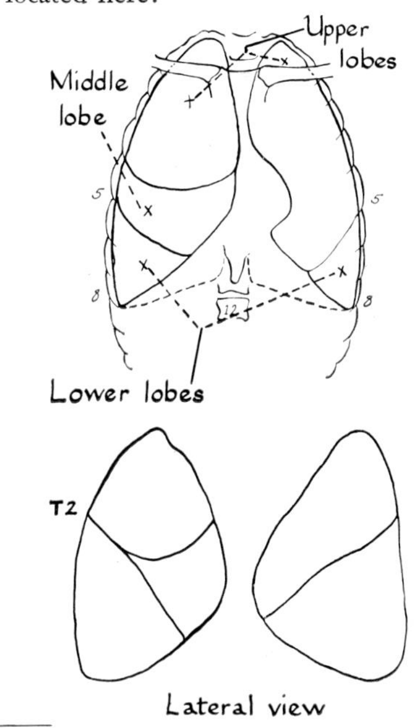

In this and some of the following chapters the illustrations have been made as diagrammatic as possible. I have often found it difficult after reading a description to look at an x-ray reproduction in a book and see what the author was trying to illustrate. To have seen a sketch first would have been a great help. I suggest you use the sketches in making a mental picture of the basic pattern and then translating the pattern to the x-ray appearance.

*W. B. Saunders Co.

but when projected on the standard posteroanterior chest film, they cover this area:

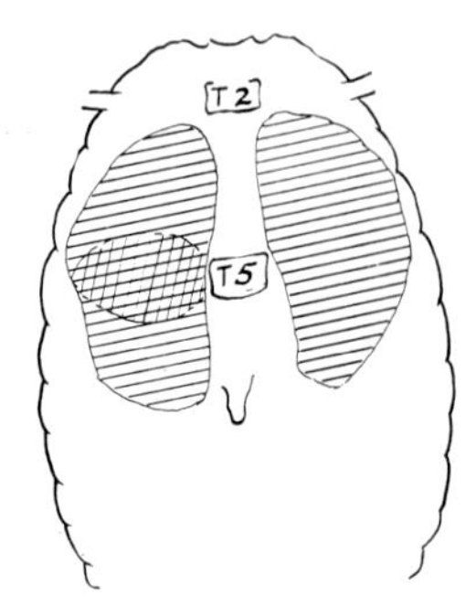

The functioning tissue of the lung itself is made up of a number of roughly pyramidal segments, with their apex pointing toward the bronchus of origin and the base toward the periphery of the lung.

The base of the pyramidal structure is often hexagonal or octagonal and may be from 3/8 to 3/4 inch across. Diagrammatically, such a segment looks like this:

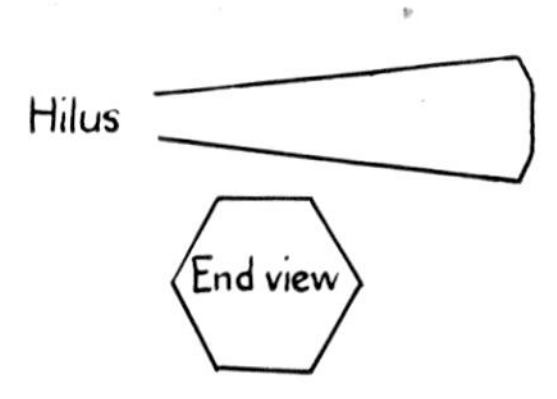

The trachea ordinarily extends downward in the midline, bifurcating at the level of the fourth thoracic vertebra in the infant and at the level of approximately the sixth vertebra in the adult.

The trachea of a young child may sometimes normally deviate to the right like this:

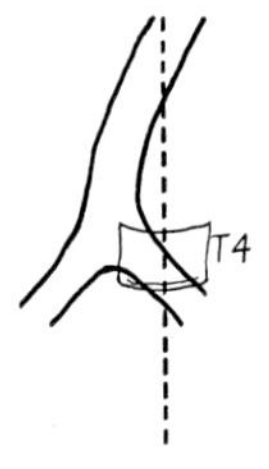

Such a deviation is a trap for the unwary.

Bronchial patterns down as far as the fourth or fifth division are well known but have little utility in office radiology. In the perfectly normal adult the visible branches of the bronchial tree are these:

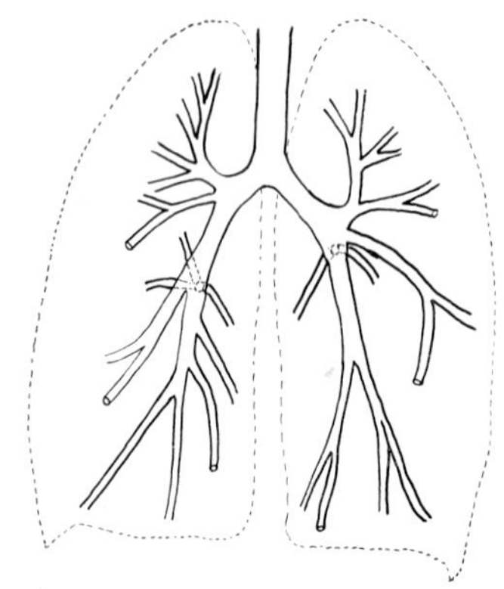

These hilar structures are seen:

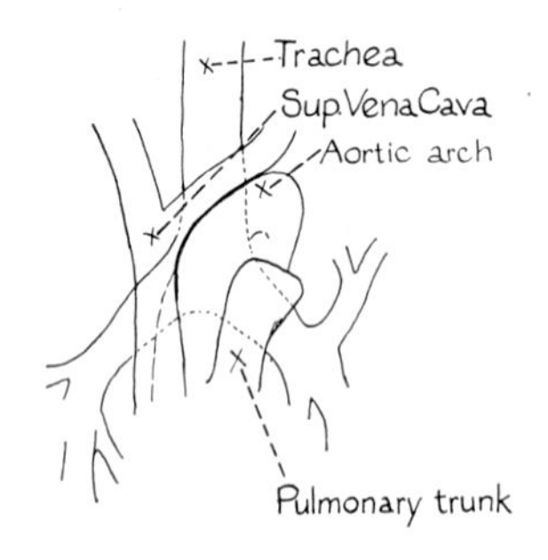

RADIOLOGIC TECHNIQUES

The standard posteroanterior chest film is far too well known to require comment here.

The straight lateral view is taken with the suspect side toward the cassette like this:

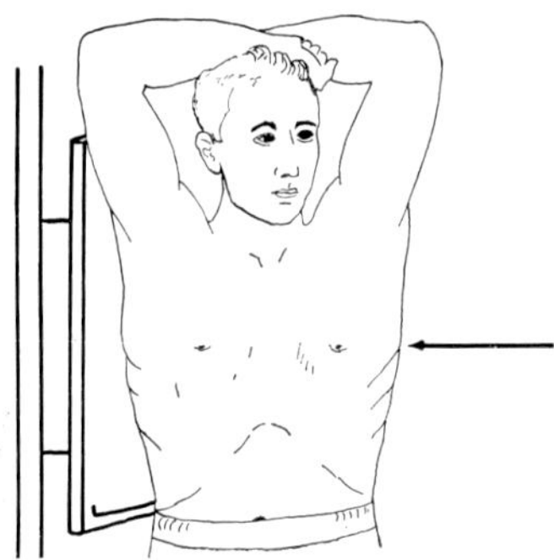

It is often of value. Here are the structures shown:

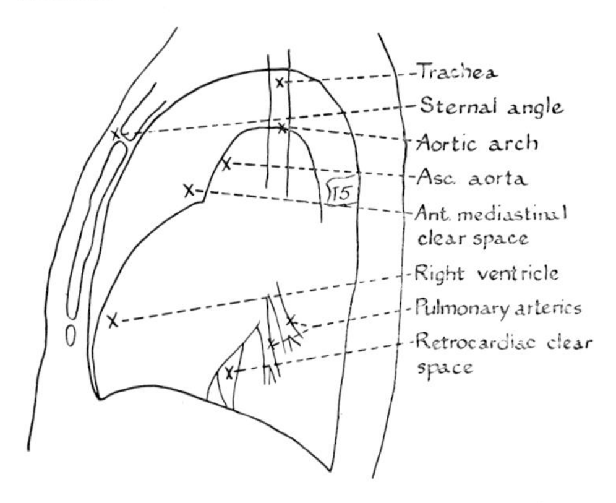

The common error is not to get the suspect side closest to the cassette.

The left and right oblique views are probably of more value in cardiology than in examination of the lung. They are occasionally indicated, however, and in those instances will be mentioned in the text. The technique for taking the views and the visible structures shown are illustrated on pages 259 and 260.

Occasionally when one suspects a lesion of the apices, the apical lordotic view is of value. The x-rays enter the center of the chest at this level:

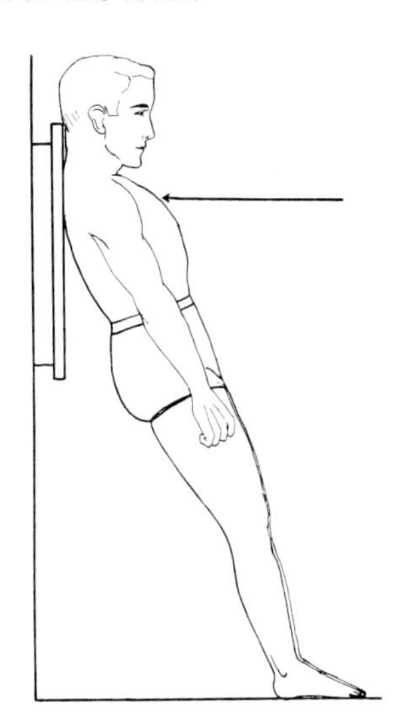

and these structures are delineated.

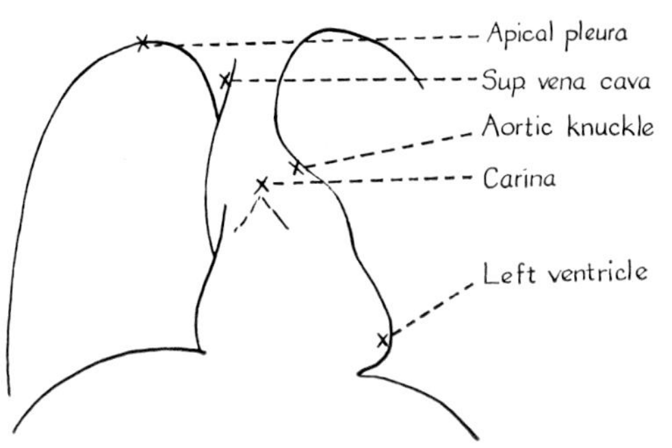

The instillation of iodized oil into the trachea is a simple procedure and may often be done in the office. Begin by anesthetizing the mucous membranes of the pharynx thoroughly, using a spray of 2 per cent pontocaine. Have the patient inhale each time you spray the solution into the throat so that some of it will be carried into the trachea and render the tracheal membrane at least partially anesthetized.

Now have the patient lean forward, letting him grasp his tongue with a surgical sponge, pulling it forward and downward as if trying to pull it out of the mouth. Use a specially designed catheter or a blunted spinal needle to drop iodized oil along the back of the tongue as shown here:

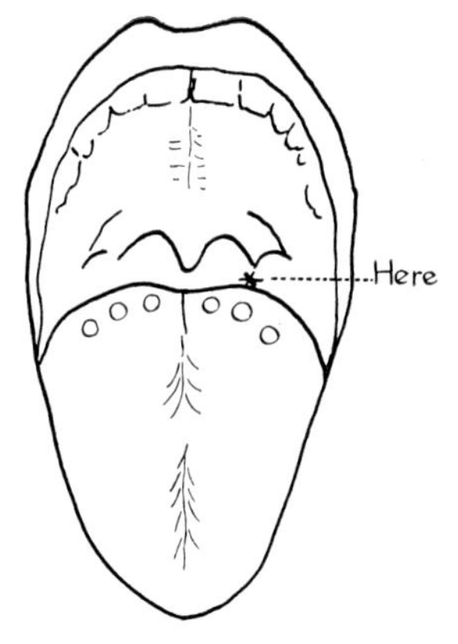

The oil will usually run into the bronchi. There can be some selectivity of location by positioning of the patient.

Little iodized oil is needed, usually less than 10 ml. being required for entirely adequate visualization in the suspected area. It is usually not wise to instill more than 15 ml. of iodized oil. The least amount possible should be used.

FLUOROSCOPIC TECHNIQUES

Fluoroscopic examination of the chest is one of the most important parts of the adequate roentgenologic study. Whereas the chest film is the old standard spot check of medicine, suffering from all the deficiencies of such a procedure, the fluoroscopic examination is a chance to see and visualize action of the dynamic respiratory processes. Thoughtful examination of the chest in this way will not only help the physician with the diagnosis, but it will also teach him the mechanics involved in both normal and pathologic processes.

It is always wise to have a definitive routine for this examination. No special order of procedure is particularly advantageous over any other. The following one is submitted without any recommendation except that we have used it and found it satisfactory.

Begin with an over-all survey of the entire chest. Have the patient breathe quietly and do not try to make any diagnosis. Simply look for gross and obvious evidences of dysfunction.

Next, have the patient take several deep breaths. Notice whether the pulmonary fields seem to be equally aerated and whether visible structures within the lung fields move freely with relationship to the rib cage. Any lateral movement of mediastinal structures with respiration should be noted.

Then close the shutter so that the visualized area is a horizontal slit about four inches wide and place it in front of the leaves of the diaphragm. Ask the patient to sniff as if he were trying to detect the odor of something burning; notice whether the diaphragmatic movements are free and equal. Obviously the contour of the diaphragm should also be marked.

Use one of the standard anatomy books to check the structure of the diaphragm. Note that it is made up of a number of muscular slips, some of which may be partially independent. A careful check will render it obvious why the "step" and double doming of the diaphragm are oftentimes normal.

Using the same three- or four-inch slit, move the fluoroscope upward and downward to inspect and carefully compare the two sides of the lung field. If one area seems not to be aerating well, close the slit even further (to one inch wide or less) and carefully compare aeration on the two sides during quiet respiration and during deep breathing. Then change the opening to a rectangle about four by eight inches and look at the hilar areas, again comparing both sides. Hilar structures usually seen are these:

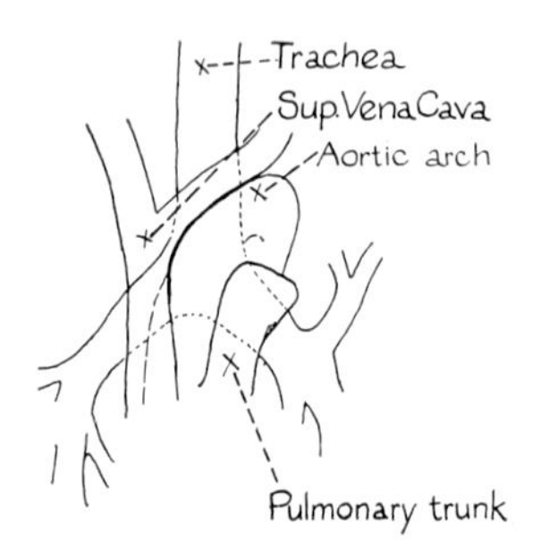

Do not hesitate to rotate the patient freely so that a good view at any suspect area may be obtained from several different angles. The two oblique positions are particularly valuable in some cases. Actually they are more often used in fluoroscopy of the heart.

A straight lateral view is of some value to show the depths of the posterior costophrenic recess and to delineate lesions lying in the lung field. If there is any question about an interlobar area or the positioning of the interlobar fissures, have the patient assume this position:

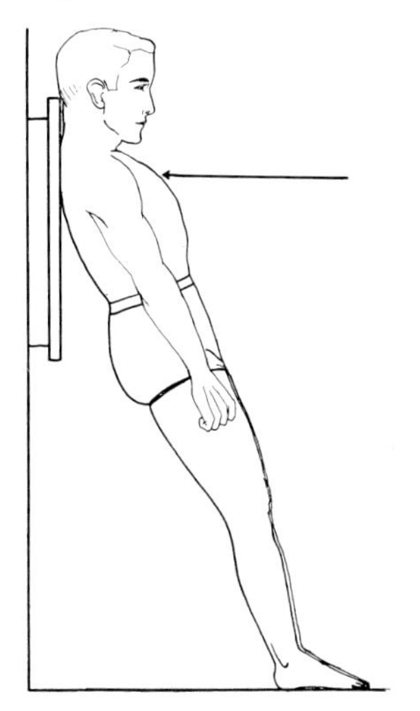

Here the rays nearly parallel the interlobar fissures and a lesion lying within the fissures becomes obvious. If your technician is not familiar with this, have her take several practice pictures.

When a lesion appears in the lung and you wish to know whether or not it lies close to the pleura or deeper within the substance of the lung, simply rotate the patient about an imaginary axis passing through the hilus of the lung like this:

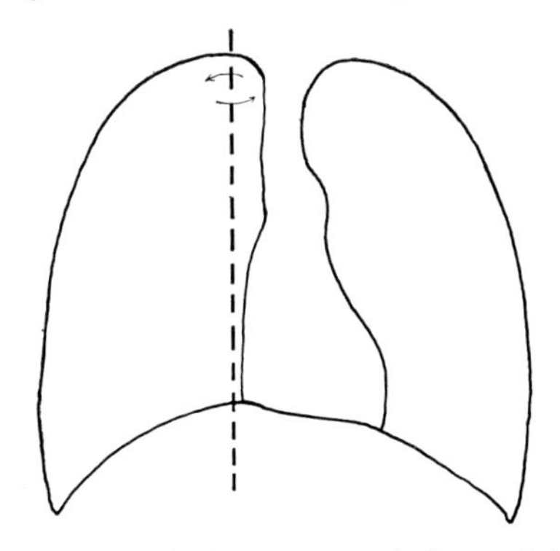

The further a lesion is toward the periphery, the more it will seem to move on such rotation, whereas a close-in lesion will appear more stable.

LOBAR PNEUMONIA

With the advent of the new and powerful antibiotics, lobar pneumonia has almost ceased to be a disease for which hospitalization is required, except in extraordinarily severe and complicated cases. Home care of even moderately severe lobar pneumonia in the intelligent patient has proved, at least in our practice, just as satisfactory as hospital care. For that reason the office x-ray sometimes comes into use.

The disease is originated when the patient gets a large dose of virulent pneumococci. They invade and set up a small focal lesion, usually in the alveoli near the periphery. The inflammatory reaction engendered causes an outpouring of fluid into the alveoli, which makes a perfect set-up for the pneumococci. The fluid is a good culture medium, for not only does it furnish them food, but when the outpouring is sufficient it actually carries them to surrounding alveoli. This method of spread by means of inflammatory exudate seems to be well proved and would logically explain why this type of pneumonia usually (but by no means always) is confined within the limits of a single lobe.

If the process continues, red blood cells escape into the alveoli and leukocytes are mobilized. New white blood cells in large quantities invade. They literally trap the bacteria against the walls of another cell, either of the lungs or in the exudate, and devour them. When this process is finished and virulent bacteria are no longer present, debris still remains in the alveolus, which must be cleaned up by the phagocytic cells. All through this process, from the earliest outpouring of the inflammatory exudate till the last scrap of debris is cleaned up, there is diminution or absolute prevention of aeration in the involved area. That is, of course, what x-ray demonstrates.

Technique

Actually before one discusses the localizing and diagnosis of a lobar pneumonia by means of x-ray, one basic question arises. Should these patients be x-rayed? My answer would be that they probably should not. Lobar pneumonia as an entity can be diagnosed clinically with absolute assurance in at least 90 per cent of the cases. In big hospitals where case following for research purposes and the accumulation of data are the major factors, then, of course, x-ray is indicated. In an office practice where a $15 x-ray means something to the patient, x-ray of an obvious case of lobar pneumonia is probably not good medical practice.

If there is an actual question as to the diagnosis, take a simple posteroanterior film of the chest. If the pneumonic process appears bizarre in extent or location, take additional lateral, oblique, or lordotic films, as indicated, to localize it.

Interpretation

A typical picture is consolidation limited sharply to one lobe or one portion of one lobe and showing a patchy, peripheral spread like this:

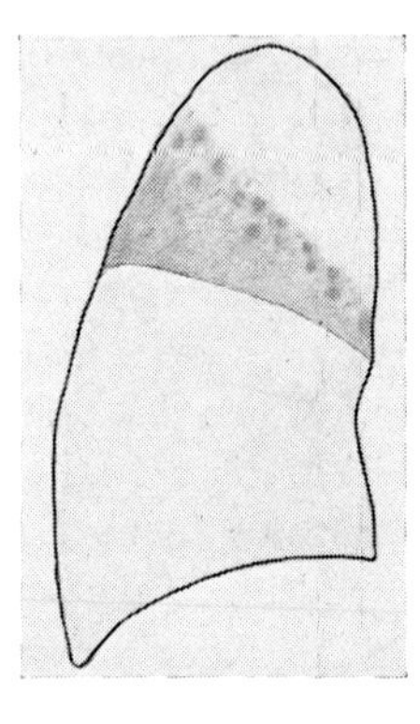

There are increased linear markings between the involved area and the hilus due to perivascular and peribronchial thickening and engorgement of lymphatic channels.

Sometimes there may be a differential question as between atelectasis and lobar pneumonia. When this is so, take a small overpenetrated film of the involved area and look particularly for vascular markings. They are clearly visible in the pneumonic process but are frequently not seen in atelectasis.

When one finds a consolidated lobe it is safe to assume that the invading organism is probably a pneumococcus, but this is by no means certain, because the amateur radiologist—and even at times the highly trained man—can make no etiologic pronouncement in regards to the invading bacteria. Lobar consolidation is usually, but by no means always, caused by the pneumococcus.

We are frequently puzzled in the office by an obviously resolving respiratory process in which diagnosis is uncertain. The picture of a resolving lobar pneumonia is specific. There is a gradual clearing of the opacity, usually beginning at the periphery and progressing toward the center of the lesion. Fine striate markings appear in the consolidated area and usually run either horizontally or toward the hilus. Within a few days to a week the opacity has cleared completely, but the fine, striate lines may remain for three to six weeks. If there has been consolidation along an interlobar fissure, there is usually thickening in this area, which remains for several months.

Errors

The most common error is probably overuse of the x-ray in the pneumonias. Rarely, an embarrassing mistake is made when a patient comes in with a resolving pneumonia and complains most bitterly of a cough. An x-ray picture may be more confusing than helpful unless a history is taken and the obvious acute respiratory infection discovered.

BRONCHOPNEUMONIA

Bronchopneumonia is not an etiologic designation. It simply indicates a way of spread. It starts with an inflammatory reaction in the membrane of the bronchioles and spreads peripherally, involving, last, the alveoli.

At least a dozen organisms have been implicated as the cause of bronchopneumonia, and unquestionably the atypical pneumonias caused by the viruses have essentially the same mode of spread. These facts offer the basis for differentiation between this and lobar pneumonia.

In the lobar type, chances are excellent that the pneumococcus is the cause. In bronchopneumonia, the pneumococcus, Friedländer's bacillus, or any number of other organisms, as well as the viruses, may be the cause. It is more difficult to make an exact clinical diagnosis regarding the bronchopneumonic process and, therefore, the x-ray is more often called into use.

Technique

The standard posteroanterior chest film will suffice for diagnosis in more than 98 per cent of the cases. However, do not forget the possibility of a small patch of bronchopneumonia behind the heart shadow.

Interpretation

Experienced radiologists can often gain some idea as to the infecting agent by examining the chest film. Ordinarily, the practitioner is not skillful enough to do this and probably should not try. The presence of typical bronchopneumonic consolidation should only indicate to him that any one of a number of organisms might be involved.

The patchy, irregular consolidation of bronchopneumonia may be found anywhere in the lungs, but in most cases it is present in the lower lobe and usually starts medially. This is a typical early case:

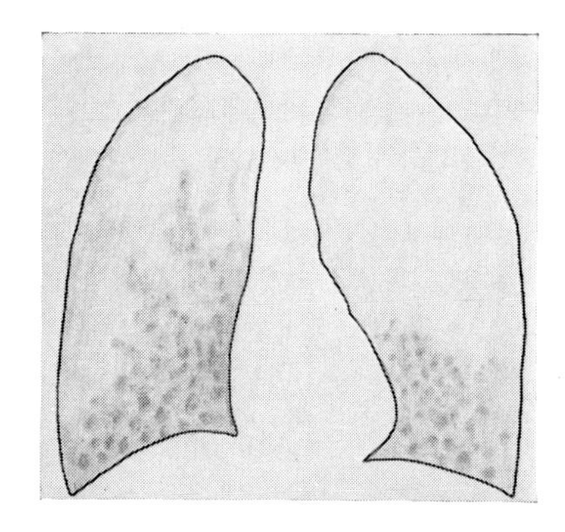

A later case with extensive consolidate areas looks like this:

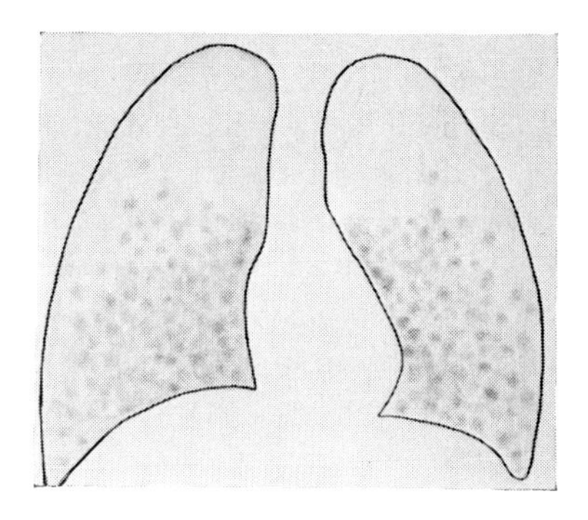

Occasionally the upper lobe may be involved with such a projection as this one:

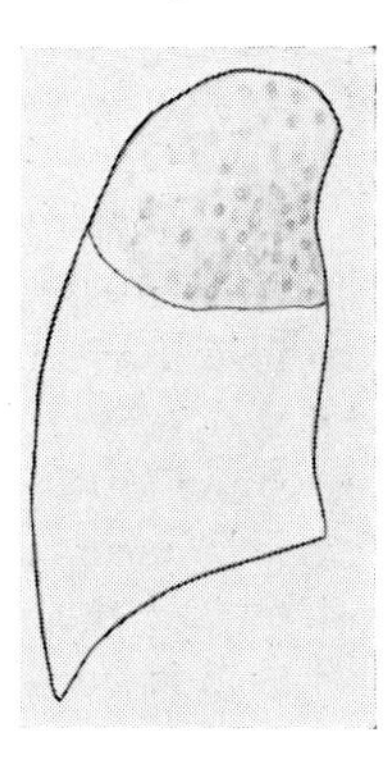

Errors

After the roentgenologic demonstration of typical patches of consolidation, one has only half made the diagnosis. In a few cases there may have to be a demonstration of the etiologic agent because of nonresponse to routine therapy.

In clinical practice one can usually differentiate the typical virus pneumonias from those caused by bacteria by considering the signs and symptoms. If this cannot be done, then one should use the office laboratory. Occasionally bronchopneumonic lesions near the apices may lead one to believe that he is dealing with an acute tuberculosis. Laboratory procedures and response to therapy will often clear up this problem, and an x-ray film taken after the original picture may dispose of it completely.

BRONCHIECTASIS

We probably see a great deal more bronchiectasis than we recognize. The disease, at least in its minor form, is relatively common, and many who complain of repeated respiratory infections actually have some degree of bronchiectasis.

In order to understand what happens in such a case one must review briefly the protective mechanism of the bronchioles. Extraneous material, including bacteria, cannot help but gain entrance into the respiratory system. There is a constant secretion of mucus into the bronchioles, much introduced extraneous material becoming stuck in the mucus and thoroughly entrapped.

The mucous membrane lining the respiratory system from the trachea down to bronchioles less than 0.5 mm. in diameter is ciliated. The regular motion of these cilia carries the secreted mucus and the trapped matter upward toward the opening of the trachea. This system is surprisingly efficient, because cultures taken from most of the alveoli are sterile.

Ordinarily, the small bronchioles are freely movable and expand or contract with changes in pressure. The process of coughing includes a dilatation and then a contraction of these bronchioles, so that contained matter is both expelled by air pressure and a wavelike motion that travels along the bronchiole itself. This, too, is an efficient aid to the expulsion of foreign material. So long as these mechanisms are intact there is little chance for invasion of the bronchiolar wall by pathogenic organisms.

Now suppose that during a severe infection there is sufficient bacterial attack and breakdown of these defense mechanisms so that not only the bronchiole wall is invaded (bronchitis), but there is also some necrosis. These necrotizing infections may actually destroy a portion of the wall and even invade surrounding peripheral tissues. When this happens there is not only some necrosis in the bronchiole, but also a complete breakdown of the defense mechanisms in the immediate area. Mucus-secreting cells are destroyed, as are cilia-bearing cells, and the loss of bronchiolar structure prevents normal results to be expected from a cough.

Saprophytic organisms invade regularly and occasionally real pathogens invade this area, so that there is little tendency toward healing. When the healing process does occur it is fibrotic in nature and does not re-create the structure of the destroyed tissue. The patient is then said to have bronchiectasis.

Extensive full-blown cases of bronchiectasis are probably somewhat rare, but minimal or moderate degrees seem much more common than anyone has thought.

Most of the severe cases can be diagnosed by means of the x-ray. Mild or minor cases, however, may take repeated, careful x-ray examinations, backed up by adequate preliminary history and physical examination. Even so, they may present diagnostic difficulty. Probably 90 per cent of the cases involve the lower lobe, but it is perfectly possible to have bronchiectasis in any portion of the lung.

Technique

In perhaps 50 per cent of the moderate cases and 10 per cent of the minimal cases, findings on the ordinary posteroanterior chest film will be sufficient to allow some diagnostic pronouncement.

If the history is consistent with bronchiectasis, one should consider seriously the instillation of iodized oil. The technique for this is mentioned on page 237.

There are some contraindications. If a respiratory infection is present or if the patient has within the past two or three weeks recovered from one, instillation of the iodized oil is not a good idea. One routine to follow is to check that the patient has been fever-free for a week, has no history of any sort of respiratory disease for a month and has had no changes in the blood count indicating the presence of infection. An occasional person is sensitive to the iodine content of the oil and such is an absolute contraindication to the study. Such persons are rare.

The first detectable signs upon x-ray examination are usually those of perivascular thickening between the involved area and the hilus. This, of course, has no specific meaning. It simply indicates that some inflammatory or infectious process is in progress. Next to appear may be patchy areas of pneumonitis surrounding the injured bronchus. These give a honeycomb appearance in the involved area, like this:

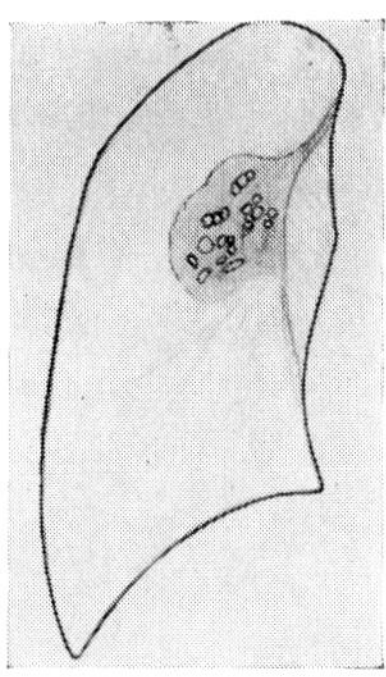

There is frequently an atelectasis of some portion distal to the involved areas, and a regional compensatory emphysema may be one of the original findings. Overdrawn schematically it would look like this:

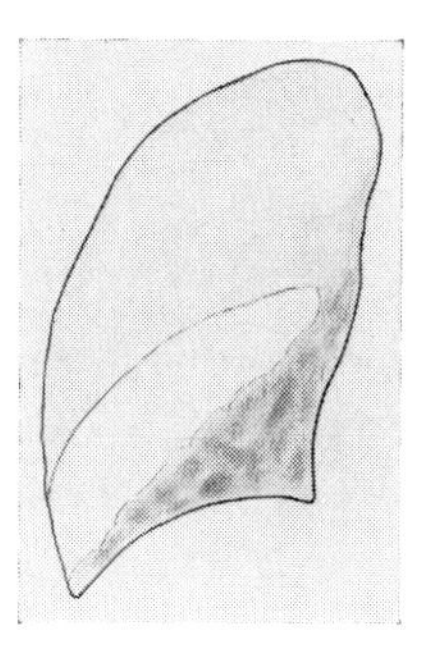

After the injection of iodized oil the cavitation about the bronchi stands out vividly, like this:

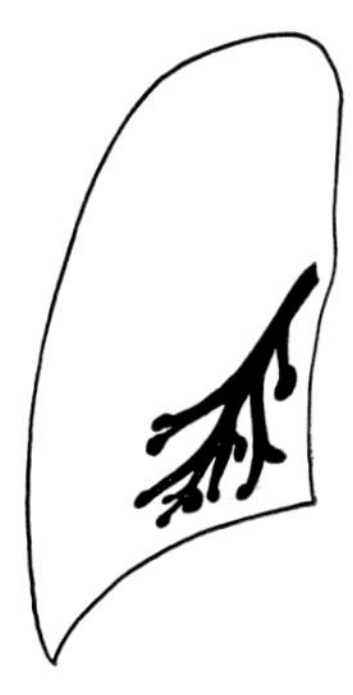

Diagnosis after such a procedure is no problem.

Errors

Bronchiectasis is not an easy disease to diagnose, even when using the x-ray. Some peribronchial thickening may occur in the presence of chronic bronchitis without actual dilation or destruction as is seen in bronchiectasis.

Sometimes the pneumonitis surrounding the involved area is so great that one gets the impression a bronchopneumonia is present. This may be true during an acute, inflammatory episode, but the chronicity of the process and the history of repeated episodes and other salient clinical points usually indicate clearly the actual pathology.

Probably the most common error is to miss bronchiectasis when present in minor degrees, not because it is difficult to see, but because the practitioner is seldom looking for it.

Comments

There is some controversy among radiologists about the prevalence of bronchiectatic changes. Some competent men believe that they are seldom seen. Others say that such lesions are among the commonest ones found in the chest. Depending upon the viewpoint of the consultant, films may often come back labeled "possible bronchiectasis" or may never come back so labeled.

It is my impression, backed up only by clinical experience, that minor degrees of bronchiectasis are frequent. I tend, therefore, to agree with the radiologic consultant who looks for and often finds minor evidence of such disease. For a time the average practitioner will do well to have any film about which there is question read by the most competent radiologist he can find.

ATELECTASIS

Atelectasis is a symptom, not a disease. Our interest should center in the process causing the collapse and the corrective measures to be undertaken.

The etiology may be divided into two great groups:

The first type is atelectasis due to an external cause, in which something serves to change the pressure relationship and thereby collapse a lobe or lobule. Examples are pneumothorax and pleural effusion. This type has little importance from an x-ray standpoint because the causative condition is usually just as apparent on the x-ray film as is the atelectasis itself.

The second type, and by far the most important from a diagnostic standpoint, is atelectasis caused by obstruction of the bronchi. When there is bronchial obstruction, air contained in the alveoli distal to the obstruction is soon absorbed by the circulating blood and the area becomes unaerated and atelectatic.

Acute obstruction may occur from the presence of foreign bodies during a respiratory infection and frequently during bouts of allergy. These are of little significance because they re-expand promptly and seldom is treatment indicated. Postoperative atelectasis is a common occurrence but is not for consideration in this discussion.

In a small number of cases chronic atelectases are usually due to pressure on the bronchus by large lymph glands or in a large number of cases, to carcinoma. In the office the chronic atelectases due to carcinoma are probably the most important of all the types seen.

Often minor atelectases occur in even trivial respiratory diseases. These small areas of collapse are not significant in themselves, but they do form an excellent growth area for bacteria. In such a case they may be the nidus from which a severe infection takes its start. They will bear careful watching.

Technique

The ordinary posteroanterior film of the chest in most cases will allow one to make a good estimation as to whether atelectasis is present. Usually when it is suspected, a lordotic chest view as mentioned on page 239 will add some information and rarely the oblique view will be needed to decide just what portion of the lung is collapsed.

In partial collapse the normal vascular markings of the area are crowded together and a compensatory emphysema surrounds the involved segment. A typical collapsed lower lobe might look like this:

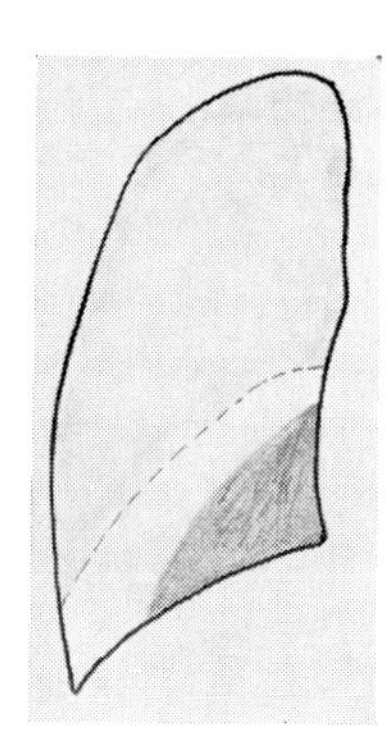

After complete collapse the affected portion of lung usually assumes a homogeneous increase in density and compensatory emphysema is even more obvious.

Whether there is movement of the mediastinal structures toward the affected side depends entirely upon the mobility of the mediastinum and the degree of compensatory emphysema. This mediastinal shift should be looked for but little in the way of interpretation should be done by the practitioner, whether it is present or not. Such determinations lie in the field of the expert radiologist.

In partial atelectasis notice the retraction of the nearest interlobar fissure toward the atelectatic area, like this:

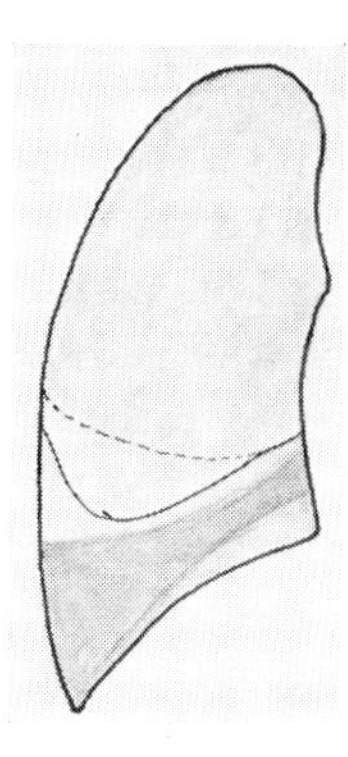

Interpretation

Patients with massive collapses of the lung will ordinarily not be seen in office practice. Small segmental or lobular atelectasis in association with no acute disease is of little significance. The important point for the practitioner to remember is that chronic atelectasis in a patient over 40 is bronchiogenic carcinoma until proved otherwise. Such patients should be referred immediately to a medical center for a complete diagnostic work-up.

EMPHYSEMA

The statement has been made that emphysema is the most frequent chronic respiratory disease seen in males over 40. In our practice this proved to be true. It is also one of the most frequently missed entities in practice.

There are two types: the obstructive and the senile. The type induced by obstructive changes is seen most often. It usually begins with spasm or partial mechanical obstruction of the bronchioles. Spasm is common in asthmatics, persons with chronic bronchitis (often due to persistent postnasal drip), and bronchial irritations, such as those found in overuse of tobacco or inhalation of irritant chemicals.

Some diseases call forth the production of thick, ropy mucus which soon becomes inspissated and effectively plugs or partially plugs the bronchioles. Intermittent partial plugging as seen in these diseases initiates the emphysematous process.

What happens from the standpoint of an individual alveolus is shown. Upon inspiration, expansive drag is exerted upon the alveolus, like this:

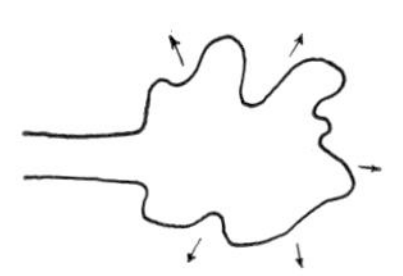

Air cannot pass through the constricted bronchiole quickly enough to meet the demands of the expansive drag, so inspiration is somewhat prolonged. The alveolus finally becomes distended but not to a great degree because distention upon inspiration must, of necessity, be brought about by inflow of air and this is limited. When the alveolus finally becomes full at the end of inspiration, pressure in the bronchioles and in the alveolus is equal. Normally, expiration is a passive process, the elastic tissue of the lung expelling air helped slightly by the passive fall of chest wall structures. Air is literally squeezed out by contraction of the alveolus, like this:

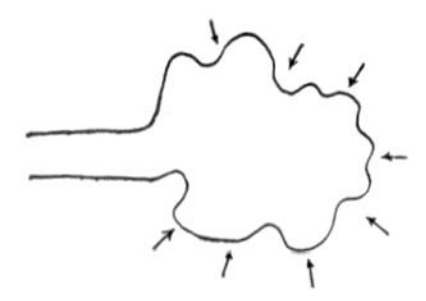

In emphysema the bronchial tube is too small to allow free escape of the air and it is squeezed out slowly as is done when deflating a toy balloon.

The patient cannot interrupt his respiratory cycle to allow full deflation to take place in its own slow fashion. Usually he gives the process a push, using the accessory muscles of respiration to force expiration like this:

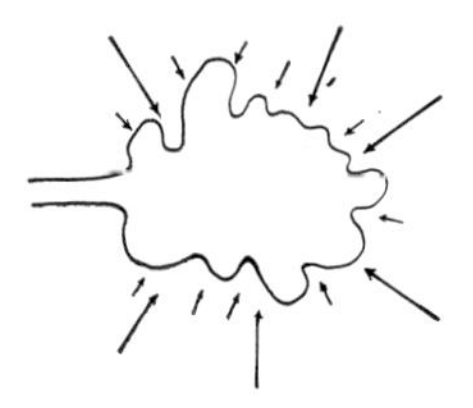

Even bringing force into play, he cannot empty the alveolus as completely as the normal person can. A little air remains trapped. Over thousands of cycles the alveolus becomes distended. Now several factors begin to operate to make the situation worse.

If the alveolus is distended enough the elastic fibers in the tissue surrounding it are ruptured. What happens can be duplicated exactly by overstretching a rubber band until it breaks. As more and more of these tiny fibrils are broken, the lung loses its elasticity and can help less and less in the process of expiration. The whole load, or a good portion of it, is thrown upon the accessory muscles. This loss of elastic tissue, along with air circulatory changes due to pressure from the distending alveoli, may operate to allow degeneration of alveolar walls with confluence of several alveoli into a large air cavity.

The effective air, insofar as gaseous exchange is concerned, is that which lies next to the alveolar wall, not that located in the center. In a distended alveolus the air in the center is practically useless for respiratory purposes. Notice the relative amount of "useless" air in these diagrams:

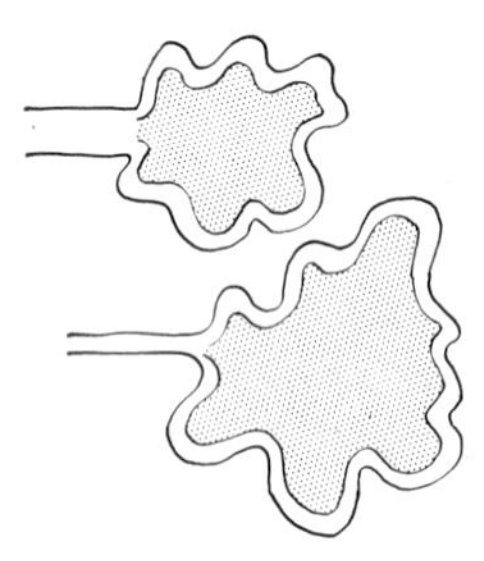

When this happens a large part of the respiratory effort is negated. To acquire the normal amount of blood aeration, a greatly increased quantity of air must be moved. In severe cases the amount that must be moved exceeds the respiratory capacity and exertional dyspnea occurs.

Another factor is the increase in carbon dioxide tension which occurs. The air trapped in some of the alveoli is quickly exhausted of its oxygen but carbon dioxide is continually moved into it. This carbon dioxide is not blown off and, if the concentration gets sufficiently high, will be reabsorbed into the blood stream. There gradually develops a slightly increased carbon dioxide tension in the blood. This reacts on the respiratory center to increase the rate of respiration and this, in turn, lessens the efficiency of the already damaged lung. A vicious circle may be created.

Actually, this sounds as if most people with emphysema die a horrible death by slow asphyxia. They do not. Most cases progress little further than annoying respiratory embarrassment, although a few go on to dissolution. Even so, the disease is a dangerous one. In the elderly, particularly, it may so cripple respiratory function that the patient will succumb to the first moderate respiratory infection that comes his way. In younger people, emphysema may force major diminution of activity.

Certain anatomic changes occur as a result of the gradual pulmonary distention. In respiration the ribs have little expansile motion. They move in expiration and inspiration, like this:

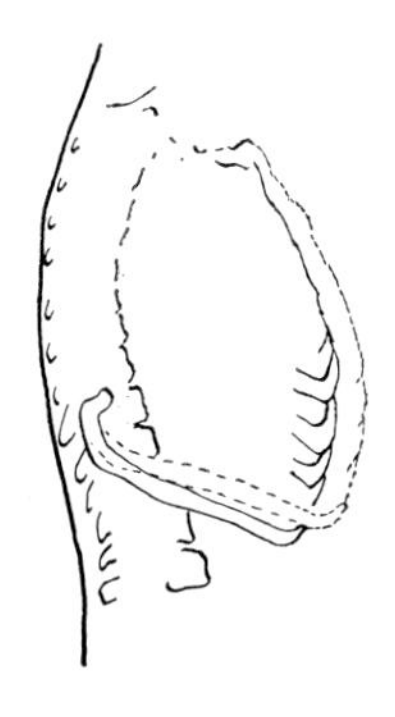

As the lungs become distended the rib cage tends to remain in inspiratory position, which enlarges the anteroposterior diameter of the chest. The diaphragm is pushed downward and the intercostal spaces are widened.

Technique

Posteroanterior and lateral films of the chest are all that are needed for diagnosis.

Interpretation

Alteration in general configuration of the chest is usually striking. It assumes an outline like this:

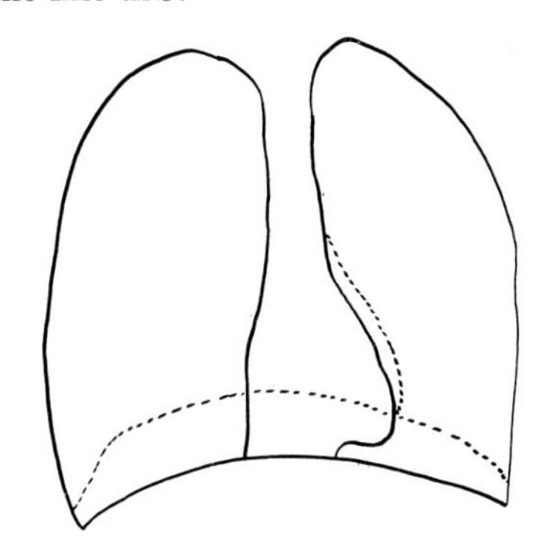

The diaphragm is usually one, sometimes two, interspaces lower than normal and the costophrenic "dip" is often nearly eliminated.

The heart shadow is usually small and narrow because the apex has been displaced downward by the expanded lung. Even so, there is often visible a clear space between the apex and diaphragm. Vascular markings at the hilus seem prominent because of the increased contrast between them and the lung fields. These lung fields are much increased in transparency; the normal peripheral markings are much reduced. Bullae may occasionally be found.

Fluoroscopy is fully as important as the film, if not more so. One notices particularly the limited excursion of the diaphragm and the unusual position and action of the ribs.

Errors

Errors in diagnosis are rare. Perhaps only one deserves any mention. In asthmatics, particularly in those who are exceptionally thin, one may err toward "overdiagnosis." Usually such people have some slight emphysema and this may become much more pronounced during or immediately after an attack.

One cannot tell accurately how much permanent emphysematous damage has been done until the patient has been thoroughly examined between attacks when breathing is essentially normal and has been so for several days.

Senile Emphysema

Senile emphysema seems to be more a degenerative disease with "accidental" emphysematous changes than a true entity. Many writers believe it is due to a fixation of the thoracic spine, with consequent limitation of the normal chest excursion. Others feel that it is purely a degenerative vascular disease. I do not know. In our own practice it was much more rare than obstructive disease. We most often were given a clue to the diagnosis by chest fluoroscopy. In such an examination one notes the great limitation of respiratory movements and can occasionally detect areas of lung that aerate less well than others.

Recently the relationship between fibrosis of the lung and this so-called senile emphysema has come under study. After careful evaluation of our cases I am inclined to believe that many cases of senile emphysema are truly the end result of repeated bouts with pneumonitis.

Certainly the patchy formation of scar tissue would duplicate all the findings we see in such a chest. Most patients, too, give a long history of repeated attacks of respiratory infection. The relationship is not yet clarified, but it would seem probable that scarring following these infections might be the etiology of senile emphysema.

TUBERCULOSIS

The practitioner should not attempt an exact diagnosis of tuberculosis on the basis of unsupported chest films until he has had extensive experience with chest roentgenology. When we can back up a diagnosis suspected from films with identification of the mycobacterium, the case assumes a different aspect. A good rule to follow is to send all questionable films to a roentgenologist for an expert opinion.

Tuberculosis is noted for its protean manifestations, and roentgen diagnosis of many such lesions is not in the purview of the practitioners. We are mainly interested in the common early lesions which may be observed in the office. These are the so-called apical and infraclavicular lesions which are usually seen in this area of the lung:

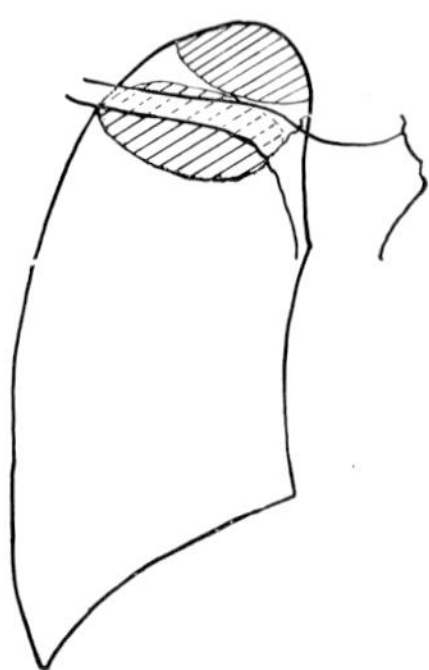

There are four types of lesions commonly seen in this area:

1. Assmann's foci. These are small round densities, usually with a clearly defined border. They are only slightly more opaque to the rays than normal lung tissue in some instances and may have to be searched for carefully. A typical Assmann's focus may look like this:

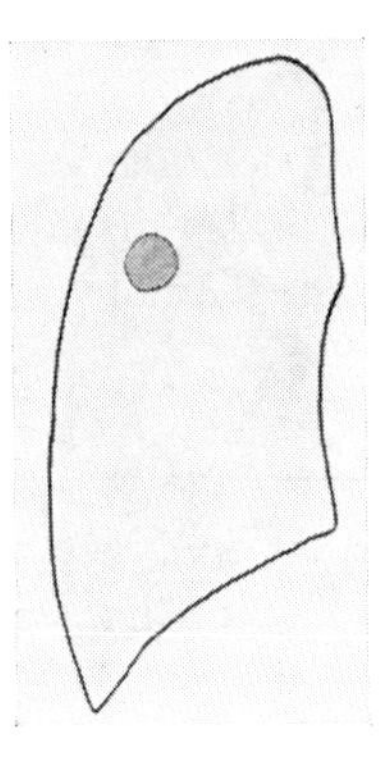

Under successful treatment the focus gradually subsides until all that remains is a fibrotic scar that may contain flecks of calcium, like this:

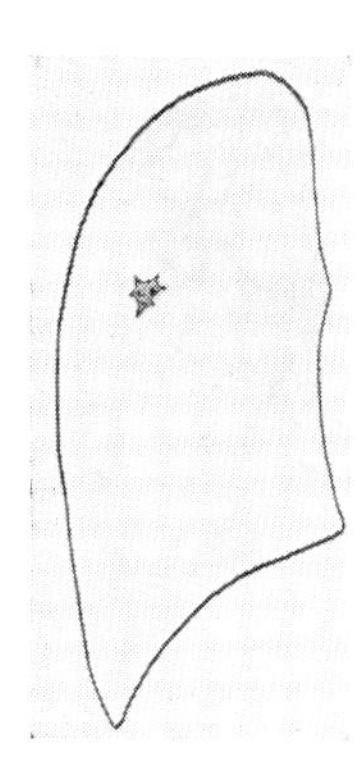

If the disease progresses, small satellite foci may appear or the original density may enlarge and break down to form a cavity. Usually the first sign of such extension is loss of sharpness in the border of the original lesion. There is a hazy corona around the original focus.

2. Segmental atelectasis. Apparently the original lesion may sometimes be peribronchiolar so that the pressure of its growth occludes the bronchiole and an atelectasis follows. Depending on the view, one of the following pictures is presented:

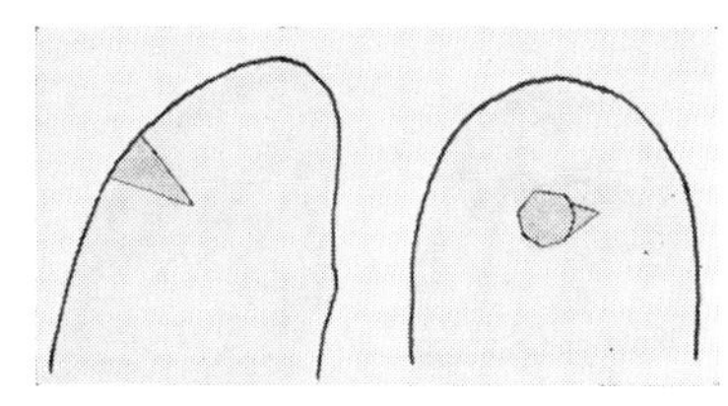

If spread occurs, typical round foci may appear near the apex of the lesion, like this:

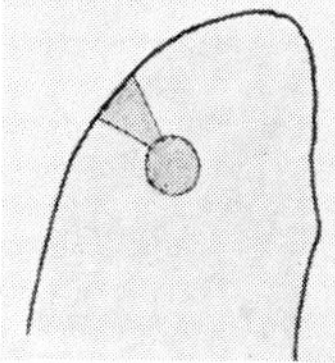

Should recovery take place, all that remains is a linear scar to mark the spot where the original manifestation occurred.

3. Groups of small round foci. These are not seen as often as the first two types. They are simply small spots, 1 to 5 or 6 mm. in diameter, which coalesce. The groups sometimes assume rosette form. Borders are sharply defined. They look like this:

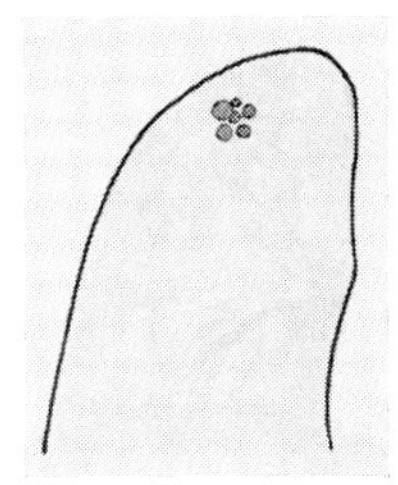

4. Soft lesions near calcified ones. This category is included only to mention that such lesions are dangerous and should not be regarded as quiescent until one is sure that they are.

Tuberculous Activity

The problem of determining the presence or absence of tuberculous activity is a major one—probably more important and more difficult than recognition of the disease. One should begin by admission that the x-ray is not a perfect means of deciding this question. Certainly a single film in the hands of an average practitioner is not very valuable. As a matter of fact, I cannot caution the practitioner too forcefully to seek expert advice on this point, both quickly and often. It takes a great deal of study to be sure of one's self in this field of diagnosis.

To understand the problem of delineating activity we must first know how the early lesions heal. In almost all cases there is some reaction in the lymphatics between the lesion and the hilus.

An early lesion is first encapsulated in a firm sphere of fibrous tissue. If this manages to contain the infectious process, it shows in the x-ray as a ring of dense tissue surrounding the involved area, like this:

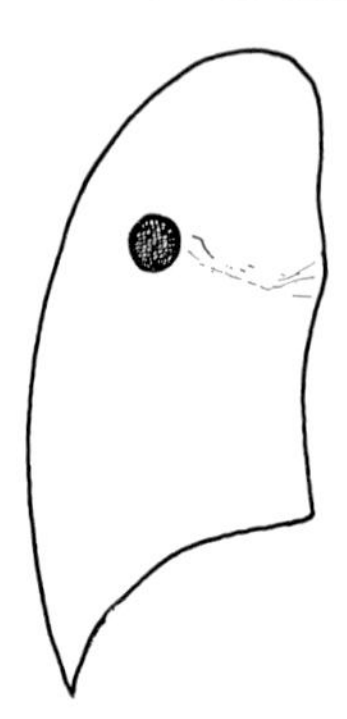

Next, fibrous tissue is laid down along the involved lymphatics between the tuberculous area and the hilus, forming a radiating network of densities, like this:

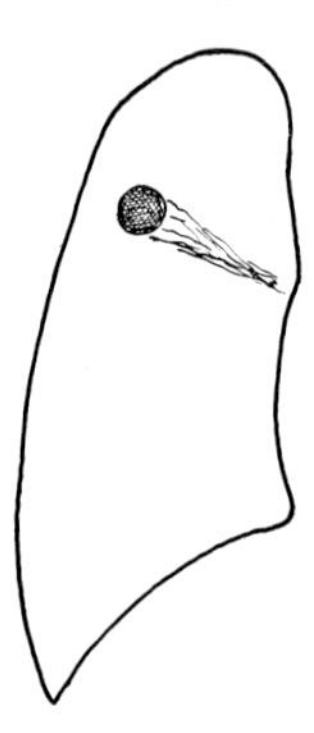

Ultimately the fibroblasts invade the actual site of the original lesion and proliferate masses of tissue. This fibrous tissue contracts until all that remains is a dense, irregular scar which sometimes contains calcium. It may look like this:

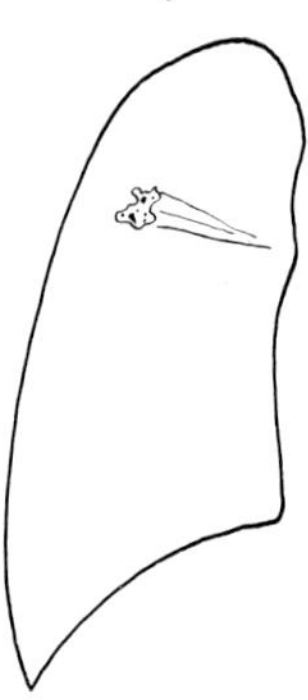

Contraction of the scar tissue along the course of the lymphatics pulls them into straight lines so that the typical "t.b. fan" is seen, like this:

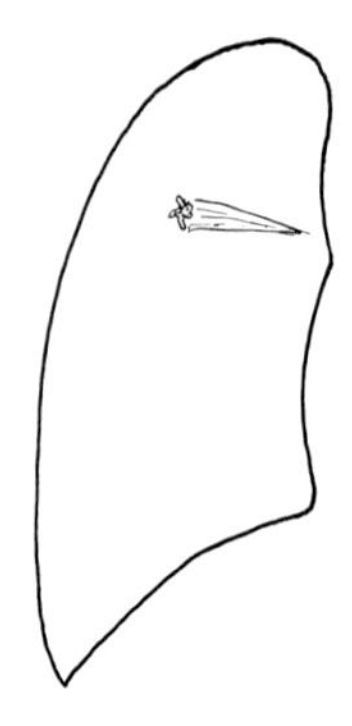

The primary lesions treated by the practitioner may contract enough to pull the nearest interlobar fissure toward them, with a resultant convexity pointing at the lesion, like this:

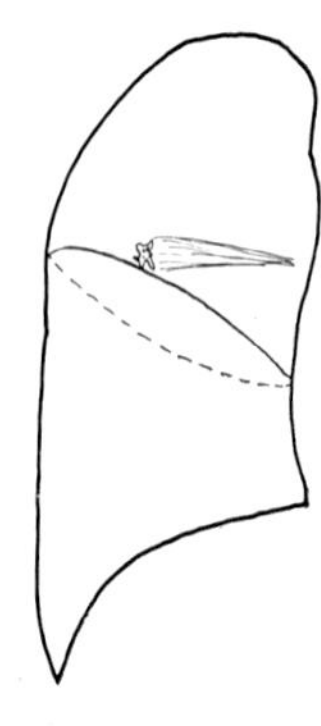

However, seldom are they big enough to result in deviation of mediastinal contents as may be seen in massive involvement.

Such is the healing process which, when demonstrated on serial films, is the best indication we have that treatment is successful. These changes do not occur rapidly. Sometimes three or four years elapse between the beginning of healing and the final destruction of the lesion.

There are all degrees of intermittent processes; however, there is only one that needs consideration. What about the "soft" lesion that stays constant, with neither spread nor healing? Apparently it is possible for a human being and the mycobacterium to live in perfect harmony, at least for a time, like two bulls in a pasture. The trouble is that the potential battle is just as much present in the man-mycobacterium association as it is in the bull-bull association. Such an unchanging soft lesion represents a constant threat and should be followed carefully for as long as ten years before being dismissed as insignificant. Even then there will be the occasional case which shows unsuspected activity. These are rare but they do occur.

Tuberculosis activity is indicated by the appearance of new soft lesions on serial films or by cavitation of existing lesions. There are some signs on a single film that indicate activity, but they are so difficult to interpret that the practitioner should not attempt to do so. Serial films are the answer.

Tuberculosis in Children

Tuberculosis in children is remarkably different from the lesion as seen in adults. The disease tends to run a much more acute course.

In far more than half the cases the lower lobes are involved with an infiltrating lesion which seems disproportionately big for the symptoms that are present. Regional atelectases are common.

Most outstanding is the tremendous involvement of the hilar glands which may present an outline like this:

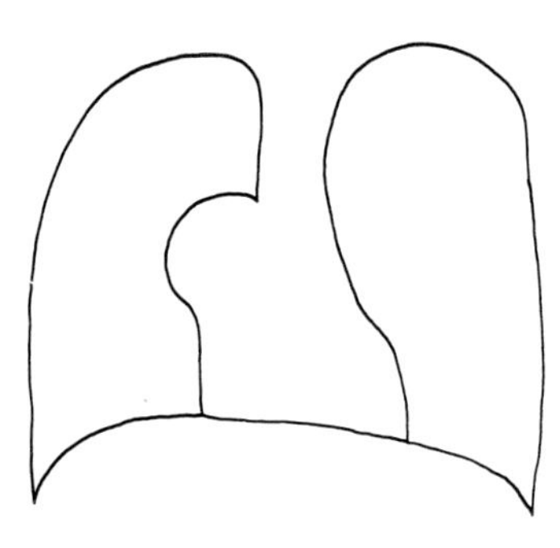

Comment

Unfortunately there is a tendency today to consider the x-ray a kind of diagnostic vade mecum for tuberculosis. It is about half as good as most physicians believe. This does not mean that it should not be used in every case, but its use does not relieve the physician of his responsibility to do a careful clinical work-up.

The x-ray is a tool and probably the most valuable one we have for diagnosis of tuberculosis but, still, only a tool. Use it for this and nothing more.

CHILDHOOD PULMONARY DISEASE

In general, x-ray findings in children are not vastly different from those in adults in the various pulmonary diseases to which they are susceptible. There is one, however, that deserves comment. It is one of the most vicious and most often missed respiratory diseases seen in children.

The entity actually goes by several names and has several possible courses. Acute tracheobronchitis is one name; acute bronchiolitis is another. What actually happens is that there is an acute inflammatory reaction of the mucous membrane of the bronchial system which may start in the trachea and extend as far distalward as the terminal bronchioles.

In young children it may result in immediate plugging of the bronchiolar passages with tenacious secretion. Death supervenes so quickly that x-ray diagnosis is essentially useless, for the child is moribund when first seen. When it occurs in a slightly older child it can be even more vicious because of the element of surprise which it may offer.

In an older child it may progress about this way: The patient is thought clinically to have a simple bronchitis—which he has—and a routine treatment is followed.

After several days at home he suddenly begins wheezing and becomes cyanotic and has obvious gross respiratory difficulty. He is rushed to the physician in serious condition. Upon clinical examination, no consolidation is found but there is wheezing and bubbly râles throughout the lung field. Since the child seems obviously too ill to be suffering from a simple bronchitis, an x-ray is promptly taken, with the idea of locating the consolidation which was not found on examination. Surprisingly, at first glance the x-ray seems negative. There is no consolidation and little increase in bronchial markings. If the film is dismissed here, chances are the child will die.

What has happened is that from the irritated bronchioles there is a profuse secretion which has become somewhat inspissated and has acted as a partial block to the free moving of air. Read now the section on emphysema, beginning on page 245, and notice the physiology involved in such blocking. The x-ray findings of bronchiolitis are those characteristic of emphysema. In a way this might be said to be exactly the reverse of those usually found in consolidated areas.

Postural drainage, the instillation of liquefying agents, and immediate bronchoscopy may sometimes be necessary to save the life of such a child.

Technique

The ordinary posteroanterior film of the chest will give much information and chest fluoroscopy will give even more. When the film is examined and the indications of this disease are found, immediate fluoroscopy probably should be done unless the child is obviously too sick to withstand such a procedure.

Interpretation

In the film look for the obvious signs of patchy emphysema, with lowering of the diaphragm and some widening of the intercostal spaces (which may or may not occur). If patchy lightening of the lung field occurs, along with some loss of the usual structural markings, use the fluoroscope immediately.

When this is done notice the limited respiratory excursion on the involved side and whether any fixation of the chest structures seems to be in the inspiration. Close the shutters down to a horizontal slit and notice the obvious change in aeration in the uninvolved lung as the respiratory cycle occurs and the limited change in the involved lung. This diagnosis, like many others, is missed, not because it is difficult to make, but because it is not taken into consideration.

Errors

The most frequent error is failure to take cognizance of this process, knowing that it may occur. The next most frequent is mistaking the emphysematous lung for a healthy one because the opposite lung obviously casts a darker shadow on the film. Most of us are worried by the serious illness of these children so that we only glance at the x-ray, looking for consolidation. When none is seen we are likely to turn quickly to some other diagnostic means.

METASTATIC TUMORS

The lungs are the most frequent site of metastasis for all tumors. When considered without differentiation as to type, over one fourth of all malignancies will show metastatic pulmonary lesions during their course.

Certain exceptions, of course, are outstanding. Perhaps the one most important to the practitioner is the fact that metastases by means of the portal venous system usually occur in the liver, not in the lung. It is, therefore, somewhat rare to find tumors of the small and large intestine metastasizing to the lung.

The following three types of pulmonary metastasis will cover nearly 80 per cent of all cases seen.

1. The nodular metastasis. This is considered to be blood-borne and results from embolization of small arteries or capillaries by groups of tumor cells. Probably because of gravity relationships, they occur most often in the bases but have been seen in any area of the lung. Since these growths start from a central focus within the lung tissue itself, they usually develop more or less equally in all directions and, therefore, cast a round or slightly oval shadow.

2. Lymphatic. The metastases usually considered lymphatic in origin show involvement of the hilar gland, sometimes with peripheral extension along the lymphatic, so that there are projections from the hilus consisting of cords of tumor cells. More often one or two cords will lead from the enlarged hilar glands to one or two larger metastatic nodules.

3. Subpleural or pleural involvement is usually manifested first of all by a nearly symptomless pleural effusion. For some reason which we cannot explain readily this is most common in carcinoma of the breast. Quite often one sees this slight pleural effusion without any distinct x-ray signs of metastatic lesions. One should always suspect metastatic tumors in such a case, and it is almost safe to assume that a metastatic tumor is present when such findings occur in a woman who has been proved to have breast cancer.

Technique

The straight posteroanterior film of the chest will demonstrate most of these metastatic lesions. Rarely, if there is a question about the hilar glands being involved, a swallow of barium during fluoroscopy will show the esophageal deviation around the enlarged gland.

Interpretation

One must begin by admitting that it is possible to infer, but not possible to diagnose, the existence of metastatic cancer from the appearance of the x-ray plate. In a patient with known cancer it is almost certainly safe to assume that the shadows are metastatic lesions, particularly if they fall typically into one of the three classes previously described.

In a person who does not have known cancer, such shadows should make one intensely suspicious that a malignancy exists. The diagnosis is such a serious one that it is best to say little until one can make a repeat film and make a diligent search for the original lesion. This of course, must be done quickly. Characteristics of the three general types are as follows:

1. *The pleural effusion* differs in no respect from the film of pleural effusion of other causes. Such films are discussed on page 256.

2. *The nodular type.* These hematogenous lesions are usually round or slightly ovoid in a plane parallel to the bronchial tree. They have sharply defined edges and are much more dense than surrounding lung tissue. They may be solitary or multiple, but most often in our limited practice we have found them to be multiple. Here are diagrammatic sketches of two typical lesions:

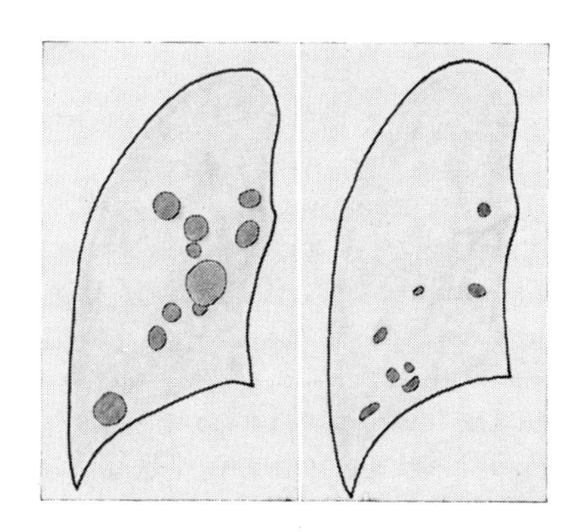

3. *The lymphatic spread type* may take one of several courses. It may involve the hilar glands at first, with slight enlargement as shown here:

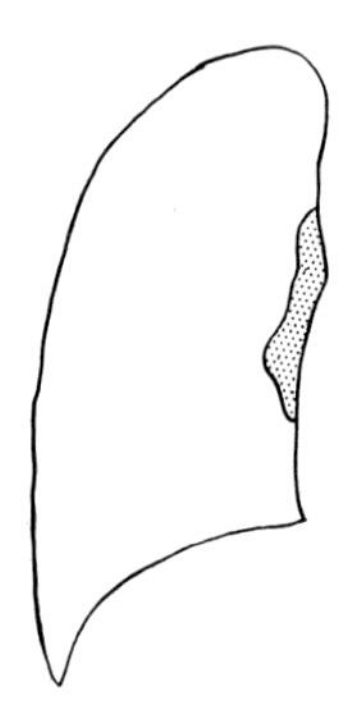

As the lesion progresses an extension along the lymphatics occurs more frequently in one lung than the other.

Even more often there are one or two solitary, rounded, peripheral lesions connected to the enlarged hilar glands by strands of dense tissue like this:

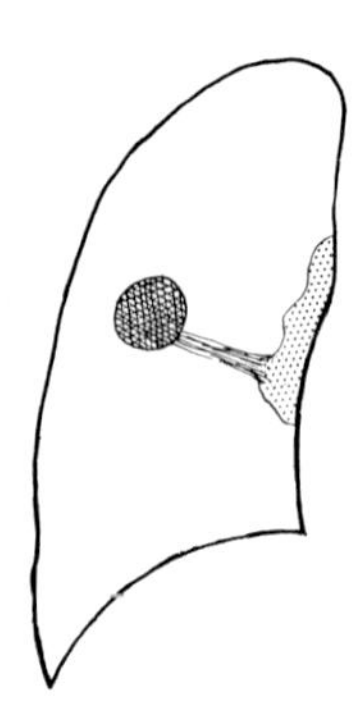

It may be extremely difficult to make a diagnosis of metastatic lesions involving only the hilar glands. If you suspect this and are not sure, send the patient to an expert roentgenologist at once. If several films are available compare them for obvious gradual enlargement of the hilar glands.

Errors

Rarely, there may be confusion with a primary tumor of the lung. The differentiation is discussed under the next heading.

Also there may be confusion as to whether or not a lung lesion is metastatic in origin. This is usually decided by a careful clinical evaluation of the case. If the point cannot be decided after such study, then the film should be sent at once to an expert roentgenologist for his opinion. Sometimes he, too, is not entirely sure that it is a metastatic tumor. It is an error to continue utilizing the diagnostic facilities of the office or the small country hospital in such a situation. Such a patient should be sent immediately to a cancer detection center for complete and detailed study.

BRONCHIOGENIC CARCINOMA

Bronchiogenic carcinoma is the common cancer of the lung seen by us practitioners. Statistical studies would indicate that in comparison with other cancers this type is becoming more frequent.

As this book is written, there is considerable controversy over carcinogenic factors, and the present theory is that in many instances bronchiogenic carcinoma is due to irritation caused by tobacco. This seems possible but is by no means proved.

The overwhelming majority of such tumors arise in one of the major bronchi within two or three inches of the tracheal carina. The growths arise in the mucosa of the bronchi, and there are seldom any symptoms for a period of time.

Extension to the hilar gland is the rule and occurs early. When symptoms do appear they are usually due either to obstructive phenomena in the bronchus or to changes brought about by the enlarging hilar gland.

In most instances when the growing tumor escapes the bronchus it merely compresses surrounding lung tissue. Later it may actively invade and destroy pulmonary architecture. It is often limited in its extension by the interlobar fissures.

Technique

The ordinary posteroanterior film of the chest is often adequate to delineate these tumors, but special positioning may be needed to show their outline more clearly and to depict their relation to the interlobar fissures.

Interpretation

The usual picture is that of an homogeneous hilar density with smooth edges. It is usually rounded, though not circular, and sharply delineated from the surrounding lung tissue. Such growths often look like this:

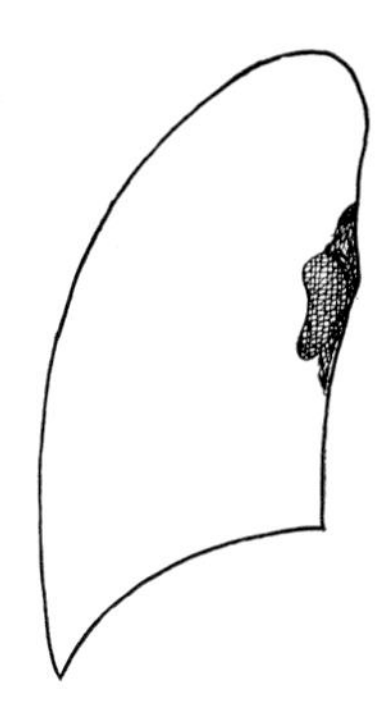

As the growth develops it may spread in retrograde fashion through the peribronchial lymphatics, giving an appearance like this:

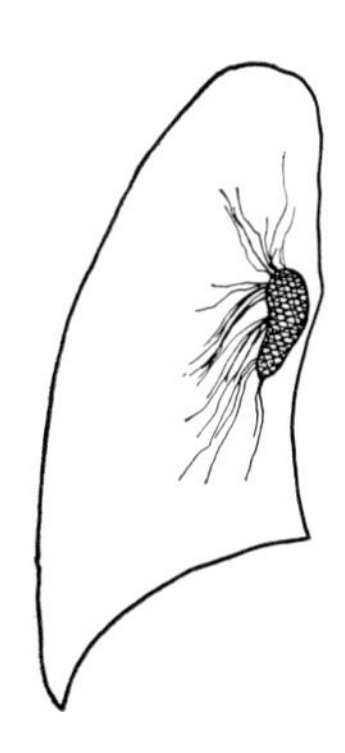

Later findings are atelectasis of the lobe and sometimes emphysema. Both are due to bronchial obstruction.

The findings in these cases are so typical that only one diagnostic problem should arise. Sometimes one does have the question of determining whether or not the growth is primary in the lung or represents a lymphatic spread from a malignancy in other locations. In most cases this is easy because of the relative location of the metastatic malignancy. In other cases where the only sign seems to be a hilar enlargement, x-ray differentiation can be most difficult. The problem can usually, but not always, be answered by careful clinical history.

Films in which a question exists should always be referred to an expert roentgenologist.

If confirmation of your diagnosis is made and the patient actually seems to have bronchiogenic carcinoma, he should, of course, be sent to a regional cancer center without delay.

Errors

Two errors occur with some frequency and should be thoughtfully considered:

The first is failure to recognize the possible significance of early hilar enlargement. This should be studied assiduously and bronchoscopy should be done if any question exists.

The second is failure to realize that either atelectasis or emphysema may occur among the first signs of bronchiogenic carcinoma. Both are, of course, due to obstruction of the bronchus.

PLEURISY

Irritative phenomena of the pleura are still relatively common, although it has become out of fashion to diagnose them. One of the most frequent pain-producing mechanisms in the human body is that produced by two inflamed serous surfaces rubbing together. When an inflammatory reaction of the pleura occurs, both visceral and parietal layers usually partake in it and any motion of one on the other is exquisitely painful. In the chest there occurs a restriction of motion to prevent this rubbing together.

Even early in the pleurisy there is some adherence between the two surfaces, although this seldom remains permanent. It is, however, the basis of the most reliable of x-ray signs.

Technique

Fluoroscopic examination is more valuable than radiographic examination in the early stages. Look for the obvious restriction of motion in a portion of the chest and for early signs of adherence.

Normally, intrapulmonary structures near the periphery of the lung change their relative position in regard to the ribs on inspiration and expiration, like this:

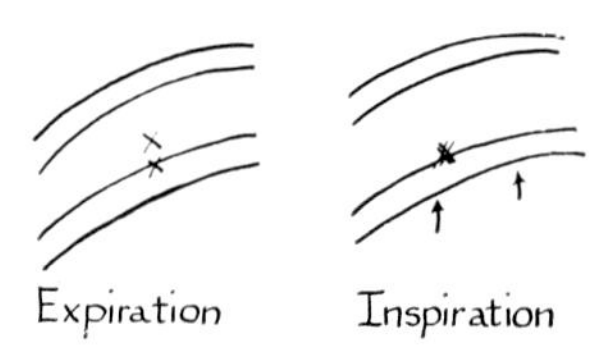

When there is adherence between the two pleural layers in addition to restriction of general respiratory motion, these structures do not change position.

Errors

The most frequent error is failure to look for these signs. They are seldom missed when carefully sought.

PLEURAL EFFUSION

Pleural effusion is much less frequently seen than it was in former years. The reason for this is probably the decrease in the number of cases of tuberculosis. Even so, an unexplained effusion is tuberculous or malignant until proved otherwise.

Since the advent of the antibiotics, effusions are no longer common with the pyogenic infections. Whereas several cases a month were seen in the average practice fifteen or twenty years ago, now it is rare to see one case of pleural effusion a year. During the last five years we have averaged 0.8 case per year.

The condition is mentioned here mainly because of its relationship to early tuberculosis. When effusion is present without clear-cut reason for its existence, one may suspect that between 25 and 50 per cent of these patients will show pulmonary tuberculosis in succeeding months.

The early appearance of fluid in the chest is essentially the same, regardless of whether the fluid be blood, a transudate, an exudate, or a purulent substance. First there is blunting of the costophrenic angle like this:

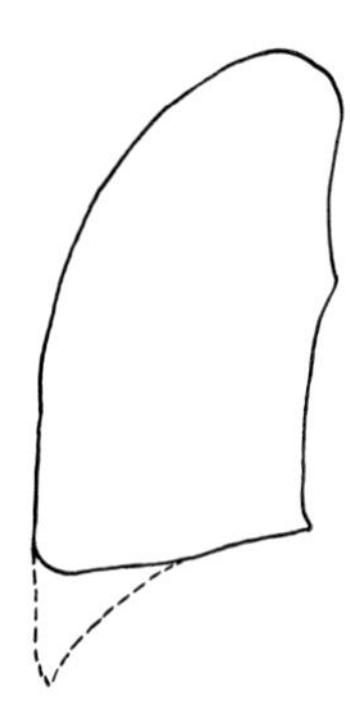

As more fluid is formed, the lung is lifted free from the diaphragm and floats on the fluid, like this:

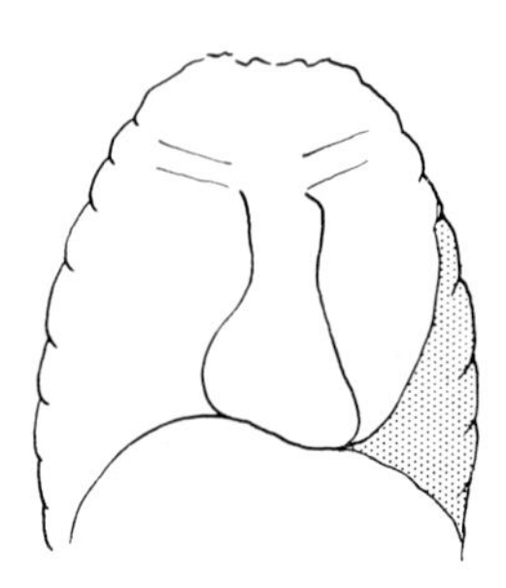

In such a case the lateral roentgenogram is particularly interesting. It usually shows that the fluid ordinarily extends further up posteriorly than anteriorly and that it enters the interlobar fissures, like this:

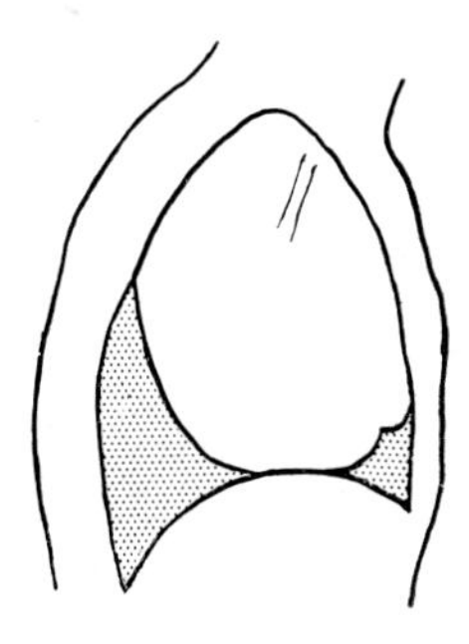

Rarely a collection of fluid will form and be isolated in a specific area of the pleura. An example would be the exudates that form in an interlobar fissure and remain trapped therein.

This happens so infrequently that it is of far more academic than practical interest. You will probably not see more than one case in a decade.

Technique

The posteroanterior and the lateral x-ray films will usually serve to allow diagnosis without further study. In cases involving fluid isolated between the lobes, an x-ray should be taken with the rays paralleling the interlobar fissure. Here is an example which was taken in the posteroanterior position:

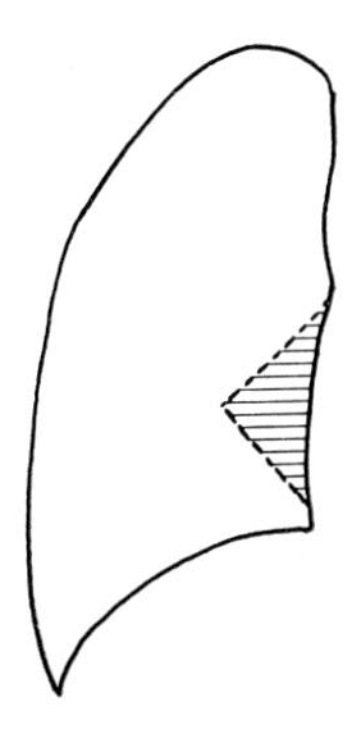

and this one in the lordotic position:

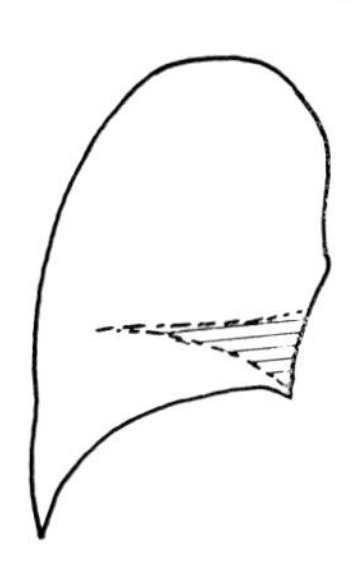

Interpretation

From the x-ray plate alone one can only say that fluid exists in the chest and then give a good estimate as to whether it is encapsulated or restricted in free movement by adhesions.

Diagnosis of the nature of the fluid usually remains a clinical problem. Expert roentgenologists can often give a canny estimate as to the origin of the fluid, as well as its type, but such diagnostic pronouncements from the film alone do not lie in the realm of the practitioner nor are they necessary.

Errors

Small pleural effusions which merely fill the costophrenic angle are missed with surprising frequency. There is no excuse for this except that one simply fails to look at the film. While radiologists never understand how this can happen, we practitioners at least can sympathize with each other.

The harried physician with twenty more patients to see sometimes is inclined to glance superficially at an x-ray film rather than to examine it carefully. Perhaps you would be interested in a technique we used in my small clinic hospital to avoid these errors. Once or twice a week we had lunch served in the x-ray room, or a view box brought to the hospital study, where, during lunch, we carefully went over all films taken during the preceding two or three days. This can be done without interfering with the busy practice and you will be surprised how much you will learn about x-ray by reading the films not only at the minute, but also in retrospect.

Interlobar effusions are so rare that we are inclined to forget the possibility of their existence, and unless reminded rather forcefully by an occasional case, we sometimes puzzle over such a film. I would suggest you obtain a textbook on x-ray diagnosis that maps out the projection of various interlobar pathologies and memorize this mapping. Then when such a lesion is seen you will suspect immediately that it is something in an interlobar fissure and order proper x-ray films to prove it.

Encapsulated effusions are sometimes easy and sometimes extremely difficult to diagnose. I would suggest that all films in which this is a possibility be submitted to a qualified radiologist.

PNEUMOTHORAX

The major pneumothoraces and the severe hemopneumothoraces which occur frequently in practice are problems unsuited to the office. Clinical diagnosis is so simple and hospitalization so necessary that it is improper to waste time even on the office x-ray in such a case.

There are, however, certain cases of partial pneumothorax due to a ruptured bulla (even one of pinhead size) which are seen in the office. Such cases may be diagnosed clinically, but a confirmatory x-ray usually shows the extent of the process and may be an excellent guide to treatment.

This accident is by no means one that applies solely to the person with obvious lung pathology. Certainly, a person with emphysema or chronic inflammatory disease of the lung is subject to rupture and escape of air into the pleura. On the other hand, most of the cases we have seen occurred in otherwise perfectly healthy people. Frequently a spontaneous pneumothorax occurs as a result of effort.

Notice that when you try to pick up something heavy, for example, you are inclined muscularly to force expiration against a closed glottis. The grunt of effort is a release of this phenomenon. Such action builds up pressure quickly in the lung and a weak spot may simply rupture.

Surprisingly, we have seen quite a few cases in young children, including several in the newborn infant. Apparently they were brought about by strain while crying but, of course, we have no way to be sure.

Technique

Ordinarily, the straight posteroanterior film will be all that is necessary to demonstrate the partially collapsed lung and air surrounding it.

Interpretation

The diagnosis will be made clinically. X-ray serves only to clarify the extent of the process and sometimes to give a clue as to why it occurred.

The expected x-ray picture is obvious. It looks like this:

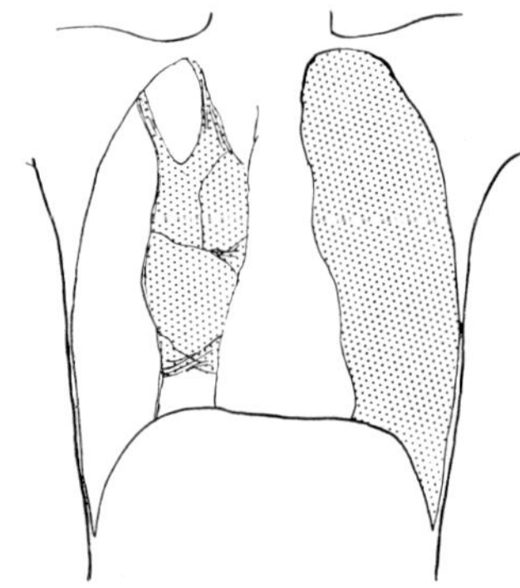

Errors

The principal error is using x-ray to make an obvious diagnosis. Another error is to subject patients with mediastinal shift and extreme respiratory difficulty, etc., to office examination, since they should be referred to the hospital.

CHAPTER TWENTY-FOUR

The Heart and Vessels

Radiography of the heart is not nearly as rewarding a procedure as many physicians think it is. Indications of cardiac enlargement, either general or regional, are often clearly manifest but are usually equally apparent or inferrible from clinical examination.

The practitioner would do well to use a minimum of cardiac x-ray. Costwise the fluoroscopic examination is much better (usually $3 as against $10) and will actually give more information. A film has no superiority as a permanent record over a series of carefully dictated notes following fluoroscopy.

THE NORMAL HEART

Positioning for radiographic examination is not greatly different from that used in fluoroscopy. In the posteroanterior view the heart borders are made up of the following structures:

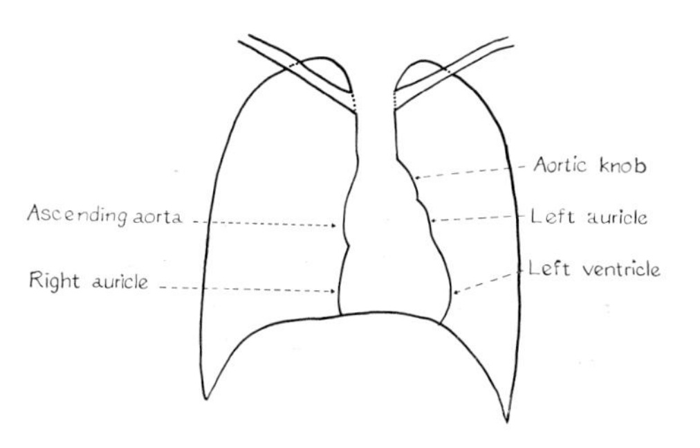

In the right oblique view the patient is positioned like this:

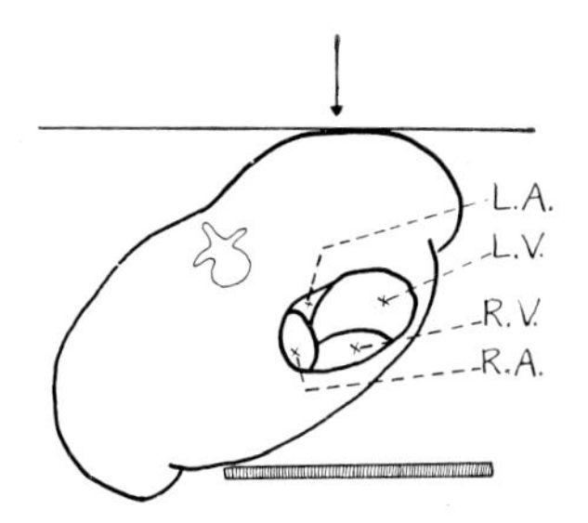

and these normal structures are seen:

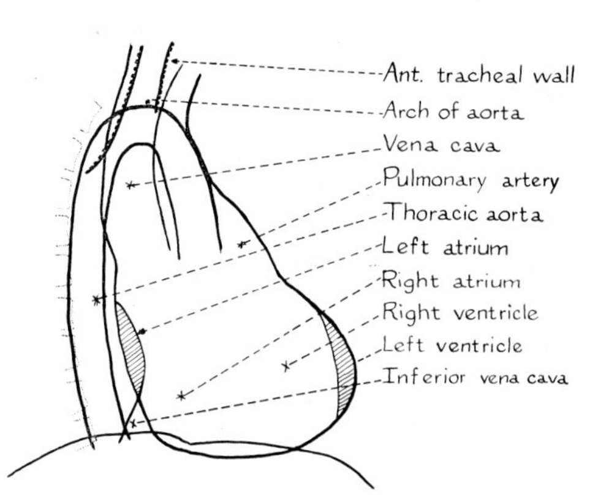

Notice particularly that the left atrium and the left ventricle make up the "edges" of the cardiac shadow. Enlargement, if localized to either chamber, will immediately become apparent in the film or upon fluoroscopy.

Left oblique views present these structures:

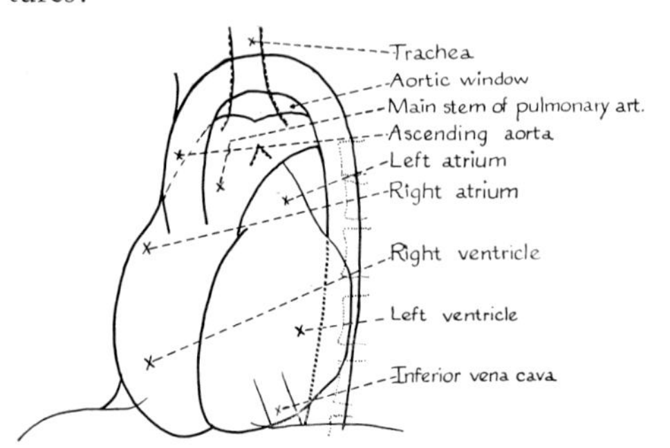

In deciding what a normal heart is, one must take into consideration the deviations in cardiac placement that may occur due to body habitus. A tall, thin man may have a long, narrow heart, like this:

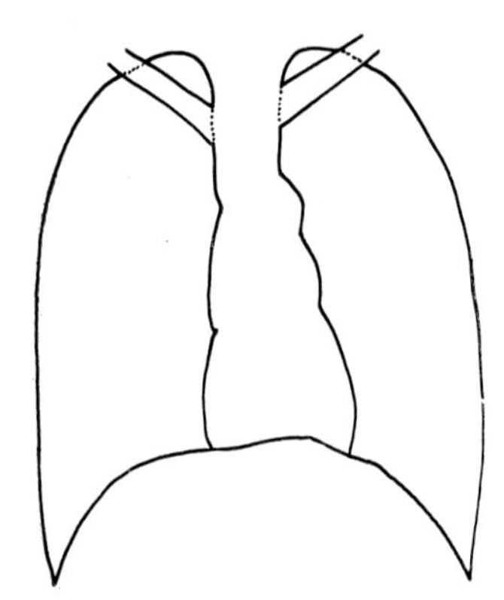

and a short, fat man may have a heart with an axis much more nearly transverse, like this:

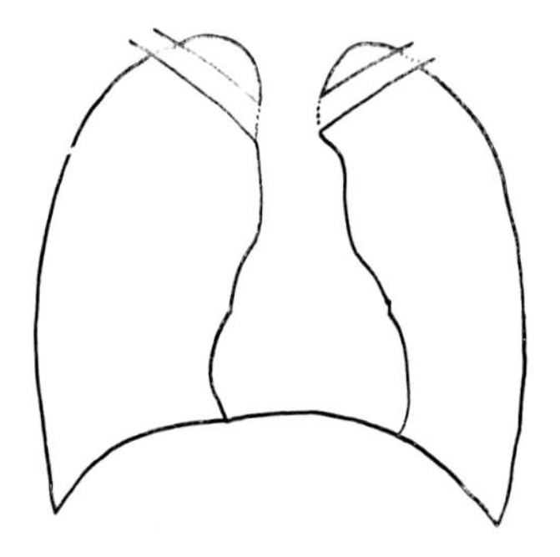

It is only in its relationship to general body build that the heart may be considered abnormal. Surprisingly enough, many mistakes are made because of failure to remember this simple fact.

CARDIAC FLUOROSCOPY

Cardiac fluoroscopy is more valuable to the practitioner than is x-ray. It permits a dynamic view of the heart in action, whereas the film is a "spot check" with abnormalities in action or inferred from heart contours.

The most important part of fluoroscopy is that it allows one to visualize the motions of the heart borders engendered by systole. Any abnormality of this cardiac action can be detected immediately. Certain factors are of parallel importance in this observation. They are as follows:

1. The point of opposite pulsations. When the ventricles contract, a charge of blood is extruded and the outflow tract of the heart enlarges as this ventricular output enters it, like this:

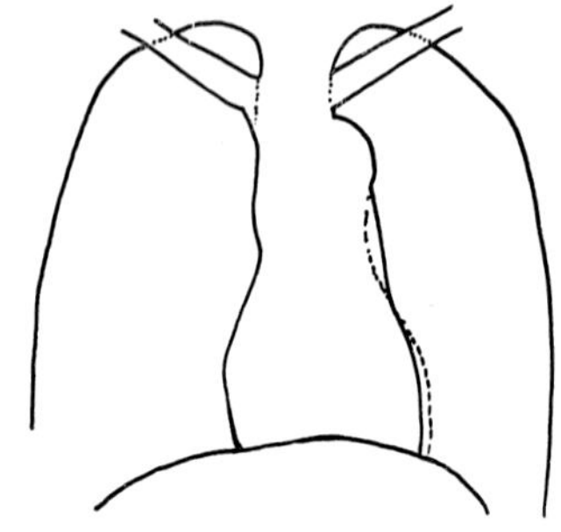

Gradually, as the blood is propelled peripherally, the outflow tract resumes its normal size. This cyclic motion gives the left border of the heart a walking beam or seesaw motion, like this:

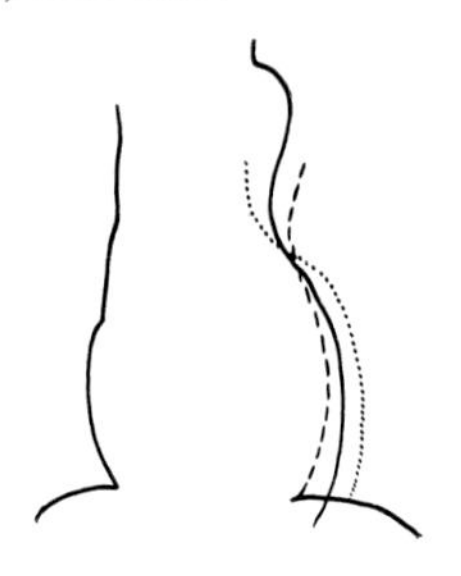

It is extremely important to identify the location of the point of opposite pulsation, which is no more than the fulcrum of the seesaw motion. This can usually be done by careful observation. Sometimes it is necessary to reduce the opening of the fluoroscopic diaphragm to a horizontal slit about one or two inches wide. One then observes the left atrial border and lowers the screen until the point becomes obvious.

In various conditions which cause enlargement of the ventricles, the point of opposite pulsation is obviously raised from the normal. There is no hard and fast rule stating where it should be, but one or two observations on the normal heart will delineate clearly the approximate area to be occupied by the point of opposite pulsation.

2. Relative strength of the pulsation. Normally the pulsations are most intense near the cardiac apex and gradually decrease in point of excursion as one follows the left cardiac border upward. The pulsations of the left border are two or three times as great as those in the right border.

A particular characteristic of the pulsation is its homogeneity. As one watches, it becomes apparent that it is obviously a part of a single movement. When a portion of the cardiac musculature is impaired in function so that it does not contact properly, it becomes equally apparent upon observation that this homogeneity of movement is lost.

After a severe infarction, when all that remains is a thin shell of scar tissue in a portion of the cardiac border, this portion may actually expand outward, while the normal muscle contracts like this:

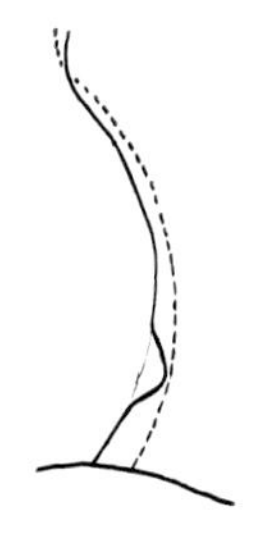

In practice such findings are rare.

If there is difficulty making out the left cardiac border or in following its action, a sheet of heavy black artist's paper may be cut like this:

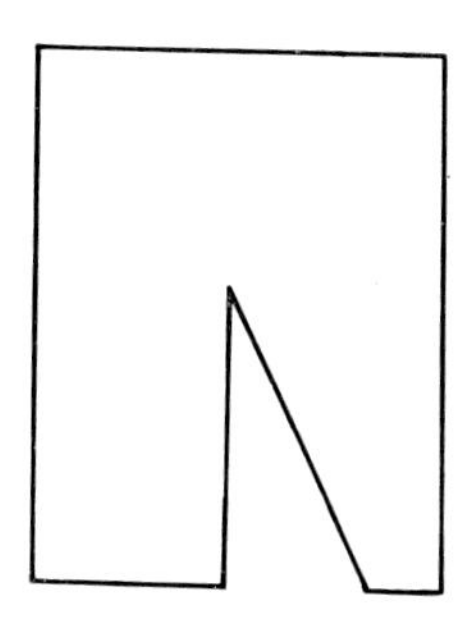

and the screen moved so that the cardiac border is silhouetted within the "V" cut in the paper.

Occasionally one may gain a great deal of information by having the patient take a swallow of barium solution, noticing any displacement of the esophagus caused by changes in the cardiac outline as it is swallowed. This procedure is done often enough in practice that it is probably wise to have a glass of barium mixture prepared during all cases of cardiac fluoroscopy.

HYPERTROPHY AND DILATATION

Cardiac hypertrophy and dilatation might be named dramatically the "protest of an overloaded heart." This condition does invariably result when the heart is called upon for work greater than that of which it is normally capable. The diseases which might cause this are, of course, legion. Hypertension is probably the most often seen and valvular disease is next in frequency.

The process may occur as a generalized phenomenon or it may occur involving specific chambers. As seen by the practitioner, it most often begins as a left ventricular process and inexorably continues until all of the chambers are involved to some degree. Depending largely upon the area in which one practices and upon the "doctor consciousness" of his patients, one will see either hypertrophy and dilatation in its earliest stages or (as I did) will see the patient after generalized involvement has taken place and each gasp seems the last one.*

If this seems hard for some younger physicians to believe, I shall have to tell you about a man who broke his arm while plowing in the field. He put it in a sling, finished his plowing, went home, spent the night with his folks, and came in to see the doctor in the morning. He said he did not want to bother me at night and waited until 5 A.M., when he "was sure I would be up."

It is, of course, easy to tell both clinically and by x-ray what chambers of the heart are enlarged.

Technique

If one wishes to use roentgenology, the posteroanterior view and both oblique projections will usually give all the information that is necessary.

A systematic fluoroscopic examination will give even more information. Begin by examining the patient with the rays passing through his chest posteroanteriorly. Note the outline of various structures and increase the penetration just a little bit to check for left auricular enlargement as mentioned below. Then give the patient a swallow of barium and note any deviations of the esophagus. This should also be done in the lateral projection.

When you have completed your observations, it is well to make a record like this: Have the patient stand with the anterior chest wall as close to the fluoroscopic screen as possible (i.e., in the normal anterior position) and use a wax marking pencil to outline the cardiac borders and the inner border of the thorax on the fluoroscopic screen. When the fluoroscope is shut off and the lights turned on, your fluoroscopic screen should look like this:

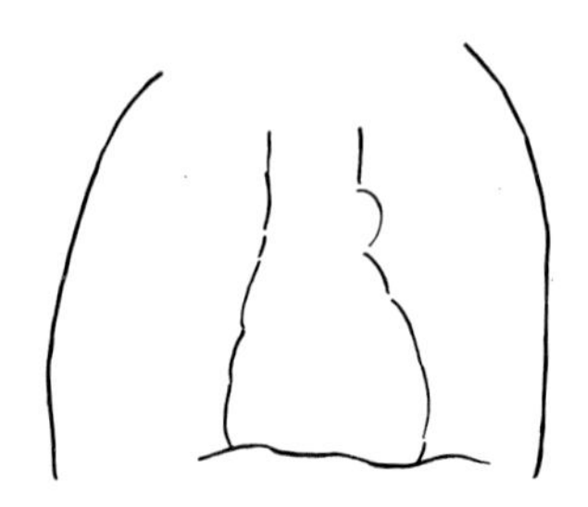

Now take a second to transfer this picture as a sketch to the patient's record and then clean the fluoroscopic screen by wiping with acetone.

This procedure is just as valuable as any x-ray in a one- or two-man practice, for it allows you not only to sketch what is seen in the chest accurately, but you can also mark down measurements from the fluoroscopic screen and have a record which certainly approaches in accuracy that offered by x-ray. Since this record has been taken from a dynamic picture, it is sometimes even more accurate than an identical record taken as a spot check film.

Interpretation

The simplest way to remember the pathologic entities involved is to say that in the blood flow tract the chamber behind the lesion is the one that enlarges. In systemic hypertension, for example, the left ventricle must bear the brunt of the increased peripheral resistance and, therefore, it enlarges. Left ventricular enlargement would also be a primary finding in disease of the aortic valve whether it is stenosis or regurgitation.

*For many years my practice was among hearty pioneer stock who believed that anyone who was well enough to crawl up to my hospital and scratch on the front door was frivolously wasting time seeing a physician. Expenditure of money for such trivial things as medical care was something one did when it was necessary to be carried in to see the doctor.

Mitral stenosis would tend to cause hypertrophy and dilatation of the left atrium and, if severe, the left ventricle and then the right ventricle. Increased resistance in the pulmonary circulation would cause primary hypertrophy and dilatation in the right ventricle, etc.

Early enlargement of the left ventricle causes moderate rounding of the cardiac contour and raising of the point of opposite pulsations, like this:

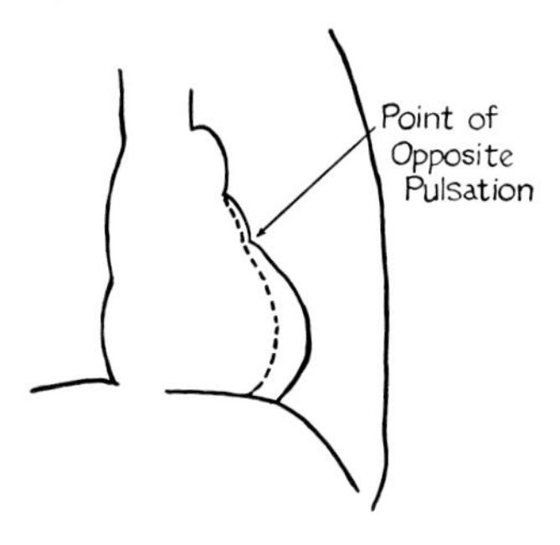

In the earliest stages the changes are so slight that they are not well seen on the x-ray film.

As the enlargement progresses, the apex extends leftward and downward so that the entire left border of the heart extends outward, upward, and downward, like this:

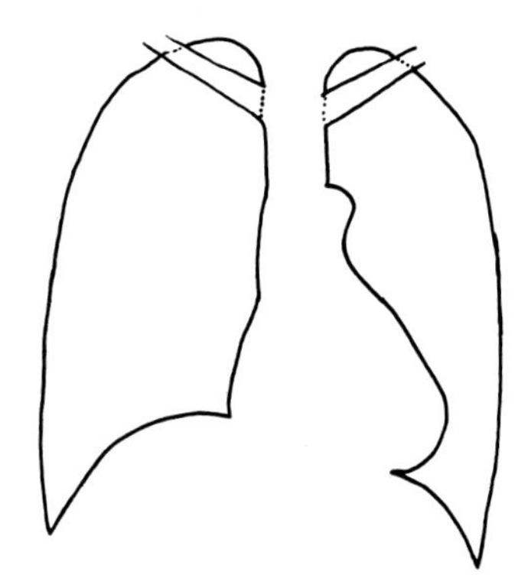

In the left oblique view there is normally a clear space between the posterior border of the ventricle and the spine. As ventricular hypertrophy and dilatation occur this clear space is obliterated and the ventricular shadow impinges upon the vertebral shadow, like this:

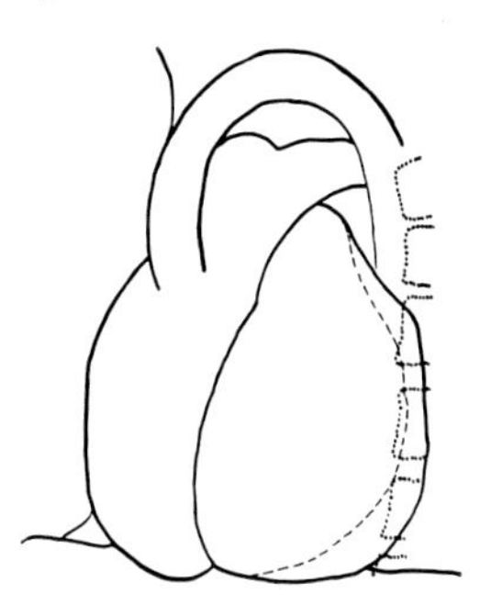

The important thing to remember is that in early stages there may be no great change in cardiac measurement. The only thing that may be seen is increased roundness in the left border of the heart and some protrusion toward the spine in the left oblique view.

Enlargement of the left atrium takes place with protrusion posteriorly and to the right. There are four signs commonly seen.

The first is a straightening of the left border of the heart in the anterior projection, like this:

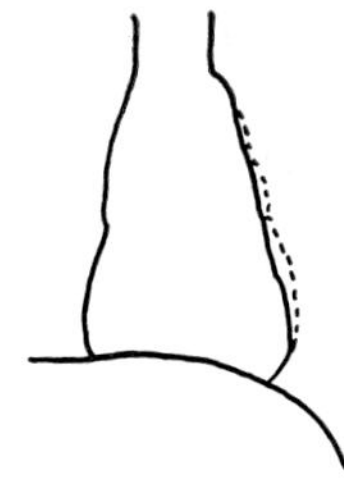

Occasionally a ball-like density may be seen behind the heart shadow, like this:

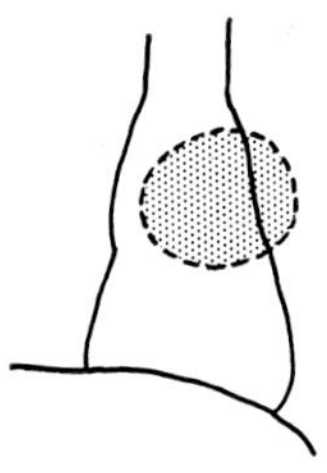

It consists of the dilated left atrium filled with blood. This is most often demonstrated on the roentgenogram and is the least important of the various signs of atrial enlargement.

In the right oblique position the enlarged atrium eliminates a portion of the space normally seen between the heart and the spine. This may be even better demonstrated by following a swallow of barium as it passes through the displaced esophagus. The picture looks like this:

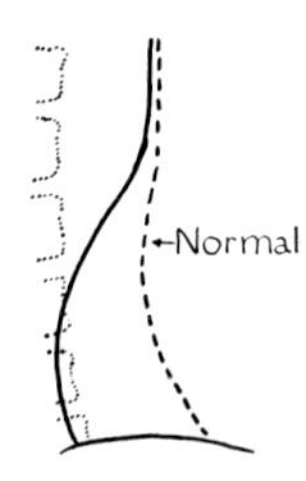

The two signs, posterior bulging in the right oblique view and displacement of the esophagus, are probably the most reliable roentgenologic and fluoroscopic signs of left atrial enlargement. Not rarely may they antedate any physical findings. When such things appear in a nominally healthy patient, proceed cautiously.

Enlargement of the right ventricle is the most difficult to diagnose insofar as individual cardiac chambers are concerned. There is a prominence and an elongation of the right middle pulmonary segment, like this:

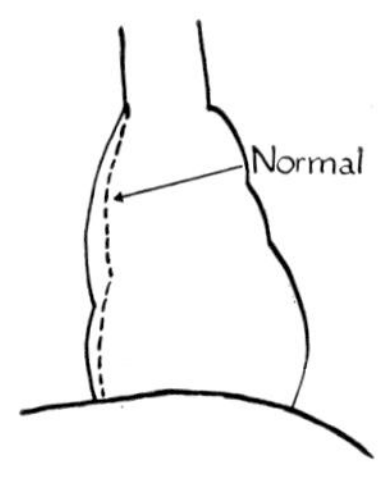

In the right oblique and lateral projections there may be obliteration or great reduction of the normal retrosternal space, like this:

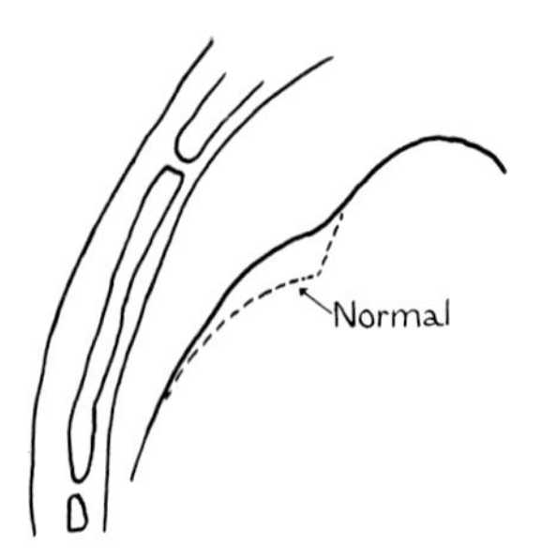

Right atrial enlargement is usually simply diagnosed by the outward displacement seen in the lower segment of the right cardiac silhouette, like this:

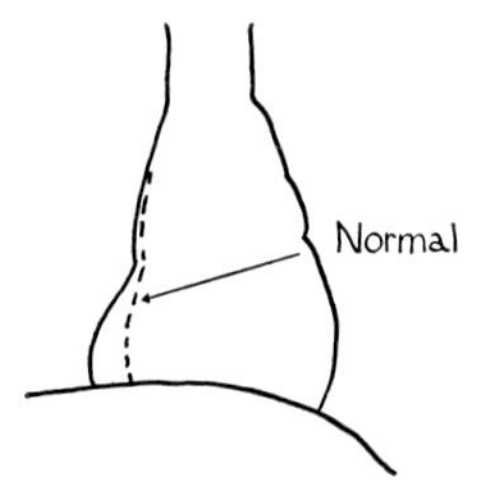

Errors

The most frequent error made with both films and the fluoroscope is to diagnose left ventricular enlargement when it does not exist. Various positions of the normal heart may closely simulate enlargement of the left ventricle in the anterior projection. If the physician will keep two facts in mind, however, it is unlikely that he will make mistakes on this point.

The first fact is that early signs usually consist principally of a rounding of the ventricular contour and not of expansion in its diameter. The second fact is that a left anterior projection will usually show that the normal heart is anterior in the chest, leaving a definite clear space between the cardiac border and the spine. This is not true in a case of left ventricular enlargement.

A good history and physical examination will often supply just as much information about enlargement of the cardiac chambers as will the x-ray. Quite obviously the x-ray is something one can see and the history and physical examination provide only something that must be inferred. Nonetheless, the good physician should have no hesitancy in accepting the obvious inference.

A severe mitral stenosis with obvious signs of pulmonary congestion means that the left atrium is enlarged. X-ray or, more particularly, the fluoroscope provides the best means at our command for estimating the size of the enlargement. This information is often of great value but seldom of lifesaving value. In the ordinary course of practice a cardiac fluoroscopy should probably be done on such patients and results computed in total evaluation. To depend upon fluoroscopy or x-ray for diagnosis in such a case is tantamount to an admission of incompetence on the part of the physician.

ROGER'S DISEASE

The interventricular septal defect known for years as maladie de Roger is one of the commonest congenital malformations of the heart that we see. The defect is usually relatively small and generally relatively innocuous. On the other hand, the patient is usually brought to roentgenology because of the harsh systolic murmur heard in this area:

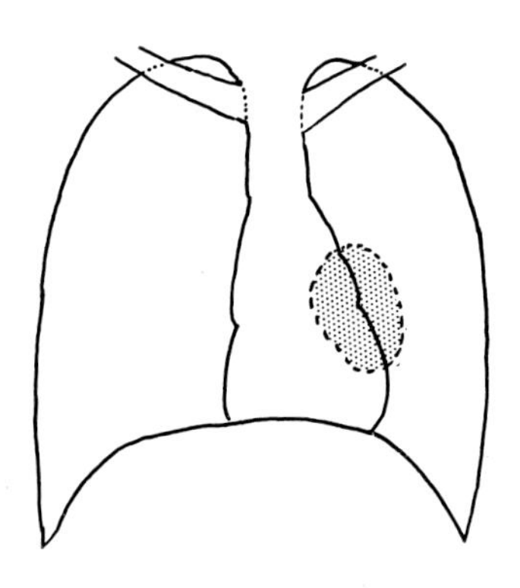

Most frequently there are no symptoms and the only x-ray finding is enlargement of the pulmonary arterial segment.

Technique

The ordinary posteroanterior film or posteroanterior fluoroscopy will give all the information that is needed.

Interpretation

There are no characteristic x-ray signs of Roger's disease. In connection with the murmur heard clinically, one usually sees some degree of enlargement of the pulmonary aterial segments, like this:

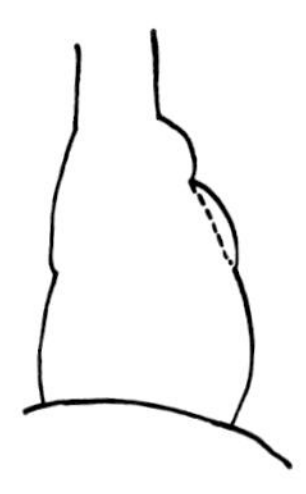

This finding is typical and, in conjunction with the clinical symptoms, is essentially diagnostic.

Massive interventricular septal defects do occur with tremendous dilatation of the pulmonary segments, but the average practitioner will not see one of these in a lifetime.

Errors

The most frequent error is to assume that the interventricular septal defect means a great deal more than it does. If there are no impairments in cardiac rate and rhythm, the patient is developing well, and the x-ray signs simply show an enlargement of the pulmonary arterial segments, chances are overwhelmingly in favor of an essentially normal life for the patient.

Admittedly, the murmur sounds horrible and the x-ray signs confirm the fact that disease exists. The prognosis depends upon careful clinical evaluation, not upon the bare fact that these signs exist.

INTRA-ATRIAL DEFECTS

The foramen ovale remains essentially open (i.e., covered only by a membrane in from 20 to 30 per cent of normal people). Defects in closure of the foramen ovale are the most common cardiac malformations seen by the practitioner.

Blood, of course, travels from the left atrium to the right atrium, overloading the left side of the heart and not sufficiently loading the left ventricle. The obvious changes take place.

There are hypertrophy and dilatation of the right ventricle and atrium, with tremendous dilatation of the pulmonary artery. The left ventricle is small and the aorta is usually small and atrophic. The radiologic signs are typical.

Here is a common picture:

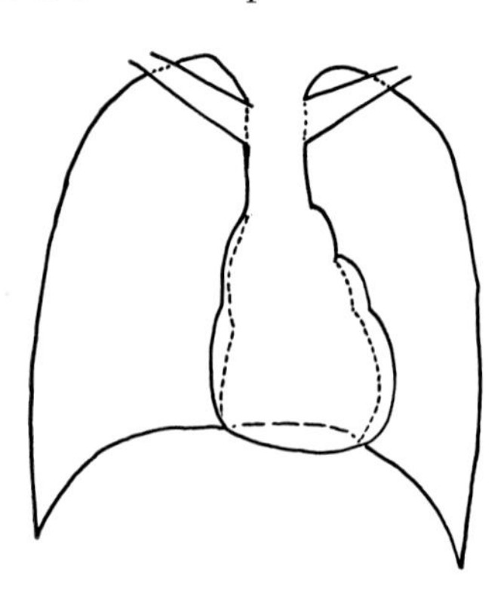

Technique

The ordinary posteroanterior film will usually demonstrate sufficient changes to allow diagnosis in connection with clinical symptoms. Occasionally, oblique views will demonstrate enlargement of the right atrium and ventricle when it is not entirely clear on the posteroanterior film. If there exists a real question, we make it a point to order the oblique studies.

Interpretation

The obvious enlargement of the right heart, along with dilatation of the pulmonary artery, is typical. Usually this pulmonary dilatation is more apparent on the right than on the left and the dilated branches may be traceable far into the lung fields. These findings in conjunction with the small aorta and obviously normal-sized left ventricle give one a tip-off that can hardly be ignored.

Errors

Errors are practically unheard of in diagnosing this condition. Diagnosis is simple and apparent in most cases, both clinically and roentgenologically. This is not true when very young babies are studied by x-ray, but it holds for adults.

CHAPTER TWENTY-FIVE

The Gastrointestinal Tract

The gastrointestinal tract is a radiologic challenge to the average practitioner. However, any physician willing to work and study can do perfectly adequate x-ray examination in the routine case. The problem is to know when to seek help.

Many well-qualified men take a viewpoint exactly opposite to the one just expressed. They say that the physician should not examine the gastrointestinal tract unless he has had long years of specialized training. As the reason for their opinion they cite the mistakes often made by those who are careless and do not realize their own limitations.

The truth of the matter probably lies somewhere between the extremes. The young general physician should learn as much as he can about gastrointestinal x-ray. Since he has little training when he leaves internship, he is not competent to do the work alone at first. On the other hand, one cannot learn by wishful thinking. Do the work for yourself but have your results checked by an expert if there is the slightest doubt. For several years this will mean that ninety-five of every one hundred cases will need to be checked.

As time passes and experience accumulates there will be less and less need for checking, until, after six or seven years, only the more obtuse cases need be sent to the radiologist. Probably the point of greatest importance is this: *Never get overconfident.* No matter how much gastrointestinal work the practitioner does, his experience is much less and his judgment poorer than that of the qualified roentgenologist. No matter how long one has been d o i n g gastrointestinal roentgenology the services of an expert should be sought for any case that is not perfectly clear-cut.

CARDIOSPASM

There is much question at present about the etiology of cardiospasm. For many years it was thought to be purely functional —a spasm involving the musculature of the lower esophagus and nothing else. Now evidence is accumulating that it may be a congenital defect in nerve cells. Nonetheless, we certainly do have adequate proof that the condition involves more than just a spasm of lower esophageal musculature.

The disease usually progresses at least intermittently for years. It begins as a spasm of the lower two or three inches of the esophagus. This may be the only manifestation for months or for several years. Inevitably there is progression, with a loss of normal peristaltic contraction in the lower half or more of the esophagus. The usual regular, smooth waves of contraction are replaced by irregular and incoordinate contractions easily visible on fluoroscopy.

As the disease progresses further, there is a loss of tone in the upper segment with dilation.

Technique

Fluoroscopy is the best means of diagnosis. Start by giving the patient a thin barium mixture and watching it transverse the esophagus. Next give a swallow or two of thick barium-water mixture and observe as it passes into the stomach.

If one is suspicious of cardiospasm at this stage but still lacks absolute confirmation, make that horror of horrors, the barium sandwich. Prepare two slices of buttered bread and with a knife apply a liberal amount of a barium-water mixture that is at least as thick as butter. "Allow" the patient to eat this delicacy while you observe the passage of the heavy barium down the esophagus.

Interpretation

In early cases one will observe a conical narrowing of the lower esophageal segment at a diaphragmatic level. It looks like this:

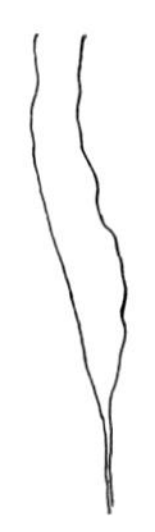

Such narrowing is often described as beak-like as it sometimes has that appearance.

For the purposes of differential diagnosis, notice whether the beak changes shape with respiration. In most cases, contraction of the diaphragm on inspiration causes a narrowing and change of contour. Relaxation of the diaphragm on expiration allows the barium to slip past the spastic area into the stomach. It looks like this:

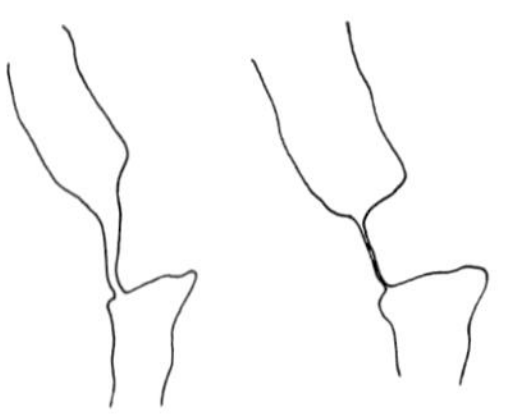

As the case becomes more advanced, normal propulsion waves in the esophagus are replaced along the lower third with irregular and random contractions which look like this:

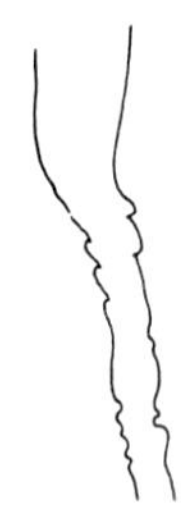

These contractions give an odd pattern of movement to the esophagus, which has been described as "shimmying" or "writhing." Neither word does justice to the actual appearance, but once seen it will never be forgotten.

In late cases dilation of the esophagus may occur. Findings, of course, are obvious.

Errors

An early interstitial carcinoma may be difficult, if not impossible, to differentiate from early cardiospasm. The defect seen in carcinoma, of course, is rigid and does not change with respiration. Neither are there major changes in peristaltic activity in the average carcinoma. This sounds as if differentiation would be easy, but it is not.

The best advice that can be given is to take a careful history and use this as one measure of making proper differentiation. If the case is one of some years' standing, beginning in the twenties or thirties, and its findings are more or less typical of cardiospasm, then it is reasonably safe to make this diagnosis.

If, on the other hand, symptoms are of recent origin and the findings are not clear-cut, showing essentially nothing but narrowing of the last one or two inches of the esophagus, then one has a problem. Make repeated observations over a sixty-day period. If you still cannot be sure, send the patient to an endoscopist for verification. The mathematical odds are probably about one thousand to one in favor of cardiospasm.

Is there a functional disease simulating in all respects, except x-ray findings, the picture we have just outlined? It is my impression that there probably is but that a careful history will show the difference between the obviously organic symptoms of progressive cardiospasm and the equally obvious psychogenic picture of incoordinate swallowing of the psychoneurotic patient. Nothing is written by the authorities on this problem, but simple observation would seem to indicate that the two entities do exist.

HIATAL HERNIA

Symptoms of the hiatal hernia commonly develop between the ages of 45 and 60 but are usually so inconclusive as to make diagnosis practically impossible from the standpoint of history and physical examination alone. This is unquestionably one of the diseases in which x-ray is the single, most important factor in diagnosis.

The problems of etiology are such that one cannot obtain a clear-cut picture of what happened. The literature is rife with theories, many of them substantiated to some degree, but none, to my knowledge, proved beyond any shadow of a doubt. For that reason we can only say here that a herniation of the upper part of the stomach into the posterior mediastinum does occur.

Over a period of time a significant number of these hernias become incarcerated so that there is some permanent fixation of a portion of stomach in the posterior mediastinum. Such hernias are not difficult to diagnose. The sliding hernias, on the other hand, almost invariably require special procedures for their demonstration.

Technique

Incarcerated hernias with a portion of the stomach fixed above the diaphragm are so apparent that the most casual fluoroscopic examination with barium will serve to demonstrate them. Special techniques should be used probably in all patients over the age of 45 who are examined fluoroscopically.

After preliminary examination in the erect position, have the patient lie on the table. Lower the head of the table 10 or 15 degrees while watching the stomach fluoroscopically. In many cases, the stomach will be seen to slide through the diaphragm and reproduce the hernia. If this does not happen, have the patient continue to breathe quietly, but ask him to raise both legs off the table. This will heighten intra-abdominal pressure and almost certainly demonstrate a hernia if one is present. Incidentally, while the patient is raising his legs he should continue to breathe quietly.

As a practical point you should remember that when a patient raises both legs from the table while in the Trendelenburg position, he may suddenly slide off and fall on his head. A pair of shoulder braces or an assistant in proper position may prevent this unusual happening.

Next, while the patient is still in the Trendelenburg position, have him take a swallow or two of moderately thick barium mixture. This will at least partially fill a hernia if one is present and make it quite obvious. It is a good idea to use a wax pencil and sketch the outline of the hernia on the fluoroscopic screen. This sketch can then be transferred to the patient's record and will provide an excellent means of permanent recording.

Interpretation

Interpretation is entirely simple. Either there is a hernia or none exists.

Errors

The procedure is practically not subject to error. The principal mistake is failure to look for a hiatal hernia in patients who might conceivably have one.

Another mistake is to assume that no hernia exists because an incarcerated one is not found in the erect position. To be relatively certain that hiatal hernia is absent one must go through all the procedures outlined above.

ESOPHAGEAL VARICES

Esophageal varices are not common. The average practitioner will see from six to ten cases a year. They result when pressure is increased in the portal venous system. The most common reason for this pressure increase is undoubtedly cirrhosis of the liver. Various splenic diseases or vascular disease may be at the root of the condition. Actually, the varicosities are not often suspected until bleeding occurs, for they are essentially asymptomatic. The majority of cases will be seen during or after a major hemorrhage. They are hospital problems in this stage. Office work is contraindicated.

Since there is no known treatment, their demonstration is of more prognostic than therapeutic significance. The pathologic dilatation usually begins in the lower segment of the esophagus and then extends upward. In advanced cases varicosities may be seen involving almost the entire length of the tube.

Technique

Give the patient small quantities of thick barium mixture to swallow and then examine him in the erect, supine, and Trendelenburg positions. The fluoroscope will often demonstrate the veins, but films should be taken in each position.

Interpretation

There are usually filling defects caused by the engorged veins. Since these veins run up and down the esophagus the defects are often linear. They look like this:

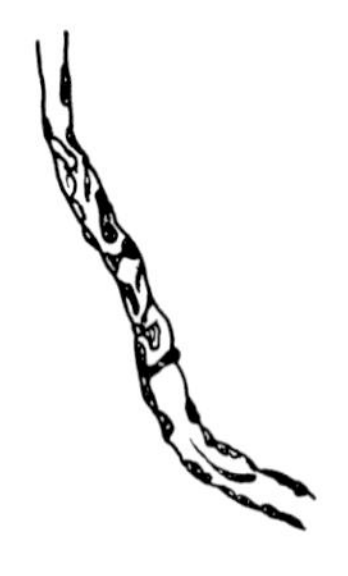

In older cases the esophagus becomes dilated and may show a slight tortuosity. In such a case the varicosities look like this:

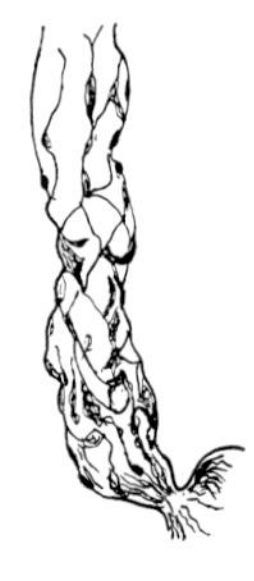

Notice that the varicosities in this picture extend distalward and actually appear in the upper portion of the stomach as well as in the esophagus. In the films, even those taken of the empty esophagus, small bits of barium may become caught in the crevices of the varicosities and present a picture that looks like this:

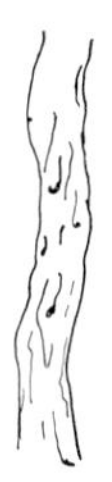

Errors

There is usually no difficulty in diagnosing a case of esophageal varices. This is particularly true of the advanced case. The common error is failure to look for them. It is true that they may not be clearly seen in the barium swallow as done in most gastrointestinal series and that one must have in mind the possibility of their existence if mistakes are to be avoided. A good simple rule to follow is that in all cases of upper gastrointestinal bleeding, examine the esophagus carefully for varicosities.

ESOPHAGEAL CANCER

There are three common sites for esophageal cancer. The upper or postcricoid is most common in women and the lower two sites most common in men, as located here:

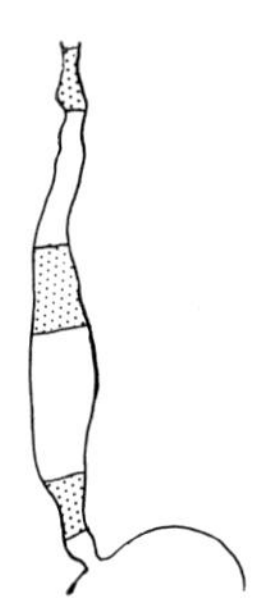

Esophageal cancer fortunately is not common. The therapeutic attack now in use is not particularly satisfactory. Ulcerative type growths are seen but the majority are either proliferative or infiltrative, both of which produce narrowing of the lumen.

Technique

The fluoroscope is more important than the x-ray in making a diagnosis, but when a typical luminar defect is found as described below, rotate the patient so that the defect is examined from every possible position. Have the patient swallow both thick and thin barium and complete your studies.

Interpretation

You will notice almost at once that the normal contractions of the esophagus are lost in the area of the tumor. The walls appear firm and rigid and thick.

The filling defect remains constant and the esophagus may be dilated above it. Frequently the stream of barium may tend to take a corkscrew motion through the obstructed area. Here are two typical filling defects:

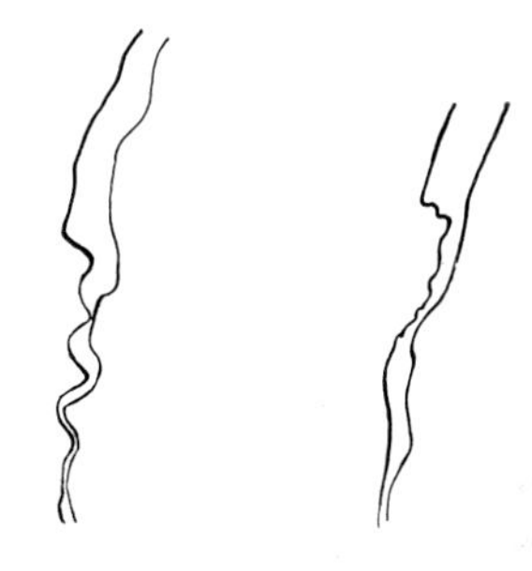

Carcinoma of the lower end may show thickening of the gastric mucosa around the esophageal opening (see page 276) and an almost horizontal positioning of the cardiac ampulla, like this:

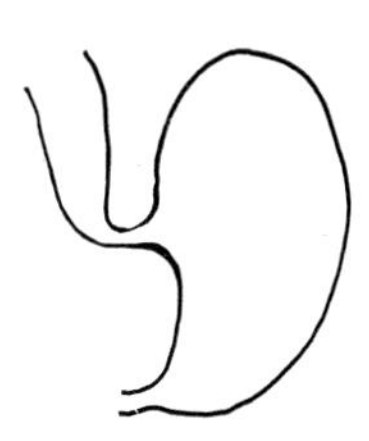

Errors

The most common error is to miss an early growth which only slightly obstructs the passage of barium or shows only a trivial diversion of the barium stream. When such things are seen they should be investigated exhaustively. If the problem is not clarified in a few weeks the patient should be sent to an endoscopist for examination and full report.

THE GASTROINTESTINAL SERIES

This section is presented here to prevent needless repetition. The technique for examining the stomach and duodenum by x-ray is standardized and is used in essentially unchanged form to demonstrate several diseases. Before detailing the technique we use, I would like to offer two comments.

First, adequate gastrointestinal roentgenology is not beyond the physician who will study and submit his results for checking. The thought that only a roentgenologist can see the obvious is ridiculous in the extreme.

If one were to take a hundred gastrointestinal series, as is done in the average practice, the physician would need roentgenologic help on perhaps five to fifteen of them, depending upon the amount of study and experience he has had. This certainly represents no plea that the family physician undertake extensive gastrointestinal roentgenology. There are and always will be many cases which require the services of an expert for diagnosis.

If you wish to do gastric roentgenology, go right ahead, but learn one fact and learn it well. When there is any question in your mind, when you are not sure what a lesion is after adequate examination (and this includes repeat examinations), always without exception submit the case to an expert roentgenologist. In such instances send the patient, not the films, to the roentgenologist.

Second, the complete gastrointestinal series is by no means always necessary. It has become a ritual which is followed to ridiculous lengths at times.

If, for example, one has a clear-cut history and physical examination indicating an esophageal lesion, perform a fluoroscopy and demonstrate the lesion exactly as directed on pages 267 to 271. It is seldom necessary to follow out the entire procedure. Most certainly it is desirable but it may not be financially feasible. This is another point where we sometimes raise the price of medicine beyond its value.

Another example would be a patient well known to you who has had a duodenal ulcer off and on for the ten years in which you have taken care of him. A simple gastric fluoroscopy at intervals will allow you to follow the ulcer perfectly adequately and it will cost the patient from $5 to $10 instead of $35 to $50 as the entire gastrointestinal series does. Such things would not work in a huge clinical practice where patients are followed as numbers and not as individuals. In the office x-ray department, where patients are people, they work with perfect adequacy.

Incidentally, it might be worth a few minutes of your time to think over the fact that big clinic practice and small office practice do not combine easily. Things that would be absolutely unheard of in a clinic employing fifty physicians are common, acceptable, and good in the small office. The opposite is equally true. Those of us in offices must do practical, front-line medicine, and if a procedure does not offer direct and unquestionable benefit to the patient at a minimum of expense, then it ill behooves us to use it.

Technique

Instruct the patient to take a laxative at noon the day before the examination is scheduled. Any of the common saline laxatives such as magnesium sulfate will probably do, although some physicians prefer the irritant laxatives and give castor oil or compound licorice powder. Then request the patient not to take any food after 6 P.M. on the day preceding the examination. Instruct him to take an enema upon arising, continuing until the return is clear, and then to report to the office at about 9 A.M. for the examination.

There are three essential points to this first examination. One should attempt to get a good visualization in mucosal relief. Second, a thorough examination should be made under compression, and, third, examination should be made during and after filling. When these have been completed dismiss the patient with instructions to take a light lunch. Make a single film at 3 or 4 P.M. for the checking of any gastric retention.

In all new patients and in all patients in which you are not positive of the nature of the lesion, both a thoroughgoing fluoroscopy should be done and a film made. If anything, the films are better diagnostic agents than the fluoroscopy. Such extensive examination is not necessary for following lesions the nature of which you are certain you know.

Most modern machines either have or can be equipped with a spot film device. As the practitioner enlarges his roentgenologic abilities, it will be found useful.

When the patient actually reports for examination, several things must be present and ready. There should be three mixtures of barium: one the consistency of soft butter, the second distinctly watery, and the third the consistency of or a little thicker than maple syrup. The practitioner should have been wearing red, dark-adaptation glasses for at least ten minutes before entering the fluoroscopic room and should remove these in the dark room and wait at least one minute before proceeding with the examination.

Various compression devices of balsa wood, felt, or wool should be available. These are obtainable commercially or can be made locally by the physician who is mechanically adept.

Begin by giving the patient a single swallow of the medium barium mixture. With your hand attempt to push it into all portions of the stomach so that the mucosal pattern is outlined. One should, of course, take films of any questionable area and should rotate the patient as necessary to get a thorough view of as much of the mucosa as possible.

Compression views may be useful at this stage but are more often of value when examining the duodenum. If the first mixed barium extrudes into the duodenum, it should be examined for defects in the mucosal pattern, both with and without compression. *Be sure* to get a thorough view of the duodenal cap from several angles and take a minimum of two x-ray films in different planes at least 45 degrees apart. Compression in examining the duodenum is almost a necessity and should not be omitted.

After maximum information has been gained from studying the mucosal pattern, both with and without compression, ask the patient to drink 6 to 8 ounces of the moderately thick barium mixture and watch the stomach fill. During and after this process, watch the peristaltic waves carefully, locating any areas in which they are absent and noticing the depth and progression of the waves themselves.

Occasionally at this stage some stomach secretions are trapped in the prepyloric area and the picture shows a barium level which looks like this:

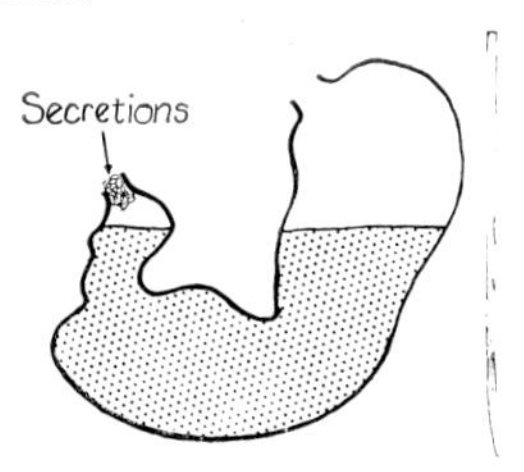

Have the patient lie down for a few minutes on his right side and gently massage the epigastrium. The stomach secretion will float to the top of the barium suspension and ultimately to the cardiac portion of the stomach when he stands up, so that barium rather than secretion occupies the prepyloric area.

You will have noticed that the ordinary examination previously described did not require the use of either the thick or the thin barium mixture. These are used principally when one is dubious about his examination of mucosal relief. Sometimes the barium does not appear to be getting into the cracks and crevices and this can be clarified by giving an additional swallow of thin mixture. Occasionally in the hyperperistaltic, active stomach the thick mixture will be of great service in demonstrating this.

In the normal person there is no retention of barium in the stomach after six hours. Particularly is this true if a light lunch has been taken two or three hours following the examination. Let me emphasize the point that we speak of a light *lunch*—not a full meal. Ordinarily we tell our patients to get a sandwich and a cup of coffee after the examination if they like and report late in the afternoon for a routine film. Retention at this time usually indicates distinct delay in gastric emptying time.

GASTRIC ULCER

There has never been a convincing demonstration of the exact etiology or precise pathologic course of gastric ulcer. We know that in the elderly these ulcers may somtimes occur as a result of arterial disease, but in the vast majority of cases (over 99 per cent) there is some psychogenic factor that operates along with and augments the various organic difficulties as a causative agent.

It can be said that peptic ulcer, both gastric and duodenal, usually originates from autodigestion of the mucous membrane by hydrochloric acid and the various gastric ferments. Whether this occurs due to changes in the usual protective mechanism induced by nerve impulses or whether it occurs as a mechanical reaction we cannot state with clarity. Be that as it may, peptic ulcer is one of the more frequent diseases seen by the practitioner. Gastric ulcers are in the minority, at least four or five duodenal ulcers occurring for each one found in the stomach itself.

The vast majority of gastric ulcers are on the lesser curvature in the lower two thirds, as shown here:

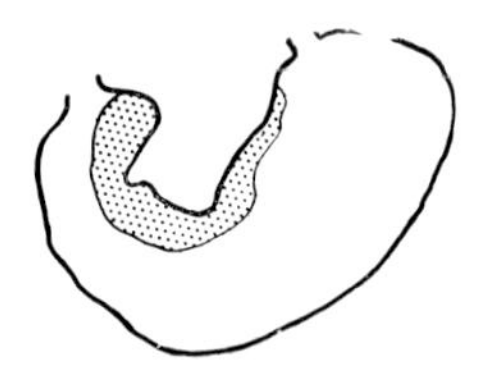

It has been rightly said that an ulcer elsewhere in the stomach should be considered malignant until definitely proved otherwise.

History and physical examination usually give such a clear-cut picture of the malfunctioning dyspeptic stomach that x-ray may become a secondary factor of great practical value but not primary to the diagnosis. In other words, after careful clinical evaluation you know that an ulcer exists or that the stage is set for the occurrence of one. When this point is reached, the function of x-ray is to demonstrate the possible existence of a crater and not whether functional disease of the stomach is present. This point cannot be made too strongly. The x-ray only demonstrates whether or not a crater exists. One depends entirely upon clinical means to determine whether or not stomach malfunction is present. A negative gastrointestinal series does *not* mean that no disease is present. It indicates that no ulcer crater was demonstrated and that none may be present. The basic disease pattern intimately associated with ulcer is determined clinically, not roentgenographically.

In the most expert hands the x-ray is probably as much as 90 per cent accurate in a single examination, and if several serial examinations are done, accuracy probably approaches 98 per cent insofar as gastric ulceration is concerned. In the hands of the practitioner who is careful and conscientious the percentage probably ranges about 80 to 85 per cent on initial examination and after repeated examinations, accuracy of 90 to 92 or 93 per cent.

I must repeat and assure you that this is accuracy in demonstrating an ulcer crater. Accuracy in diagnosing functional disturbances of the stomach should approach 100 per cent without x-ray.

Technique

After a preparatory fluoroscopic survey of the chest and abdomen, give the patient a swallow of barium and examine the esophagus as mentioned on page 268. Utilizing this single swallow of barium or a little more if necessary, apply pressure in order to push it into all parts of the stomach, using the whitewash technique. If this is carefully done and the patient examined from several angles, one should be able to see a good portion of the gastric mucosa.

Compression should be used to identify the rugae on anterior and posterior walls. There are several positive findings of ulcer at this stage of the examination, one being an extension of the barium from the normal stomach contour outward, usually forming a button-shaped protrusion, like this:

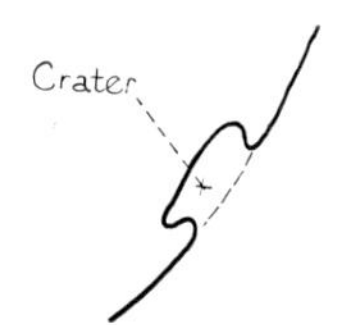

The protrusion is most often on the lesser curvature of the stomach or near it, and slight rotation of the patient in either direction will often bring it sharply into focus.

Occasionally an ulcer will be seen face-on when compression is used. It looks like this:

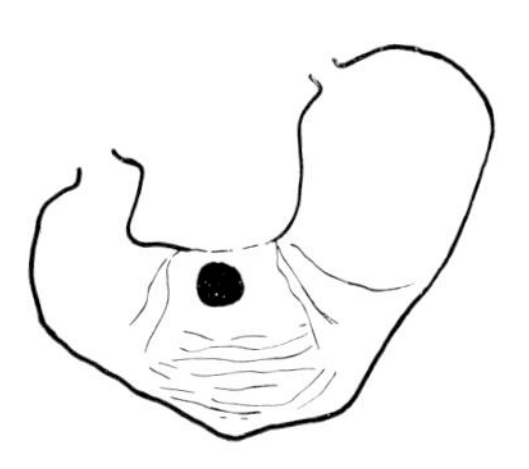

The typical corona, which is so often mentioned and is due to scar tissue contraction, may not be seen in the more acute phase of ulceration. Later, ulcers show these typical radiation of rugae from the crater, like this:

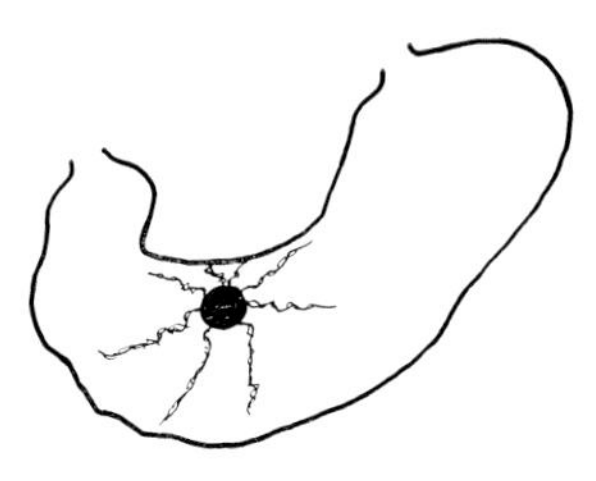

When maximal information has been obtained from the examination following the small amount of barium, and proper films have also been taken, have the patient swallow enough of the barium mixture to fill the stomach. At this stage the most pointed sign of ulcer is that of spastic incisura. This causes the typical "B" appearance accurately proclaimed as a sign of ulceration. The stomach looks like this:

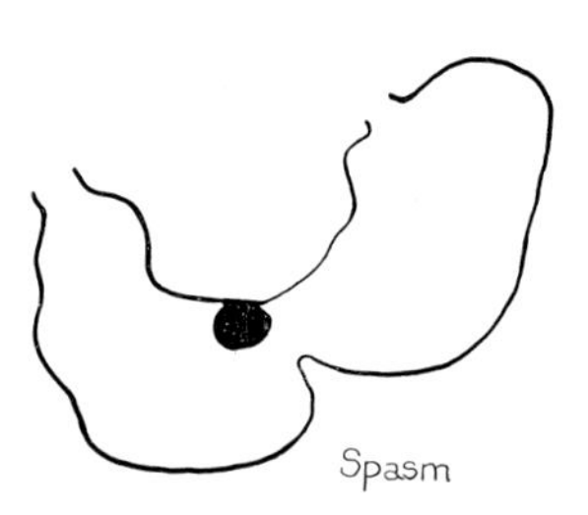

While the stomach is full one looks for hyperactive peristaltic waves which are deeper than normal and move more rapidly than normal toward the pyloris. When such waves are present they are a sign of irritation but by no means a positive sign of ulcer. Only rarely does one fail to demonstrate a typical ulcer crater if it is present. Probably most of these failures are due to poor technique, to the ulcer being filled with debris, blood clots, etc., or to ulceration in an unsuspected area where careful examination is not done.

By no means do all perforations of gastric ulcer come to surgery. Probably the majority of them do not. Frequently we see a walled-off pocket resulting from perforation and subsequent isolation of the extruded material. Such a lesion looks like this:

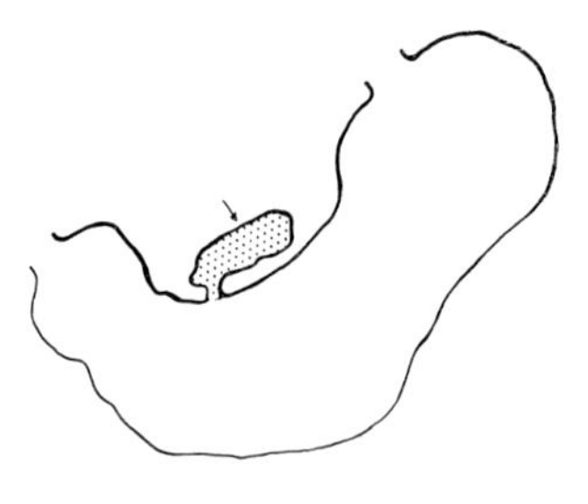

Since it is fixed in position by inflammatory reaction or scar tissue, the lesion remains extremely constant throughout the examination and usually throughout subsequent examinations.

As soon as one knows where to look for the ulcer it is usually found with facility on repeat examination. The signs of healing are typical. The crater first changes from a punched-out ulceration, with slightly overhanging edges, to a "V." It then gradually disappears, although scarring with malformation of the rugae may remain.

Errors

A common error is to spend insufficient time placing the barium so that a clear-cut view of all parts of the stomach is obtained. Anybody can see the typical deformity of ulcer if he simply takes time to make sure that a complete examination is done. Another common error is to place far too much dependence upon obvious clinical signs.

Typical ulcer lesions that do not respond should be seen immediately by a qualified roentgenologist for evaluation.

GASTRITIS

The roentgen diagnosis of chronic gastritis is so mixed up at present and so poorly coordinated with clinical studies and gastroscopic examinations that the practitioner will do well to stay out of the controversy.

If gastritis is suspected it is probably best to send the patient to an expert roentgenologist for a diagnostic survey. Even then, results are usually unreliable from the practical standpoint of guiding therapy and prognosis. We are constantly learning more about the diseases affecting the mucosa and some mucosal layers of the stomach, but until our knowledge is more extensive, exact diagnosis is unlikely.

CARCINOMA OF THE STOMACH

The stomach is the commonest site of internal cancer in men. This well-known fact is sometimes taken to mean that carcinoma of the stomach is rare in women, which is by no means the case. In females, however, it is exceeded in rate by cancer of the uterus and of the breast.

The growth is vicious because of its insidious character. Some months and rarely as much as two years may pass between the onset of the growth and the appearance of symptoms. During this early stage a chance x-ray film is about the only way that the growth is likely to be diagnosed.

The rate of surgical salvage is discouraging but by no means so low that the outlook is hopeless. For this reason every effort should be made to diagnose early cases. The lesions occur most frequently near the pylorus, as many as 85 per cent of them being found in the distal half of the stomach. Most of them begin in the mucous membranes. No way of diagnosing a purely mucous membrane lesion is available to the practitioner at present. It is only after an invasion of the muscular coats has occurred or after a mass projecting into the lumen has been formed that diagnosis is possible. The first signs are usually increased rigidity of the gastric wall and an absence of peristalsis in the involved segment.

A large number of these growths infiltrate the stomach wall so extensively that they constrict the lumen. A much smaller number project into the lumen regionally.

Technique

The ordinary technique used for the gastrointestinal series is entirely adequate *if carefully done.* In a person of cancer age with gastric symptoms one cannot emphasize too pointedly that every portion of the stomach must be visualized. Every deviation of the barium stream, no matter how trivial, must be explained either by the practitioner or by an expert consultant to whom the patient is sent.

Interpretation

Before one even attempts to discuss the interpretation of fluoroscopic findings and films, one point must be made entirely clear. There is little or no advantage to be gained in diagnosing an inoperable carcinoma of the stomach.

What we must try to achieve is diagnosis at a stage early enough to allow adequate surgical attack. In our own practice this has meant meticulous examination for the common early findings of cancer and immediate referral to an expert roentgenologist, if any are found. If the roentgenologist is unable to confirm the presence of cancer but does confirm the presence of the signs we see, a gastroscopist and a surgeon are asked to see the patient.

An aside here: We have always performed our own gastric resections for ulcer with excellent results. However, a small hospital or clinic has absolutely no business attempting either the definitive diagnosis or operation for cancer. I conceive our job to be screening those patients who present themselves and to make immediate referral of any case that is suspicious of malignancy.

Often the first sign is an aperistaltic area of the stomach wall. All that is required to demonstrate this is careful observation while several peristaltic waves pass down the wall toward the pylorus. A wave like this:

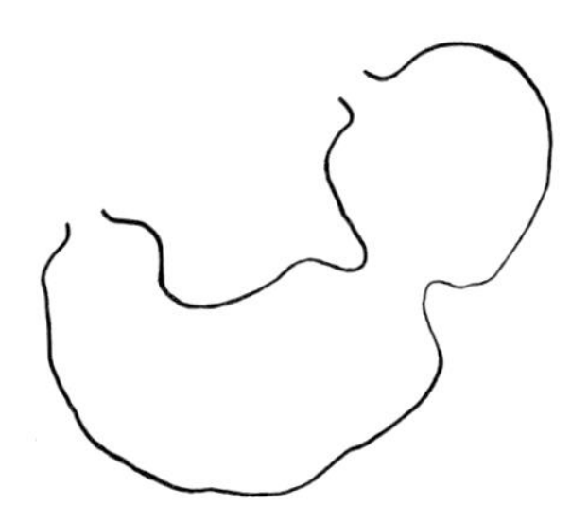

fades out when it reaches the aperistaltic area like this:

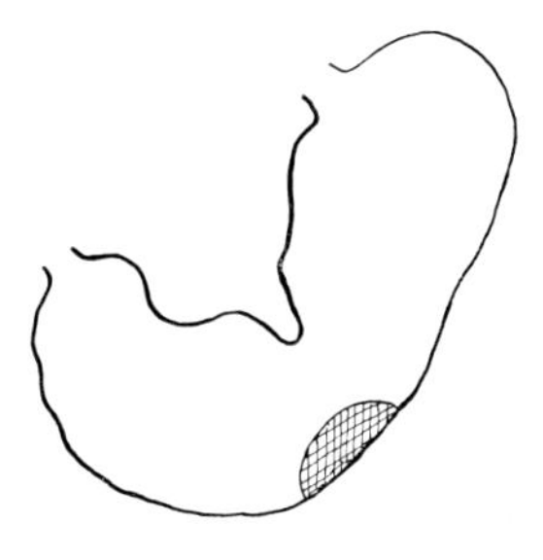

After passing the area of the growth it resumes its progress at normal intensity.

At other times there will be an area of the stomach wall that seems rigid. In the early part of the study, when you push on the abdomen with the gloved hand the stomach will bend inward under your fingers, like this:

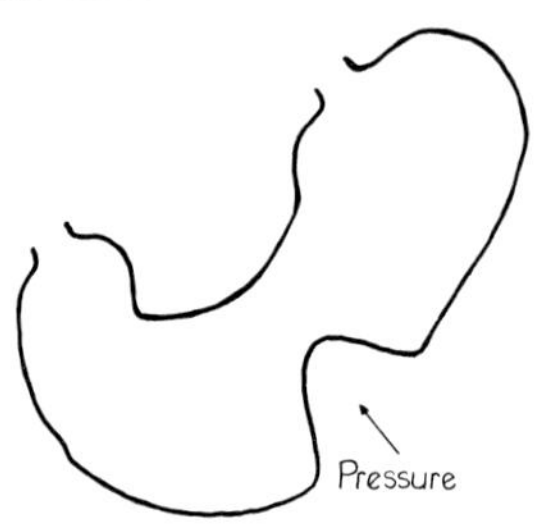

If there is a hardened plaque in its walls this bending is of slight extent or may be absent altogether. The picture looks like this:

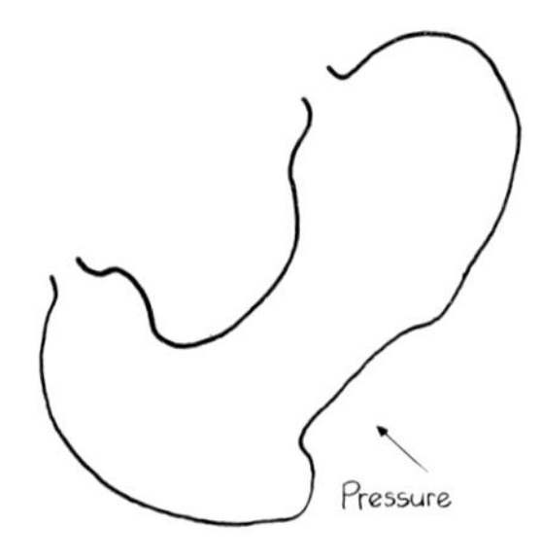

To me, one of the principal characteristics of cancer is the constancy of the defect which is seen. A typical napkin-ring deformity of the pylorus, which looks like this:

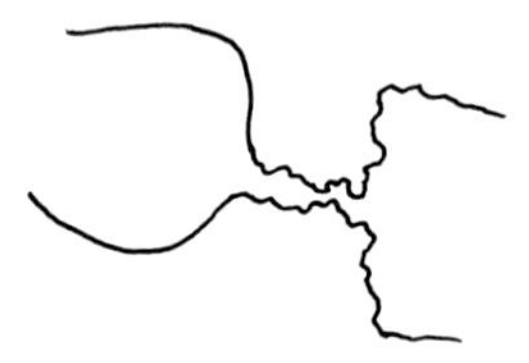

will remain constant not only throughout the original examination but will also be equally constant when a re-examination is done several days later. We make a practice to both sketch and film any deformity and to repeat the examination in forty-eight to seventy-two hours. If it is still there, evidence is almost overwhelming that a malignancy is present.

The napkin-ring deformity is common. A diffused infiltrating growth may narrow the lumen of the entire lower portion of the stomach. The typical "X" deformity of cancer looks like this:

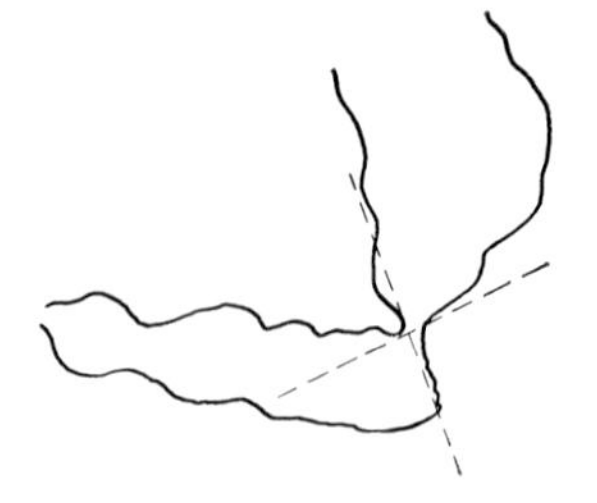

in contradistinction to the "B" deformity of ulcer.

Sometimes certain types of carcinoma extend into the lumen of the stomach without infiltrating the walls to any great extent. Such growths simply show a filling defect with typical irregular or spiky edges, like this:

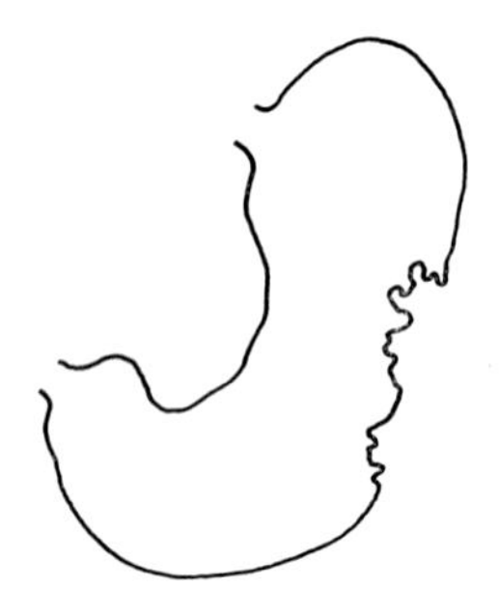

The constriction and filling defects vary so greatly that it is impossible in a brief book to list even a few of the different appearances seen. If you will simply remember that any alteration in the contour of the stomach which is rigid, aperistaltic, and not obviously due to spasm may be caused by carcinoma, you will be safe. No case showing such findings should be passed on without referring the patient to an expert roentgenologist.

Errors

The most common error is failure to make the examination in great enough detail to detect the obvious signs. There is no real difficulty in demonstrating a moderately advanced carcinoma of the stomach if one is meticulous in x-ray examination.

The second error, and by far the worst one, is to ignore the trivial findings of early carcinoma. The one most frequently ignored is the peristaltic jump which has been previously mentioned. In this, an area of the stomach is rigid and aperistaltic and no other finding is seen. When it is observed in both original and repeat examinations the case should be considered carcinoma until proved otherwise. Even this early finding is not particularly difficult to demonstrate if one watches carefully the progression of the peristaltic waves. It may, however, take four to six minutes of careful observation to pin point the area involved and to be certain that a peristaltic jump actually exists. The practitioner must have no compunction about repeating these examinations several times if necessary for positive demonstration.

DUODENAL ULCER

It has been claimed that duodenal and gastric ulcers are essentially separate diseases with little or no common relationship. In our practice it has seemed that both are psychogenic in the vast majority of instances and only involve a slightly different etiologic mechanism. This, however, is an argument for the experts, not for the practitioners.

Duodenal ulcer is one of the most common lesions to which the male human being is subject. As the tensions of our daily life inevitably increase there seems to be an almost parallel increase in the number of duodenal operations. Clinical diagnosis of the dyspeptic, hyperacidic changes leading up to ulceration of the duodenum are exceptionally easy. A carefully taken history and physical examination, with an occasional gastric analysis, will demonstrate this predisposing condition in well over 90 per cent of cases.

The x-ray then assumes the responsibility of deciding whether ulceration has actually occurred or whether it is impending or healing. Diagnosis of the basic condition is a clinical matter and not one for x-ray decision. In other words, the x-ray will tell whether or not a typical ulcer picture has progressed to the extent of mechanical change. It will not tell you whether or not the picture exists. That is a matter for clinical decision.

Technique

Technically, examination of the duodenum is more difficult than examination of the stomach. One has less control of duodenal filling and the lesion may be obscured unless the examination is both rapid and accurate.

During the first stages of gastric examination, when the mucosal folds are made out, a little barium may be extruded into the duodenum. At this time one must look for the typical distortions of the duodenal cap caused by ulceration. It is imperative that this examination be made in all planes and both with and without the use of compression.

As the duodenum fills, rotate the patient once again in order to see the edges of the filled cap from all angles. This sounds easy but it is not always possible, particularly in fat patients whose duodenum swings upward sufficiently to "hide behind" the costal margin.

Interpretation

Demonstration of an ulcer crater in tangential view is no different in the duodenum than in the stomach except for one difficulty. True tangential views may be difficult to obtain. The ulcer is most frequently seen on compression. It shows up as a rounded area of barium that is not squeezed away between the folds of mucosa when compression is made. It may look like this:

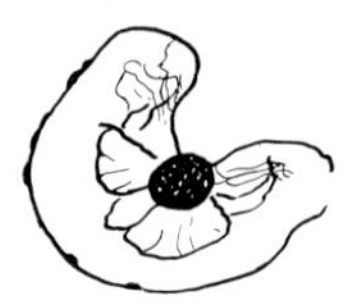

When such a picture is seen, tangential views should be checked immediately in order to demonstrate the pocket while still full of barium. Then manipulate the compression so that you distribute the barium in the duodenum and make another observation. If the coin-shaped plaque of barium is still present, chances are overwhelming that an active ulcer is its source.

A new ulcer will show this crater without great change in the surrounding mucosa. An older ulcer will show scarring and often a typical star deformity, with the mucosal folds pulled in toward the ulcer crater, like this:

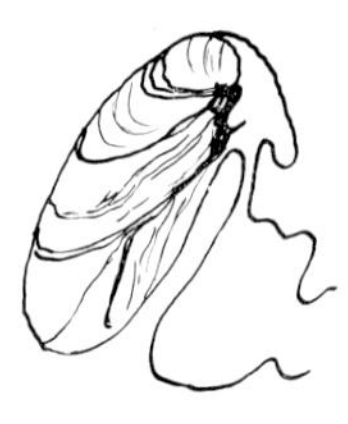

The duodenal cap in the normal individual has a smooth snake-head contour when full, like this:

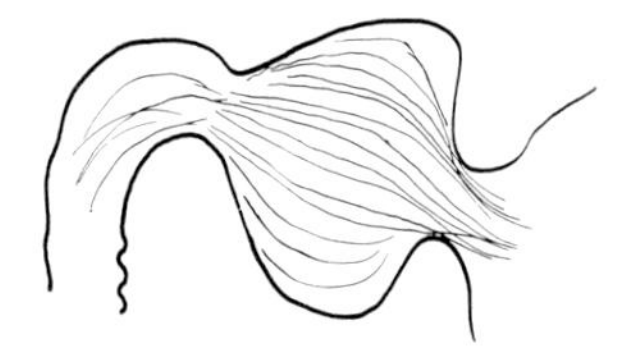

The mucosal pattern under compression is regular, with smooth waves rather than sudden angular changes representing the folds.

The spasm and edema of an active ulcer and the scarring of an old ulcer greatly change the configuration of the cap. This is a typical spastic cap:

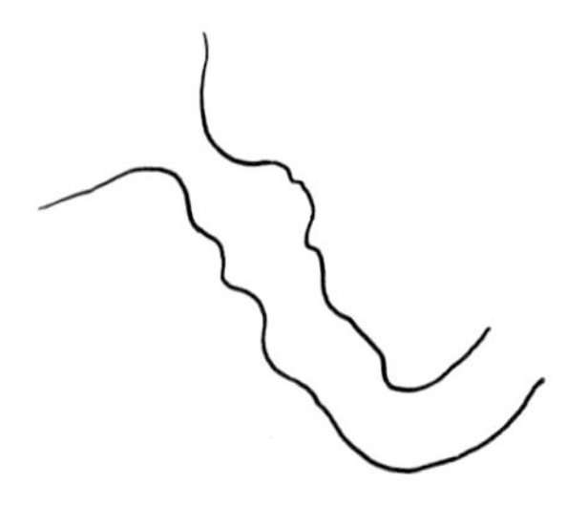

This is a typical picture of edema and spasm:

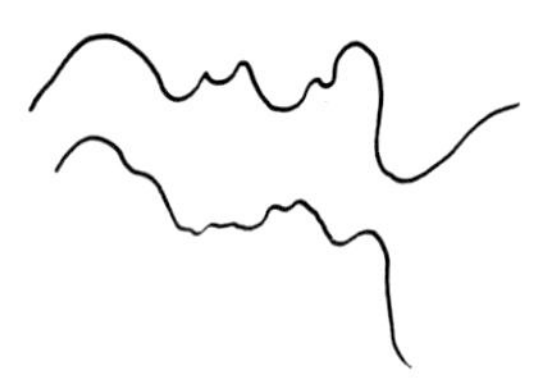

This is an ulcer-scarred duodenal cap:

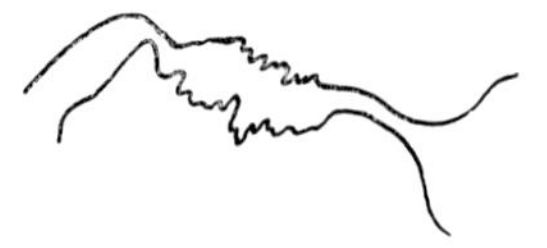

There are secondary changes in the stomach often seen in the presence of duodenal ulceration. The most frequent is hyperperistalsis, with deep peristaltic waves succeeding one another rapidly and giving an entirely correct impression of extreme overactivity.

Another finding is increase in the thickness of gastric rugae, along with the greater curvature. They appear enlarged and swollen, which is entirely true.

Healing of a duodenal ulcer is extremely difficult to observe radiologically. If all signs disappear, obviously the ulcer is healed. However, this is excessively rare.

Almost without exception, some deformity of the duodenal bulb will be present and this deformity cannot be said with any certainty to be the result of old ulceration. In our own practice we are inclined to accept clinical evidence as a much more certain sign of healing than roentgenologic evidence.

We practitioners have the wonderful opportunity of observing not only the x-ray changes but also the clinical changes in the patient. The correlation of the two greatly enhances the potential worth of each.

To repeat, even the most expert roentgenologist cannot be sure that a duodenal ulcer is healed unless all signs disappear. Since the scarring and some deformities of the bulb may persist for years or even for life, clinical evidence probably outweighs the evidence to be gathered from x-ray.

Errors

There are two common errors. The first is to fail in demonstration of pathology because of insufficient care in examination. This is usually lack of proper compression and examination in multiple planes.

The second error is to put too much faith in the x-ray picture. Duodenal ulceration is hard to demonstrate at best and a certain number of cases are going to be missed in spite of the most meticulous examination. Also, the primary changes leading up to ulcer may be present without actual ulceration having taken place. May I use a ridiculous illustration? Let us suppose that a rifle two miles away has been centered on a patient and the trigger pulled. You know this and you know that the chances of the bullet missing are about 50-50. You check the patient for a bullet hole, find none, and say, "Nope, you are all right. Nothing wrong with you," and forget it. About that time the bullet hits. The patient will think somebody a fool, and possibly rightly so. In such an example the x-ray picture simply tells whether the hole is present or not, not whether a bullet has been fired at the patient or whether he is going to be hit or missed.

PERFORATED VISCUS

Partial perforations, fistulas, and other more rare conditions are referred to in standard textbooks on x-ray diagnosis.

When an open communication is established between the intestinal tract and the general peritoneal cavity, a portion of the normal gaseous content of the intestine escapes into the peritoneum. Unless trapped by adhesions this air will rise to the highest part of the peritoneal cavity and will make itself known by typical x-ray appearances.

This is a most important point to remember, since a number of patients with perforating ulcers will be first observed in the office.

Technique

Ask the patient to stand or sit erect for a period of five or ten minutes before the x-ray is taken. Then place him in the regular chest position and make an ordinary posteroanterior exposure of the chest, usually with a slight increase in kilovoltage.

Interpretation

Escaped air will have pooled between the diaphragm and the liver and between the diaphragm and the stomach. The typical appearance of air under the diaphragm is this:

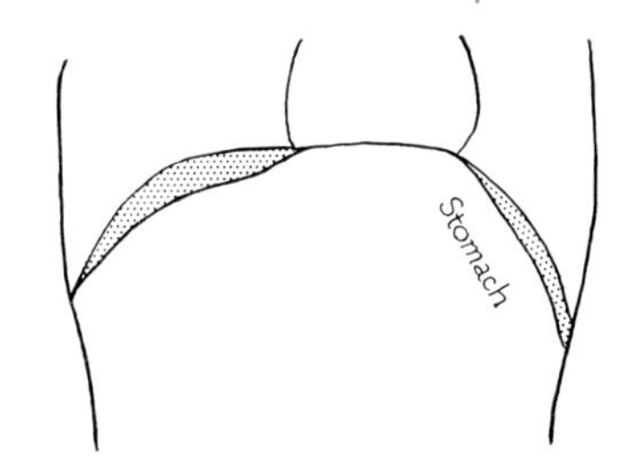

Such a finding is easily interpreted. It is an indication for exploratory laparotomy.

Errors

Errors in interpretation are practically unknown. The only error is failure to take such a film when clinical indications for it exist.

OBSTRUCTION OF THE SMALL INTESTINE

Complete obstructions of the small intestine are seldom seen in the office. At least they should not be observed longer than it takes to make proper arrangements for admission of the patient to a hospital. Office x-ray should not be done.

Partial obstructions, on the other hand, are usually matters which can be diagnosed in the office preceding the initiation of proper treatment. In the average practice the majority of these are caused by constricting bands which result from previous intra-abdominal disease or manipulation. The problem that exists is to find the approximate site of the partial obstruction.

Technique

Place the patient in the erect position, and allow him to remain in this position for approximately twenty minutes before x-rays are taken. Then make a plain flat plate while the patient is still erect. Usually this will be all that is necessary.

Interpretation

The distended loops of intestine with their fluid levels are usually seen quite clearly. This is an example of such a picture:

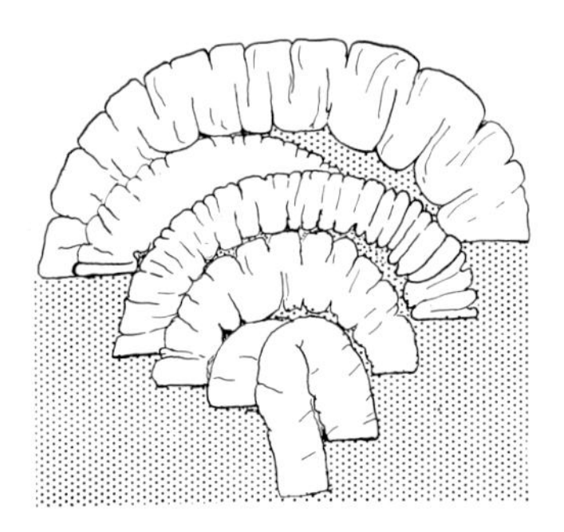

There are two common methods of locating the site of the obstruction. The first is to count the number of distended loops and calculate in your mind about how much of the intestine must be involved in the specified number. The second is to observe carefully the pattern of the distended bowel and correlate these patterns with known x-ray patterns in the various areas. This is a typical jejunal pattern:

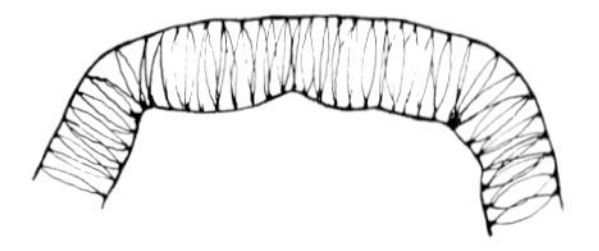

It gradually fades into the terminal pattern of the ilium which looks like this:

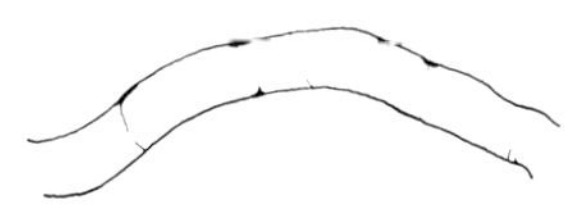

Some qualified x-ray men give barium to such people, which will demonstrate the partial obstruction with great clarity. Most of us, however, do not follow this practice for obvious reasons.

Errors

Errors are infrequent. Rarely a case of partial obstruction may be confused with a reflex ileus. If one cannot differentiate the two on the basis of x-ray (and it is usually possible), then clinical signs will often make clear the distinction.

The statement is often made that air is not found in the normal small intestine. The assumption is therefore followed that if air occurs in the small intestine, some degree of partial obstruction must be present. In the patient who is erect and walking around, this is probably true. It is distinctly not true of patients who have been in bed for twenty-four hours or more. Swallowed air in the bedfast patient rises to the pyloric portion of the stomach and is rapidly extruded into the duodenum and small intestine. In such a patient one may visualize small boluses of air throughout the small intestine without there being any degree of obstruction.

Remember well that partial obstruction of sufficient degree to bring the patient to the physician will show distended loops of intestine with fluid levels.

REFLEX ILEUS

In many diseases, both intra- and extra-abdominal, there may occur an unbalanced action of the sympathetic nervous system. One manifestation of this unbalanced action is paresis of the intestine. When trivial in degree this can be diagnosed clinically and historically without recourse to x-ray. Rarely it may be severe enough to be a presenting symptom.

After thirty-six hours or so there is usually an intra-abdominal effusion accompanying the distended intestine. This makes x-ray differentiation much easier.

Technique

Films may be taken in either the erect or prone position. However, when reflex ileus is suspected, the films probably should be taken in both positions.

Interpretation

The principal characteristic one notices immediately is that the entire intestine from the uppermost portion of the jejunum through the entire colon is somewhat distended with air. This is not a usual finding in organic obstruction except in lesions of the lower sigmoid and rectum, which can be demonstrated clinically or by barium enema.

Of course, a barium enema should not be given to a patient suspected of reflex ileus.

When an effusion has occurred, the prone picture will show separation of the distended portions of the intestine by the fluid, like this:

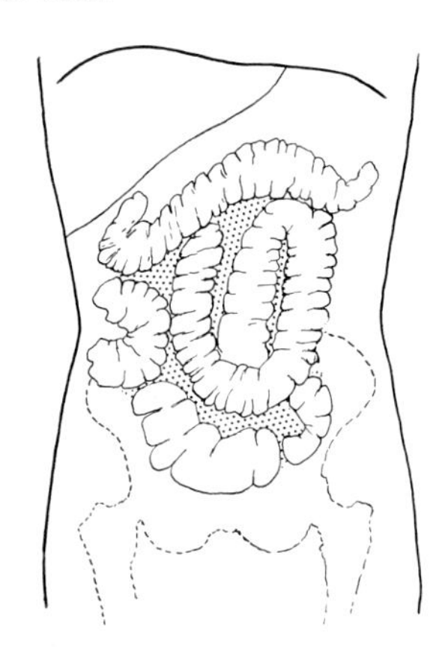

In the erect position the intestine will float on top of the effusion and look like this:

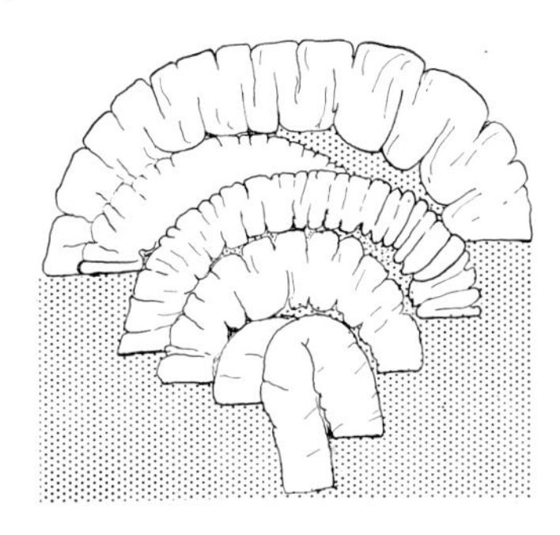

Errors

To begin with, one must realize that the effusion mentioned above often accompanies paralytic ileus, but by no means is this always so.

Actually these patients should not come to x-ray. The outstanding characteristic of reflex ileus is so easily checked clinically that x-ray examination is seldom necessary.

THE BARIUM ENEMA

The barium enema is a standard technique the world over for the examination of the colon. A number of routines are suggested by various writers on the subject and there is probably little difference in total information obtained, regardless of the particular routine followed. The one we use is as follows:

Instruct the patient to eat lightly the day before the examination and do not give any kind of laxative. In the evening before retiring instruct him to take a plain water enema.

Upon arising the next morning he should not eat breakfast. Instruct him to take at least four enemas with plain water, using a little more water each time. If the return from the fourth enema is not clear, he is to take still another. Most people resent this extremely but will comply when reminded of the fact that the barium enema will be a waste of money unless they have completely emptied the colon before it is done.

Have the patient report to the office at 9 o'clock where another enema should be given by the nurse. For approximately an hour allow him to evacuate at will before the barium enema itself is given.

Make up a watery suspension of barium sulfate (about two pints) and place in a routine enema can. Prepare a long enema tip. Before insertion of the tip perform a routine abdominal fluoroscopy with the patient recumbent. One important purpose of this is to detect any signs of air in the colon. Usually none is visible, but if several large pockets are seen, ask the patient to evacuate again before the examination is begun.

When this is achieved insert the enema tip and allow a little of the barium to run into the rectum. Here is a point where many barium enema techniques fail. The colon must be filled slowly, a little at a time. If you allow at least two minutes between introduction of small amounts of barium, the normal contractivity of the lower bowel segments will force the barium back up the colon without undue pain or discomfort to the patient. A barium enema that is literally poured in may engender discomfort, bowel spasm, and an almost uncontrollable desire to defecate.

While the barium is running in, make periodic fluoroscopies with hand compression to outline any lesions that are seen. This is one of the most important parts of the examination and must never be neglected. At this stage the patient may be turned from side to side to gain full visualization of the sigmoid loop and to delineate any pathology that exists in it.

When the colon has become filled, examination of its segments should be made by plain fluoroscopy, compression, and roentgenology.

Then ask the patient to expel as much of the barium as possible. Give him at least five to eight minutes to do this—do not constantly hurry him. Then make an examination of the collapsed colon which will still contain enough barium to outline the walls, mucosal pattern, and most lesions that might be present.

Occasionally an air contrast enema will be of service. Fill the colon with air under fluoroscopic control and allow the patient to evacuate. This may have to be done several times to remove enough barium so that the contrast becomes sufficiently great for adequate diagnostic purposes. The number of times is controlled by fluoroscopic observation.

SIMPLE COLITIS

Mucous colitis, simple colitis, and the "irritable colon" are probably all the same thing. They represent, as near as we can tell, a psychogenic disturbance which is manifested principally by spasm of the colon and hyperactivity of its mucous membrane.

The condition is best diagnosed clinically, but a barium enema usually gives great comfort, for these patients believe it is "absolute proof" that no dangerous disease of the colon exists.

It has been said that human life may be divided into three great overlapping stages: (1) worrying about food, (2) worrying about sex, and (3) worrying about bowel function. It would almost seem that the last two are related in some, not readily definable, way. We see—at least we think we see—a number of young women in the 30- to 40-year-old group who, having some sexual maladjustment, present themselves with complaints related to the colon.

Be that as it may, the practitioner will find that at least half the barium enemas he does are performed to rule out more serious lesions in obvious cases of "irritable colon." This is unnecessary since we know that the irritable colon is essentially undiagnosable by means of roentgenology.

Technique

The routine barium enema as described in the preceding section is entirely adequate. As a matter of fact, palpation will often do fully as much to make the diagnosis as will any roentgenographic study.

Interpretation

Usually a portion of the colon will show spasm and loss of normal markings. Most frequently involved is the descending portion, which looks like this:

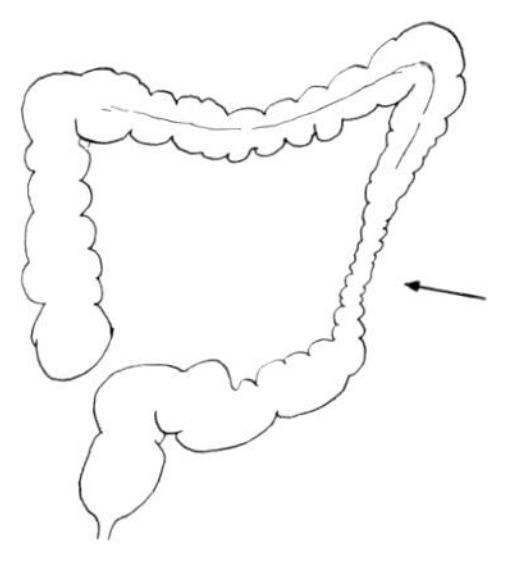

If the mucous membrane pattern is delineated after evacuation, it will be much more complex, showing various branchings and arborizations (probably due to circulatory changes) than is usually seen. A typical area looks like this:

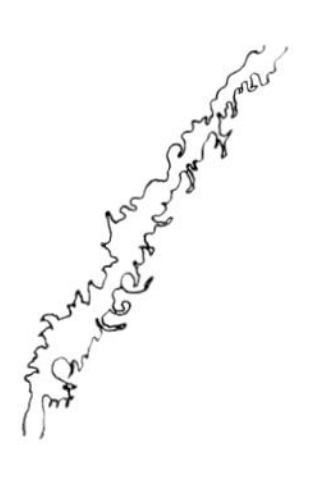

Most often, mucosal pattern change will not be seen. Whether it is not present or simply not seen because of the inadequacies of the barium technique, has never been decided.

Errors

You must remember that the same colonic change described above is often found in persons who seem perfectly normal and have no symptoms of any kind. It is often pointed out to the patient as a "spastic colon" and this is tagged as the root of all her trouble.

Actually, an irritable colon must be diagnosed clinically, not roentgenologically. What one can achieve by x-ray is to rule out the presence of more serious lesions. Here is a good place to digress for just one minute to speak to the young physician.

You will hear horrible stories of the carcinoma of the colon that was missed because the diagnosis of irritable colitis was made. These stories will be rendered with great howling and gnashing of teeth, but you will not hear the other side of the story. You will not hear about the 30,000 people who were made colonic invalids for life by the discovery of some trivial lesion that had absolutely no bearing whatever on their symptoms. You will not hear of the people who live their lives in fear of the crippling disease or imminent death from carcinoma because somebody misdiagnosed a shadow as a polyp and literally scared the daylights out of the patient.

You cannot be warned too carefully about the missed organic lesion, but these misses are rare. By and large, they are less important than the constant parade of iatrogenic cripples that we see every day because some physician made up his mind he was going to find an organic lesion and found it whether it was there or not. The office x-ray is a great offender on this very point. Guard against such errors.

ULCERATIVE COLITIS

Ulcerative colitis is a disease of unknown etiology, although the statement has been made frequently in recent years that it appears to belong to the collagen group. It usually starts in the sigmoid colon with infiltration of the submucous coats of the bowel.

Ulcers gradually appear and the infiltrations continue until the resulting fibrosis causes a fixation of the colonic walls. Rigidity appears and is responsible for some of the features seen on x-ray examination. Gradually islands of the mucosa are lost and sometimes only partially replaced. Polyps frequently form. The disease progresses until the colon becomes a rigid fibrous tube with little or no functional mucous membrane.

Technique

The ordinary barium enema is not the best way to delineate ulcerative colitis but other techniques are probably beyond the office x-ray department. The carefully done barium enema along with proper clinical and laboratory study will result in accurate diagnosis in the majority of these cases.

Interpretation

One looks first at the sigmoid colon. In the early stages of the disease it is usually slightly spastic, and the edges of the barium shadow are fuzzy instead of clear-cut, like this:

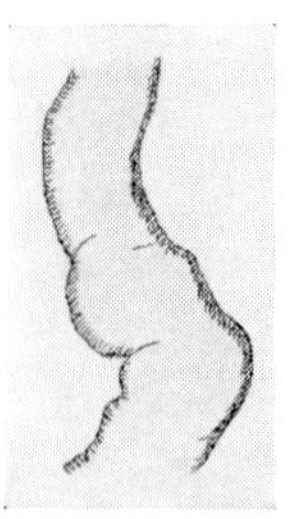

This is due to the fact that barium penetrates the tiny ulcer craters. This penetration is seen both on fluoroscope and film.

As the disease progresses, ulcers may coalesce and become larger, giving the involved area of the colon a double-contour appearance, like this:

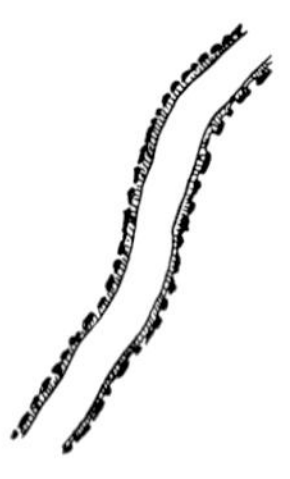

Still further along in the course of the disease, the bowel assumes a rigidity, and the enema is seen to run in much more quickly than in normal subjects. It has been accurately described as having a lead-pipe appearance. The mucous pattern in this stage is distorted beyond any reasonable recognition and may look like this:

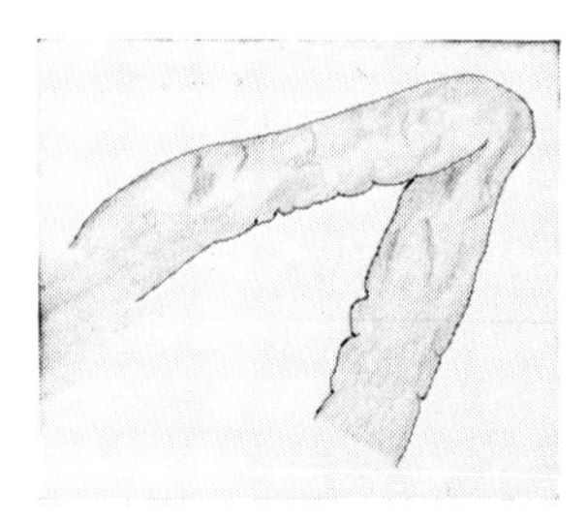

When the enema is expelled, the colonic walls fail to collapse, once again adding to the lead-pipe appearance of the colon.

Errors

Rarely the early stages of the ulcerative colitis may be confused with amebiasis or other diseases which cause colonic ulceration. This is more easily clarified by accurate laboratory examination of the stools than it is by roentgenologic examination.

OBSTRUCTION OF THE COLON

As a matter of practical consideration, any organic obstruction of the colon is a malignancy until proved otherwise. In complete obstruction, x-ray examination is of little help in delineating the exact status of the obstructing lesion, but it is useful in defining its approximate location.

Technique

A simple flat plate of the abdomen, with the patient in the erect position if possible, is usually all that is needed.

Interpretation

Colonic obstruction shows no signs vastly different from those of small bowel obstruction (page 282), except that the mucous membrane pattern of the colon is prominent among the distended loops of intestine. It looks like this:

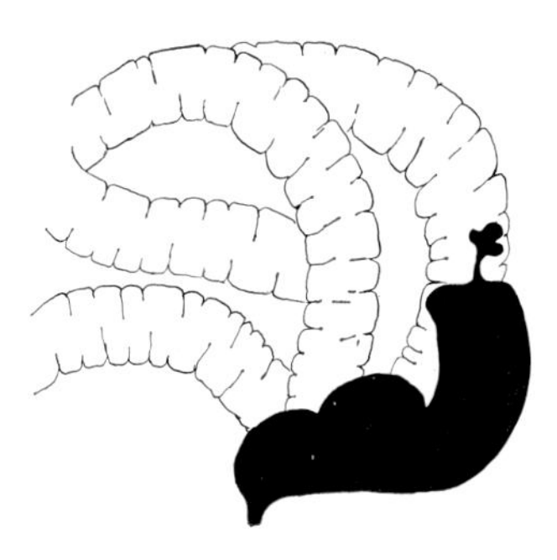

Errors

The diagnostic criteria and procedure is so simple that errors are practically nonexistent.

CARCINOMA OF THE LARGE BOWEL

Cancer of the large bowel is an exceedingly common lesion. It occurs most frequently in the rectosigmoid area, with secondary frequency in the right colon.

Fortunately the growth is slow growing and tends to metastasize late. For this reason the surgical attack is moderately successful if undertaken soon after the diagnosis. It will result in the saving of some lives, which is not always the case in other types of intestinal carcinomas.

In many cases adequate diagnosis of this lesion is in the hands of the practitioner alone. Adequate and skillful use of the office x-ray, along with a suspicious mind, will serve to pick up many an early carcinoma long before severe symptoms drive the patient to a full clinical study.

It is particularly important for the practitioner to remember that patients who have had one carcinoma of the colon have, statistically, a far greater chance than the ordinary person of having a second one at a later date. The removal and apparent cure of one carcinoma makes repeated x-ray examination a necessity.

Technique

The ordinary barium enema will demonstrate the majority of all large bowel cancers, with the exception of those appearing low in the rectum. These are, of course, in reach of the palpating finger and may be easily visualized by the sigmoidoscope, so that x-ray should not be employed for their diagnosis.

If the anterior view of the sigmoid is doubled in such a way that the course is not visible so that both the left and right oblique positions may have to be used to give complete delineation, *this procedure should never be omitted in a barium enema examination.*

Interpretation

Diagnosis is made by demonstration of luminal defects. There are two types of defect commonly seen. The most frequent is the irregular ring defect which looks like this:

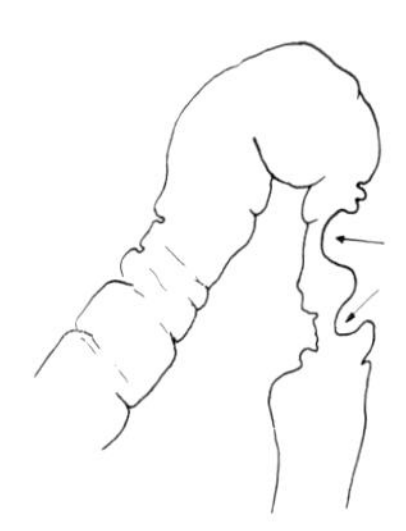

Notice that the lumen is encroached upon from all sides and that the remaining passage is somewhat eccentric. Notice, too, that the involved segment is somewhat irregular and that the bowel proximal to the segment is somewhat dilated. On fluoroscopic examination it would be seen to be somewhat hyperactive. This is often true even when there are no symptoms indicating partial obstruction.

These two illustrations represent other typical lesions:

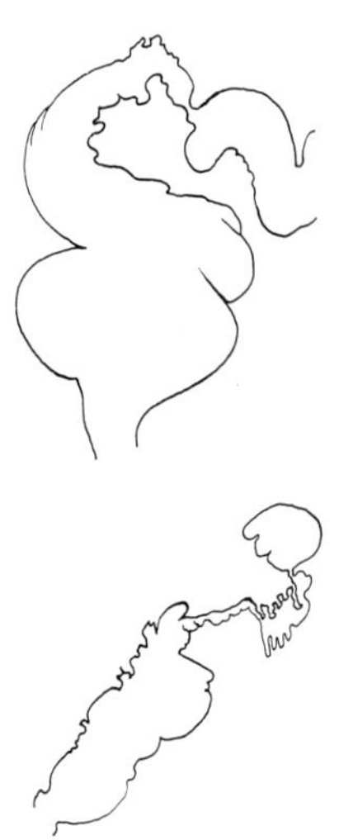

Another common defect is called by many radiologists the fingerprint defect, and looks like this:

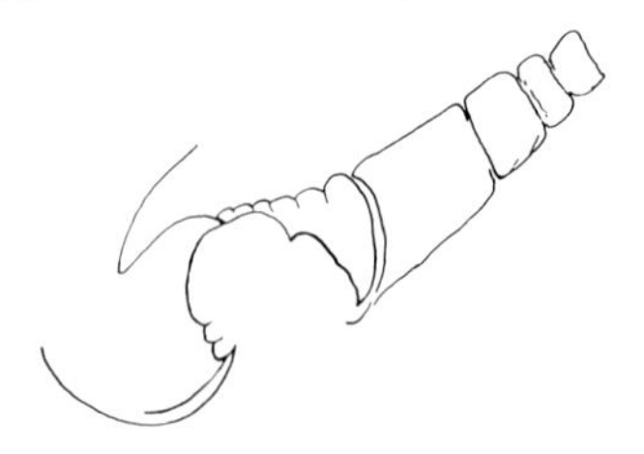

Occasionally, after evacuation of the barium, the tumor will be outlined by a thin film, like this:

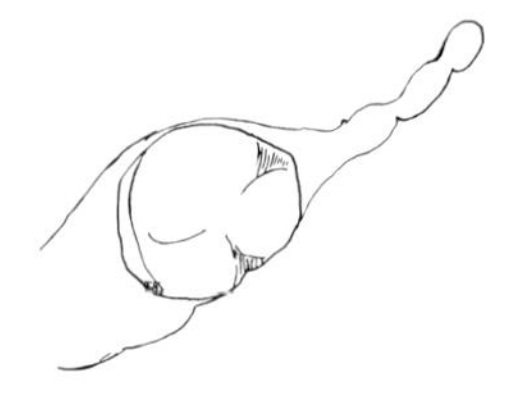

Errors

Filling defects of the colon are seldom missed. Occasionally a regional spasm, particularly that associated with diverticulitis, will be temporarily confusing. The spasm, however, has smooth edges, like this:

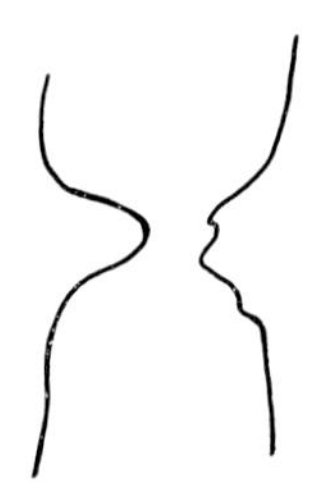

and will usually relax after a day or two of intense therapy, whereas a filling defect from cancer will remain constant.

DIVERTICULA

Diverticula are actually pulsive hernias of the mucous membrane through weakened areas in the muscular coats of the large bowel. Exactly why they occur is not known. From 5 to 10 per cent of normal persons over the age of 40 may show some evidence of diverticulosis.

Diverticula begin as small spikelike protrusions of mucous membrane in the bowel wall, like this:

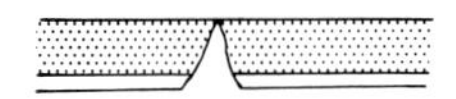

The sac then enlarges and diverticula assume a typical flasklike shape:

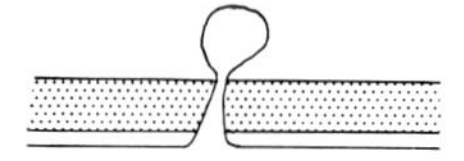

In a certain per cent of cases there occurs an inflammatory reaction involving the diverticula and the surrounding bowel wall. Ordinarily a group of diverticula in one particular segment of the bowel are involved in the reaction.

These small herniations are most common in the sigmoid area of the colon, but may be found throughout its length.

Technique

The standard barium enema technique will demonstrate a majority of diverticula.

Interpretation

The demonstration of diverticula in itself has little significance. The important point which must be made roentgenographically is to differentiate diverticulosis, which does not cause symptoms, from diverticulitis, which definitely does engender discomfort.

When simple diverticulosis is present, a routine designed to prevent inflammation in the pouches may be prescribed by the physician. Diverticulosis looks like this:

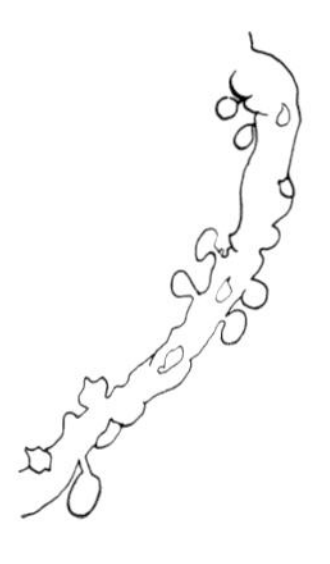

Notice that changes in the bowel wall itself are minimal. This is a similar case with diverticulitis:

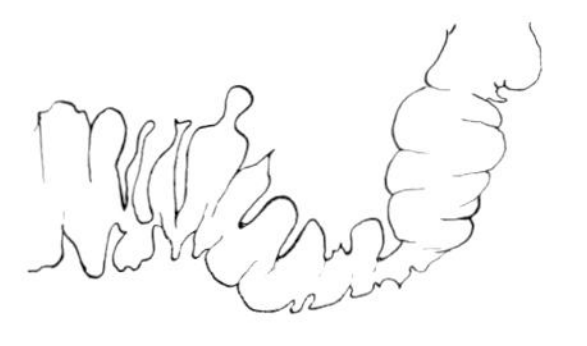

Notice the uneven, irregular character of the bowel lumen which is engendered by spasm from the inflammatory process. Notice, too, that there is some narrowing of the bowel which might conceivably be mistaken for carcinoma.

Particularly notice that the differentiation between diverticulosis and diverticulitis is not made by any change in the hernial sacs. It is made by the characteristic changes which are either present or absent in the bowel itself.

Errors

The most frequent error is to confuse an area of diverticulitis with carcinoma. The differentiation is actually difficult and sometimes cannot be made until one observes the roentgenologic changes engendered by a few days of treatment. Under intensive therapy the inflammatory reaction of diverticula will, of course, improve, whereas the defect in carcinoma will remain absolutely constant. Even with this method of differentiation there will be an occasional case in which question still remains.* These patients should be referred to the expert roentgenologist without delay.

*You have noticed the excess of cautions which have been voiced throughout these pages. I believe they are needful. Careless x-ray is worse than useless. It may often be dangerous. Let me repeat, even to the extent of annoying you—be sure of every technique and abandon no film until you are entirely certain you can explain every finding that is shown. Only when used in that way does x-ray become a worthwhile tool.

CHAPTER TWENTY-SIX

The Biliary Tract

Adequate cholecystography is well within the range of the office x-ray. We use the following preparation routine:

Give the patient a saline laxative the morning before x-rays are to be taken. Epsom salts works well but be careful of overdosage to avoid drastic purgation. The evening before the examination request the patient to take a normal meal and to include two eggs as a part of it. Just before retiring he is to take six tablets of Priodax. If a half teaspoonful of baking soda in a glass of water is taken along with these tablets, there is less danger of gastric upset. This dose of baking soda and water should be repeated upon arising in the morning and once again about one hour before reporting for examination.

Instruct the patient that on the morning of the examination he is to take enemas at home until the return is clear. Administer another enema upon his reporting to the office. Sometimes it is necessary to give 0.5 ml. of Pitressin to be sure that all colonic gas in the area of the gall bladder is expelled.

Take gall bladder films with the patient in a comfortable position, making the actual exposure at the end of expiration. If necessary, a ball of mechanic's waste can be used to push the gall bladder gently away from the spine. In doing this one must be extraordinarily careful not to use sufficient pressure to compress the organ.

If the gall bladder is visualized in the first film and shows concentration of the dye, then give the patient a glass of homogenized milk with two raw eggs beaten into it. Ten minutes after this mixture is ingested take two more films, one straight anteroposterior and one with the patient rotated 15 degrees to the right. Take another anteroposterior film two hours later.

If the gall bladder is not visualized, schedule the patient for a recheck series in twenty-four hours and give him more Priodax. At least eight to ten tablets should be taken.

CHOLECYSTITIS

This term cholecystitis covers a multitude of sins. Of course, the literal translation is "inflammation of the gall bladder," but like so many other inflammations it can be of many and diverse origins.

Patients with acute cholecystitis should not be treated in the office and certainly should not be x-rayed while using Priodax. Chronic cholecystitis is usually an office problem, at least for a time.

Discussion of the disease is not a matter for this book, but I suggest you read up on it thoroughly in any of the good textbooks available.

Technique

The technique mentioned above is adequate.

Interpretation

The normal gall bladder is supposed to be well visualized within twelve to fifteen hours after ingestion of Priodax. It should be seen contracted and nearly empty in the film taken two hours after ingestion of the milk and eggs.

Most standard textbooks say that a nonvisualized gall bladder—particularly after an increased dose of Priodax—is positive indication of organic gall bladder disease and many such texts recommend immediate surgery. I take the liberty of disagreeing.

When a gall bladder does not concentrate the dye it indicates some functional impairment in the gall bladder mucosa. *What* functional impairment is impossible to say from examination of the x-ray alone.

We have seen a significant number of these patients in whom the gall bladder utterly failed to concentrate, but who, one year later, showed a normally functioning gall bladder.

It is our opinion that x-ray helps in the diagnosis of gall bladder disease to the extent of showing positively that something is wrong with the gall bladder. What is wrong must be determined clinically. It is our belief that concentrating power or lack of it has absolutely no bearing on whether surgery should be done. Again, it indicates that there is some change in the function of the mucous membrane.

It is only fair to tell you that the majority disagree most heartily with this view and believe that a nonfunctioning gall bladder on x-ray is almost equivalent to a diagnosis of chronic cholecystitis.

Errors

If meticulous technique is used the only errors that could creep in are those of interpretation. As you know from reading the above, I disagree with the majority opinion about interpretation and, therefore, my comment on errors would be essentially worthless. Again, I suggest you read one of the standard textbooks, such as *Practice of Medicine,** *Textbook of Medicine,*† or *Principles of Internal Medicine.*‡

GALLSTONES

Nobody knows why gallstones form, but they are exceedingly common. By the age of 60 years, between a fourth and a third of the women examined will have gallstones and possibly one of every eight to ten men.

Of these persons with cholelithiasis at least 50 per cent will never have any symptoms which could be attributed to gallstones. About 25 per cent will have trivial symptoms of dyspepsia which might possibly be attributed to the gallstones although probably not actually due to them. Of the remaining 25 per cent, 15 per cent will have symptoms which may be due to gallstones and 10 per cent will have symptoms unquestionably due to the stones. As near as we can tell from our own practice, this means that about 15 to 20 per cent of the persons who have gallstones actually have some symptoms positively due to the presence of the stones.

All this is presented in order to show that the presence of gallstones by x-ray is a finding that may be helpful but that, in itself, it is insignificant. The problem

*Meakins, J. C.: The Practice of Medicine, St. Louis, The C. V. Mosby Co.

†Cecil, R. L., and Loeb, R. F.: Textbook of Medicine, Philadelphia, W. B. Saunders Co.

‡Harrison, T. R., and others: Principles of Internal Medicine, New York, The Blakiston Co.

which must be decided is whether the symptoms are due to the gallstones that are present. This must be decided clinically.

Technique

Only a relatively small per cent of gallstones is visualized on a flat plate of the abdomen. Most are transparent to the x-ray and require cholecystography for demonstration. A typical picture of stones after cholecystography may look like this:

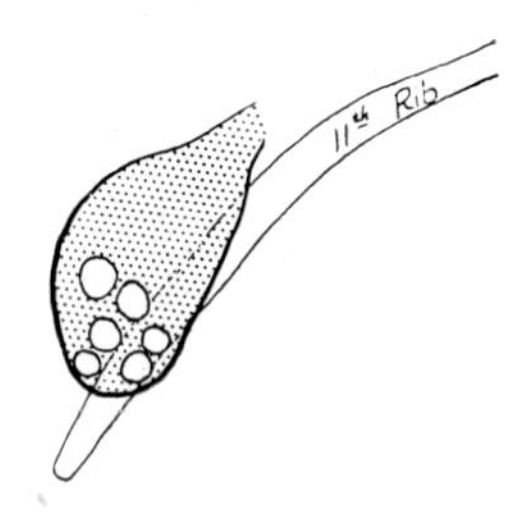

Frequently stones are associated with a nonfunctioning gall bladder, which makes their diagnosis by means of roentgen examination unlikely, to say the least.

Interpretation

When stones are found the problem facing the physician is to decide whether or not these stones are causing symptoms and whether or not the symptoms warrant their removal. This is a decision made entirely upon clinical grounds without much aid from the x-ray.

Insofar as interpretation of gall bladder shadows is concerned, either the stones are present or they are not, and nothing further is needed.

Errors

Often it is somewhat difficult to decide whether stones are actually in the gall bladder or are in other structures. Since the gall bladder lies far forward, rotation of the patient may give some information about this.

Occasionally calcification in costal cartilages may give a slight bit of trouble, but fluoroscopic observation of typical respiratory movements will clarify this point at once.

Comment

In summary, it is our distinct impression that gall bladder x-ray may be decidedly helpful. On the other hand, diagnosis, prognosis, and decision as to surgery regarding gall bladder disease are almost entirely a clinical matter.

CHAPTER TWENTY-SEVEN

The Urinary Tract

Excretory urography is within the range of every office, and retrograde examination of the urinary tract is an office procedure if the physician knows how to use the cystoscope. Cystoscopy with catheterization of the ureters is not a difficult procedure and it is something that many practitioners should know how to do. The complete technique is outlined in my book, *Office Procedures.** Interpretation of the resulting films requires detailed study.

It is imperative that the physician know well the anatomic range of the normal kidney before he attempts diagnosis from these films. In the following illustration notice the medial convexity and lateral concavity at the ureteral pelvic junction.

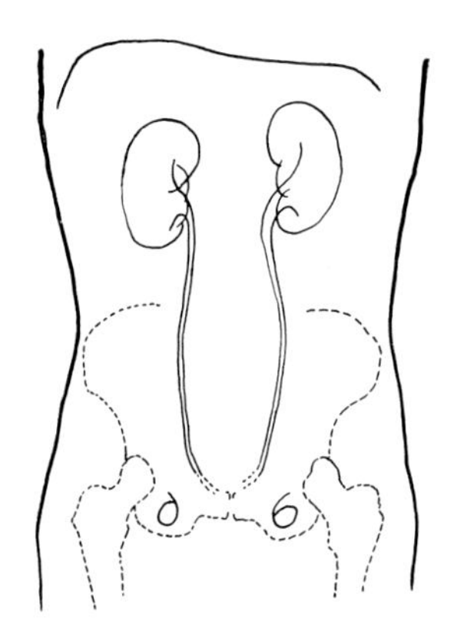

*Williamson, Paul: Office Procedures, Philadelphia, W. B. Saunders Co.

Next notice that there are usually three major calices, like this:

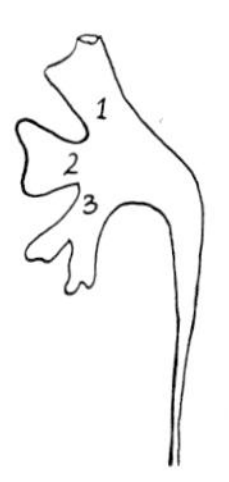

From these major calices spread four to six minor calices, like this:

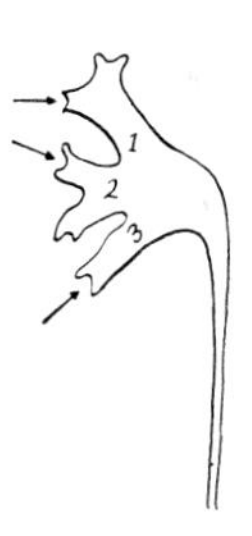

Notice the minor calix, much like the bell of a trumpet, is indented in its center by inward projection of the renal pyramid.

Normal anatomic variations from this picture may be extreme, but the general shape and formation of the pelvis and the major and minor calices will hold true. As the practitioner does excretory urograms he should be constantly on the alert for variations within the limits of normal. We have found it valuable to make sketches of these variations simply for emphasis.

Preparation for urography means first of all that the patient's intestine must be as nearly free of gas as possible. Ask the patient to take a saline laxative the night before reporting for examination and to take several enemas (until the return is clear) immediately upon arising the morning of the examination. Before proceeding with the examination itself, take a flat plate of the abdomen.

Check the flat plate for gaseous content in the bowel and for certain shadows which may aid in the diagnosis of renal disease. In the first place, the renal shadows should be clearly discerned and the shadows of the psoas muscle should be plainly seen, like this:

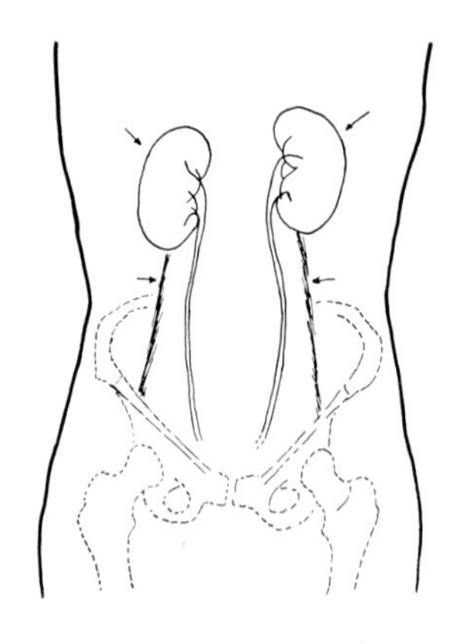

If there is any question about the existence of concretions which may be in the pelvis of the kidney, take either an oblique or a lateral picture before the dye is given. This, of course, will show clearly the location of the suspect shadow in its relationship to the kidney pelvis.

When these procedures have been accomplished and when the colon has been freed of gas (sometimes 0.5 ml. of Pitressin is needed), proceed with cystography and retrograde pyelography or administer the proper intravenous dye.

If the intravenous procedure is to be used, compression is made over the lower ureters. We use two small cotton felt pads, 2 by 3 inches, placed as shown here:

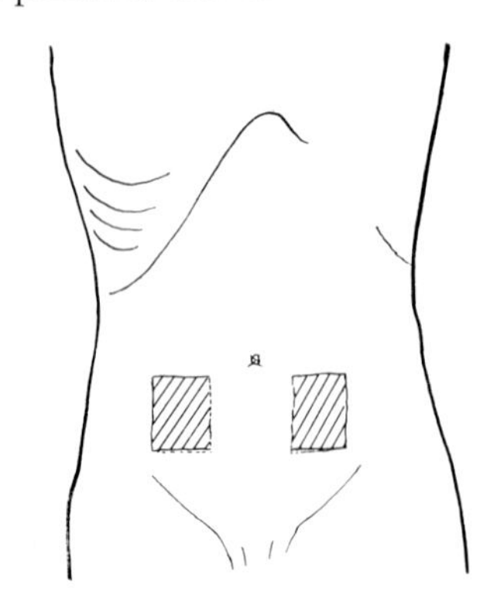

Cover these with a 4 by 6 inch cotton felt pad at least 2 inches thick.

Apply a compression band, beginning the compression gently and continuing until the patient remarks about the pressure. Then release it slightly and administer the dye. We use Diodrast or Neo-Iopax and administer it exactly according to the directions which accompany each package.

There are those who do not use a compression band and who say it is not necessary. Certainly they get good pictures. We think we get better results when we use one, however.

Place the patient in approximately a 5 degree Trendelenburg position and take films at five-, fifteen-, and twenty-five-minute intervals after the original administration of dye.

If the examination has been sufficiently complete after twenty-five minutes to obtain the necessary information about the kidney, remove the compression. Have the patient stand erect for approximately three or four minutes and then take a 14 by 17 film for outline of the bladder and ureters.

UROLITHIASIS

Stones in the urinary tract are common. Since so many theories are available as to their cause that a book could be written on the subject, it is not expedient that we discuss it here.

Clinical syndromes associated with urinary tract stones are so well known that the diagnosis may be made upon the basis of history, physical examination, and microscopic examination of the urine in the vast majority of cases.

Even so, x-ray plays a major part in the care of these persons, for by means of roentgenology the stone can be located, its movements readily charted, and accessory conditions, sometimes causative and sometimes resulting from the stone, usually determined.

Stones which are transparent to x-ray can often be delineated by intravenous or retrograde urography.

Technique

The standard kidney-ureter-bladder (KUB) or flat plate of the abdomen will often serve to show opacities which are at least thought to be in the urinary tract. Kidney stones can usually be differentiated from other opacities by checking a lateral picture and noticing that stones in the kidneys cast their shadows in line with the lumbar vertebrae like this:

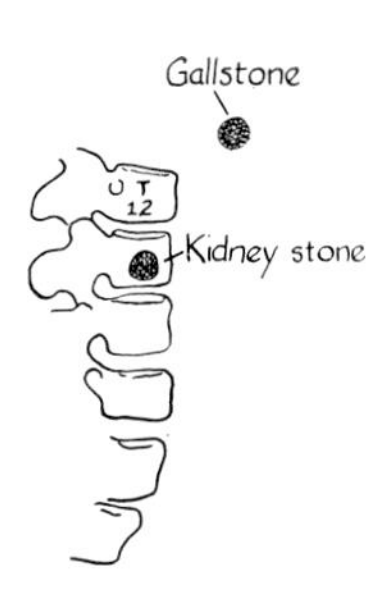

Occasionally it will be necessary to resort to pyelography as mentioned on page 294.

Opacities thought to be in the ureters can often be diagnosed by putting a radiopaque catheter into the suspected ureter and taking one x-ray, then rotating the patient slightly and taking another. This is a vein stone which was originally thought to be in the right ureter:

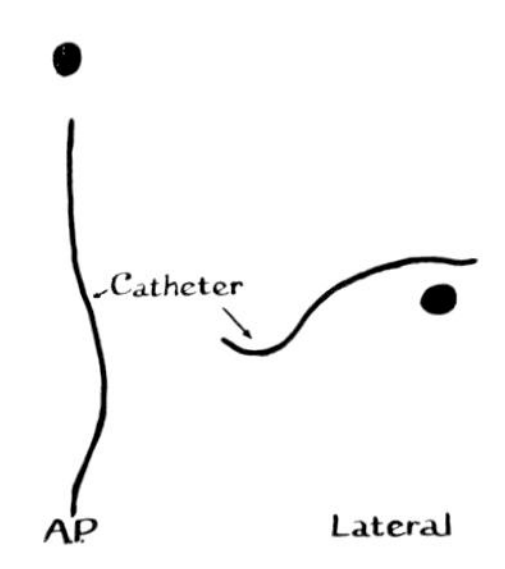

Bladder stones are often seen on the straight KUB film, but they are more easily examined by means of office cystoscopy, making x-ray of little importance in such cases.

Interpretation

Interpretation is simple since stones are either present or absent. Occasionally a negative shadow in the renal pelvis may be confusing, for one cannot be certain whether it is a stone or a tumor projecting into the pelvis. Such films are better evaluated by an expert radiologist and, if necessary, urologic consultation should be sought.

Errors

Probably the most frequent error is to base a diagnosis of stones on insufficient clinical examination and only one film which shows an opacity in the general area of the urinary tract. If one is to make a positive diagnosis on the basis of x-ray, the films must be taken in a sufficient number of planes to be sure that the opacity does lie within the tract.

PYELONEPHRITIS

Ascending urinary tract infections which attack the kidney may be divided roughly into three stages:

In the first stage the urine in the pelvis of the kidney serves as a growth medium for the organism and there is only a mild infectious or inflammatory reaction of the membrane lining the kidney pelvis. There are no x-ray signs characteristic of this stage of the disease.

In the second phase there is actually some moderate invasion of the mucous membranes and kidney substance immediately under them. When this stage is reached there are some changes which can be appreciated on the film.

The third stage may be said to begin when there is marked invasion of the substance, the infectious process extending well out into the parenchyma. This is rarely seen but is readily appreciable on the x-ray in the few cases in which it occurs.

By far the greatest number of urinary tract infections seen by the practitioner are acute or stage 1 infections. There are absolutely no findings upon pyelography and no finding during or following such an acute infection to indicate necessity for the use of the x-ray. As a matter of fact, films are worthless in such a case.

If infection continues in spite of adequate therapy and the patient shows obvious systemic signs of continuing infection, the pyelography may be an excellent means of diagnosis.

Technique

Either the intravenous or the retrograde pyelogram may be used, but in most of these cases the intravenous method is entirely satisfactory. We take retrograde films only when infection has been severe and long continued.

Interpretation

In the early stages there is usually some minor pelvic or caliceal dilatation which may be so slight that it is difficult to detect. The edges of the calices, instead of being clear-cut, show a fuzzy appearance in outline, like this:

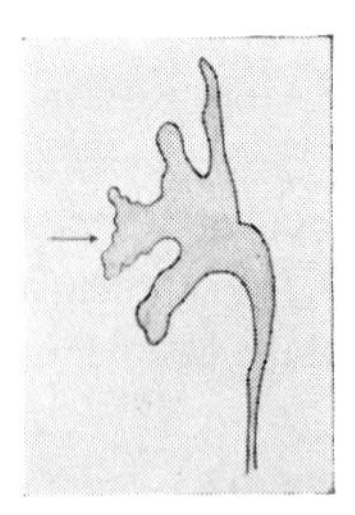

The third stage is simply a continuation of the second, with increasing fuzziness in outline, increase in dilatation, and occasional penetration of the medium into the medullary substance of the kidney at the site of an abscess. These are the common findings in chronic infection:

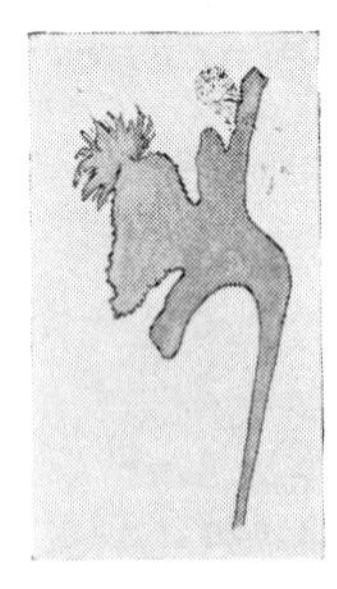

Errors

The most common error is to pass up the early changes because the edges of the calices are not carefully examined. Sometimes it is necessary to observe the film carefully with a magnifying glass to discover the earliest signs. Other than this, errors in diagnosis are extremely rare.

HYDRONEPHROSIS

Hydronephrosis is a pathologic accumulation of urine in the kidney, due to obstruction and back pressure. The back pressure causes an enlargement of the pelvis of the kidney either by ballooning out the pelvis itself or by destroying kidney substance with the ultimate formation of a hollow sac where there was once a kidney.

We do not know why in one case the hydronephrosis attacks the kidney substance and in the other balloons up the pelvis.

Obstruction to the urinary outflow is the only known cause. Causes are legion but we might mention some common ones.

In babies, posterior urethral valves may obstruct and cause hydronephrosis of both kidneys. Unilateral malformations of the ureter may do the same thing. In adults, intermittent obstruction from scarring, fibrous bands, stones, an inferior polar artery, and many other more rare entities are seen. Older men who have had prostatic disease for some years, with partial obstruction of the vesicle outflow, may show a bilateral hydronephrosis.

Late cases may be diagnosed clinically, both by the peculiar dull, nagging pain and by finding the obvious renal mass. Early cases can scarcely be diagnosed without the aid of x-ray. It is in such disease that the office x-ray can prove its value.

While intravenous pyelography will make it possible to obtain a great deal of information, it has been our experience that in adults the retrograde method is by far superior. The ureters are catheterized and both kidney pelves gently filled with Neo-Iopax. When this has been accomplished we usually whittle a match to a point and put it in the end of the ureteral catheter to prevent leakage of the contrast medium. Sometimes a safety pin will fit into the bore of the catheter and serve the same purpose.

Technique

A plain KUB plate is usually all that is needed for diagnosis.

Interpretation

In early cases one can detect signs of back pressure in the minor calices. The pyramidal portion which invaginates into the calices is slightly flattened by the back pressure and the neck of each calix is thickened. The first minor sign is the change from this:

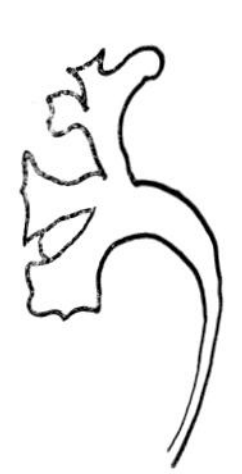

to this:

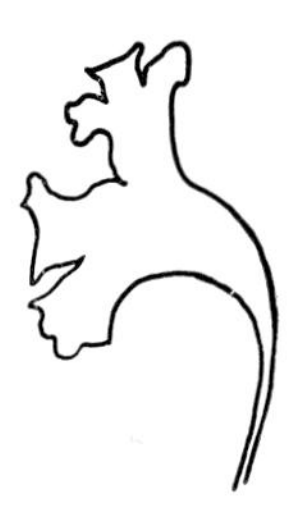

As time goes on, the pyramids are flattened and the calices may even become clubbed.

Enlargement of the kidney pelvis itself is apparent, and when things have reached this stage one decision is necessary. Is the hydronephrosis invading the renal substance or is it ballooning out the kidney pelvis?

If the hydronephrosis is invading the renal substance the calices are widely dilated and have no recognizable anatomic characteristics whatever. They extend as gross, clubbed channels far back into the renal substance, like this:

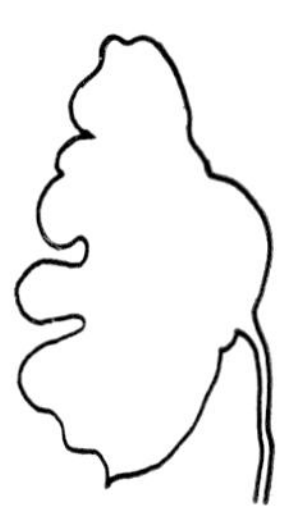

If, on the other hand, the renal pelvis is mainly affected by the disease, it is grossly dilated, but the calices retain some of their normal architecture and the kidney appears to be perched to one side of the ballooned-out pelvis, like this:

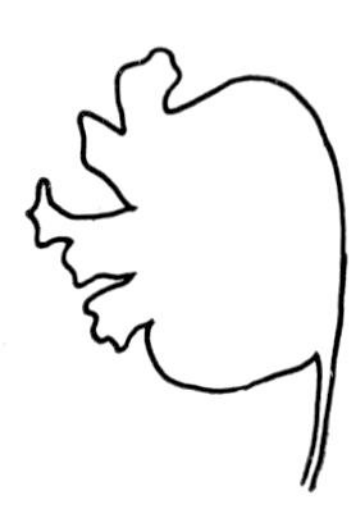

The site of the obstruction can often be delineated or clearly inferred from the x-ray film. If, for instance, the site is at the bladder mouth or lower, both kidneys will be involved. If the site is in the lower ureter the involved ureter, as well as the kidney on the same side, will be dilated. If the difficulty is at the ureteropelvic junction, only the kidney will be involved, the ureter remaining relatively normal. For this reason, these films are almost invariably diagnostic and easy to read.

Errors

Errors lie almost exclusively in the interpretation of early hydronephrotic changes. If one does not look carefully at the minor calices, the early changes engendered by back pressure may be passed up entirely.

KIDNEY TUMORS

A discussion of tumors of the kidney can still strike sparks in almost any medical meeting. Classification is by no means settled and etiology of even nonmalignant tumors is the subject for much weighty controversy. The practitioner should not attempt to make a definitive diagnosis of kidney tumors by means of x-ray.

If one can be certain that an abnormal growth exists in the kidney and not worry about what kind it is, he will do well. Such patients should then be referred to more expert hands for diagnosis.

Technique

One can obtain much information from either retrograde or intravenous pyelography, and probably both should be done if there is any question about the existence of a tumor.

Interpretation

There are seven or eight signs which may be taken as indicative of the presence of tumor:

1. Elongation and skinniness of the calices. The illustration below shows a normal kidney and one with obviously elongated calices for comparison:

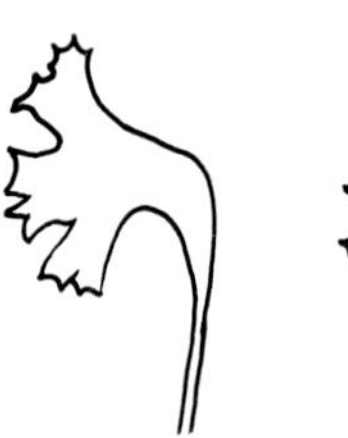

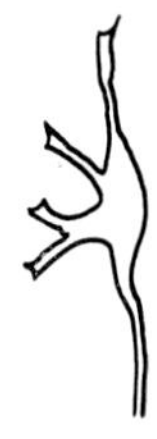

2. Obliteration of the calices. The partial or complete obliteration of the calix is evidence of a tumor until proved otherwise. In demonstrating this, do not forget that positioning may have considerable effect on the filling of the calices. Therefore the patient should be shifted about so that every opportunity may be given for a suspect area to fill. This is a typical illustration:

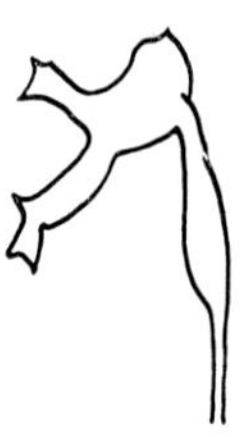

3. Regional dilatation of the calices. If a certain area of the kidney is obstructed by a tumor, then the system proximal to that

area will dilate. Here is an example:

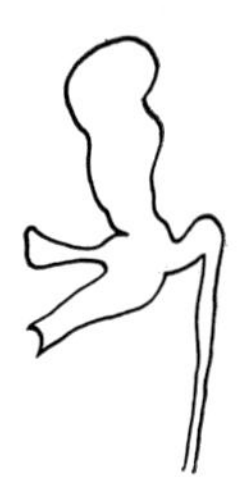

4. Displacement of the pelvis or the calices. Any type of tumor may push aside a portion of the kidney, with gross displacement. This is an example:

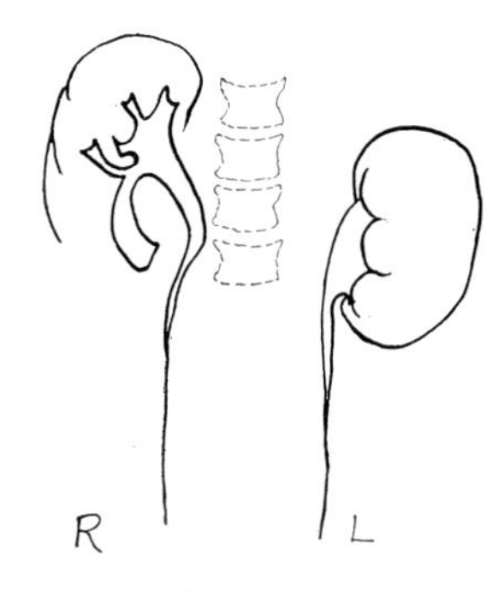

5. A filling defect in the pelvis. Rarely tumors may be manifest early only by a constant filling defect in the renal pelvis. This cannot always be differentiated from a transparent renal stone, and several examinations with various positionings may be necessary. This is an illustration:

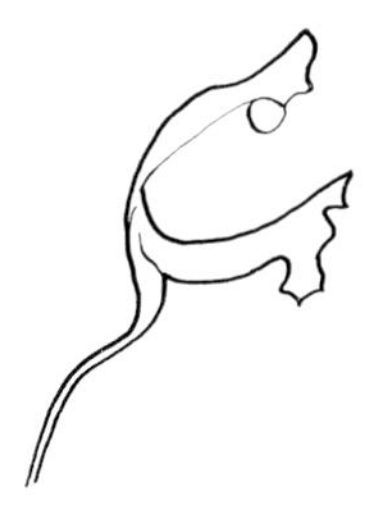

6. Nonfunctioning of the kidney. Late in the course of renal malignancy the kidney itself or the circulation to it may be so completely destroyed that it does not secrete. When intravenous pyeolgraphy is done, no dye appears in the involved kidney. This is by no means a sign of malignancy or anything else. It simply proves that the kidney is not functioning.

7. Displacement of surrounding structures. A barium enema may show the colon displaced by a mass in one kidney, like this:

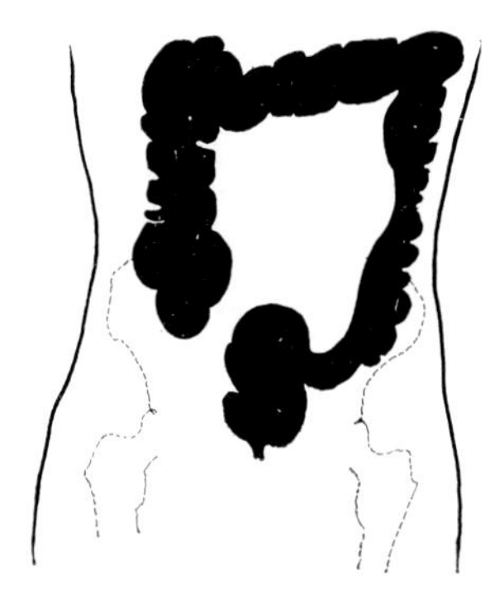

Or a glass of barium may show displacement of the stomach, like this:

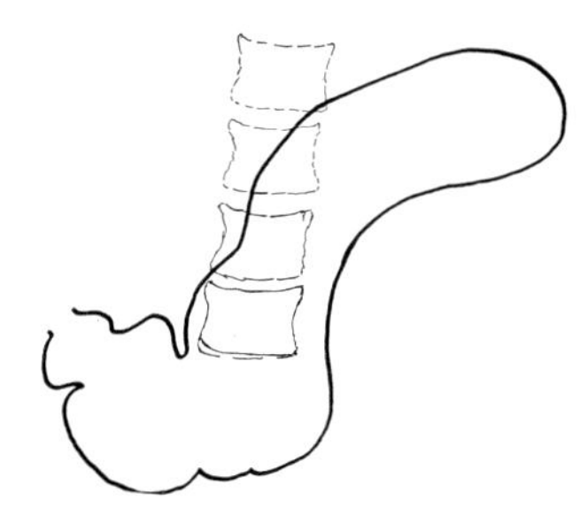

Sometimes a barium meal is a good means of clarifying the origin of a large intra-abdominal mass.

Errors

If one looks carefully for the above signs, few errors will be made in diagnosing the presence of some kind of renal tumor. Differentiation is entirely another matter. It is an error for the practitioner to go further into the diagnosis of renal tumor.

HORSESHOE KIDNEY

More than one out of every one thousand persons has this renal anomaly which may be mildly or extensively symptomatic. The kidneys are joined usually at the lower pole and fail to go through the rotative process in development, so that the pelvis is lateral and the main substance of the kidneys medial. Ordinarily such kidneys are lower than usual and the lower calices may extend far downward and point toward one another.

Technique

The excretory urograph is efficient in the diagnosis of these lesions.

Interpretation

A single glance at the film shows the failure of rotation. Instead of being like this:

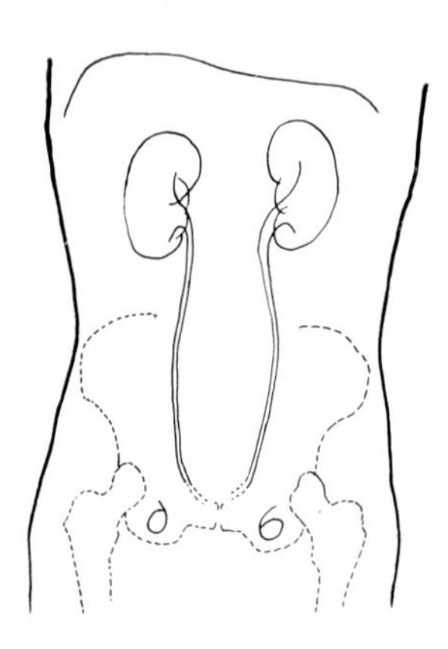

the kidneys are like this:

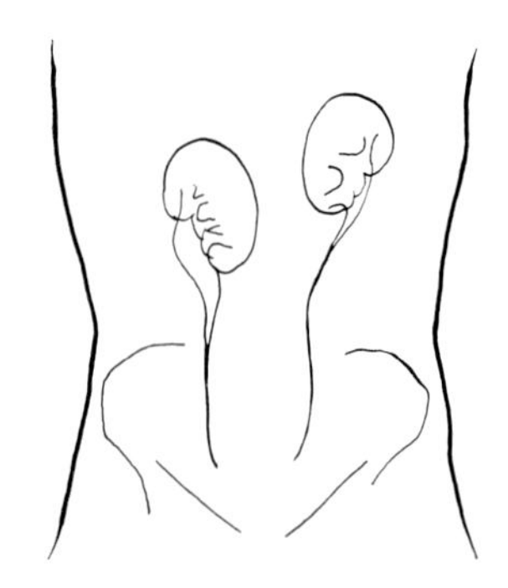

Notice that the kidney pelves are larger and somewhat closer together than normal and that the lower calices point downward and inward.

Often in such cases the outline and the isthmus connecting the two kidneys can be clearly seen.

Errors

None.

General Comment

X-ray of the urinary system is frequently indicated in office practice. Unfortunately, it is frequently neglected. By all means put your office x-ray to work solving urologic problems.

CHAPTER TWENTY-EIGHT

Gynecology

The principal office use of x-ray in gynecologic disease is hysterosalpingography. Using this simple technique with ample precautions will provide a great deal of information without subjecting the patient either to much discomfort or to more than the minimal risk. The actual procedure consists of filling the uterus with Lipiodol under moderate pressure and observing the distribution of the injected substance, both fluoroscopically and roentgenographically.

Technique

The actual technique of placing the cannula and making the injection is a medical problem, not one which comes within the purview of the office laboratory and x-ray group. Methodology may be found in my book on *Office Procedures.**

The injection is usually made with the patient on the x-ray table, the cannula having been inserted by the physician and held in place by the office nurse while the necessary eye adaptation takes place. To proceed, inject 1 or 2 ml. of Lipiodol and observe the results with the fluoroscope. If there is no sign of a dye invading the venous system (see below), inject another 2 ml. Repeat this maneuver until ample visualization of the uterus and tubes is secured. Usually the total amount of opaque medium used will be less than 10 ml. When this amount has been injected under fluoroscopic control and you are positive that none of the dye is appearing in the veins, proceed with an x-ray film.

Immediately print and examine the film. If the opaque medium is not seen to pervade the tubes and spill into the pelvic cavity, inject a slightly increased amount, but be sure the injection pressure at this period never exceeds 250 mm. of mercury. Then take another x-ray. If there is still no medium in the pelvic cavity, you may assume closure of the tube or tubes.

Interpretation

Interpretation is a matter of evaluating filling defects and lack of "spill" into the pelvic cavity when a medium enters the tubes. A normal film looks like this:

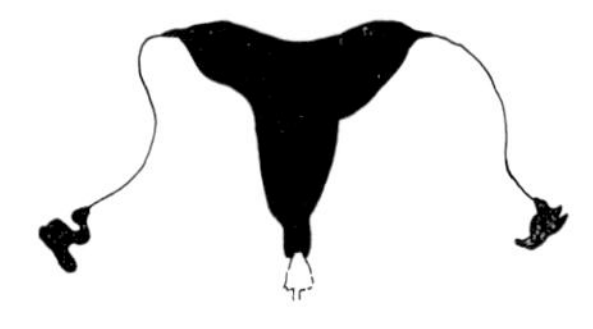

These are probably endometrial polyps:

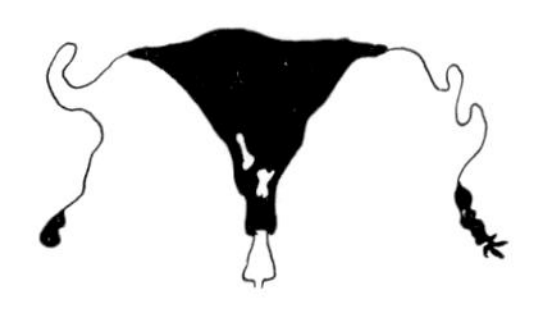

*Williamson, Paul: Office Procedures, Philadelphia, W. B. Saunders Co.

This is a typical fibroid uterus with great distortion of the uterine cavity:

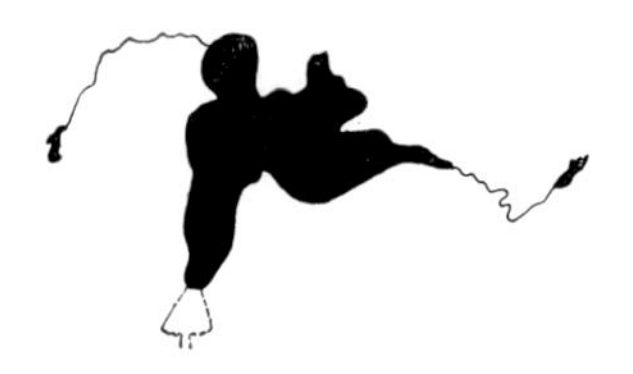

This is a hydrosalpinx of the left tube:

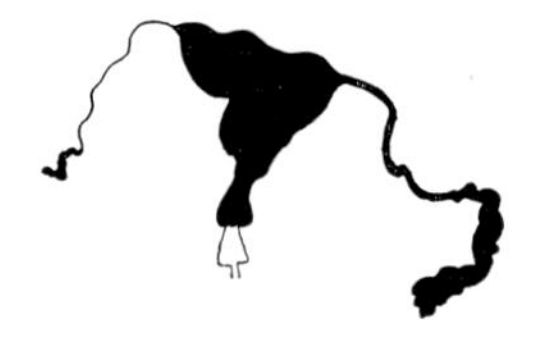

This is bilateral obstruction at the ampulla:

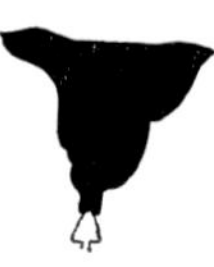

Errors

There are two absolute contraindications to the injection of the opaque medium. The first is any sort of active tubal inflammatory disease and the second is a strong suspicion of intrauterine malignancy. These are not relative contraindications; they are absolute contraindications. No information offered by the hysterosalpingogram can be worth the risk involved to the patient if these conditions exist.

During the actual injection, one observes with the fluoroscope to detect intravasation of the medium into periuterine veins. Infiltration is first seen immediately lateral to the uterus, as shown here:

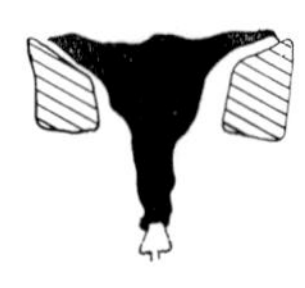

The material rapidly spreads through the venous plexes in the broad ligaments (much more rapidly than it ever enters the tubes) and may be seen here:

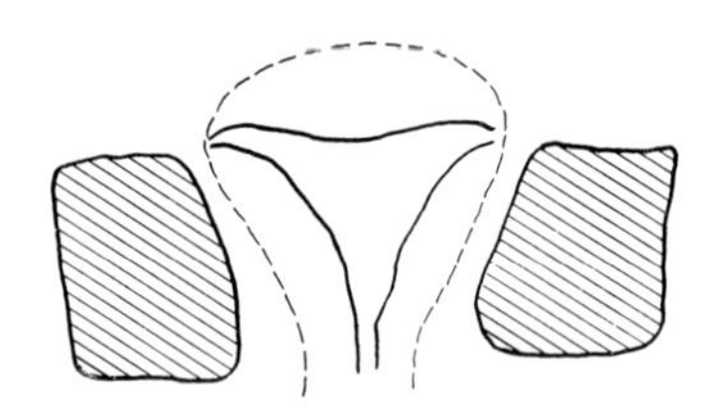

When there is the slightest sign of this happening, the injection should be stopped immediately.

We should perhaps mention that hysterosalpingograms have been attempted during early pregnancy, usually with disasterous results so far as the pregnancy is concerned. Of course, this, too, is a contraindication.

CHAPTER TWENTY-NINE

Fractures and Dislocations

The commonest use of the office x-ray is in delineation of the results of trauma. The average practitioner will take four or five pictures of traumatized areas a day.

If you will allow me, I shall repeat a statement that I have probably phrased too often: the x-ray can be a liability rather than an asset in cases of trauma. Particularly is this true if the x-ray is operated by the unthinking practitioner who subscribes to the idea that "either there is a fracture or there is not."

By no means does the x-ray show all fractures. Only occasionally does it show soft tissue injuries and soft tissue injuries may be just as serious as a broken bone. In the clear-cut fracture the x-ray is of great service and should be utilized. If it is negative it does not necessarily mean that no injury is involved, and at times the injury may even be serious. All injuries should have clinical evaluation and not depend upon negative x-ray evidence.

In this section we will consider only the common injuries which are often seen in the practitioner's office. More comprehensive textbooks are available for the rare entities. Most of the patients with these rare conditions will be treated in the hospital and not in the office.

Phalangeal fractures are so simple to diagnose and the x-ray usually so clear-cut that we have deliberately omitted consideration of them.

THE CLAVICLE

The clavicle both suspends the shoulder and serves to keep it a constant distance from the trunk, like this:

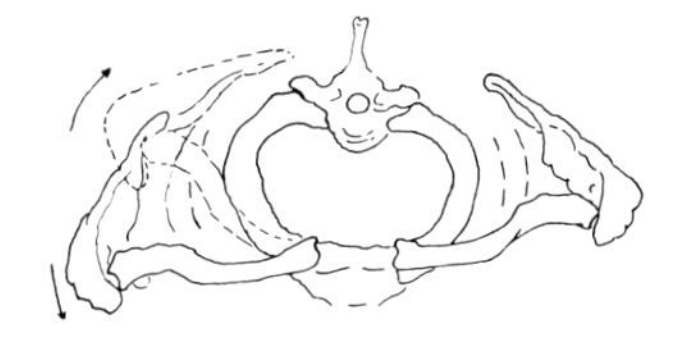

Most fractures occur in the middle third. If the fracture is complete, the shoulder literally drops away from the trunk. Shoulder muscles tend to rotate the outer fragment in such fashion that its broken end points upward and backward, like this:

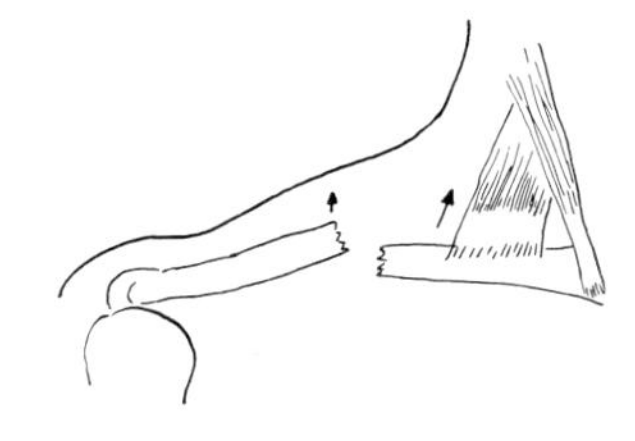

These fractures are by far the most common fractures of childhood and are seen with some frequency in adults. They usually occur in the middle third of the bone as a result of a fall on the outstretched hand. In children, from 60 to 70 per cent of the fractures will be incomplete.

The x-rays are scarcely needed in diagnosis of a complete fracture. The clavicle is subcutaneous along its whole length and fractures are readily palpated. In children with greenstick fractures, the history, coupled with the point of tenderness, is usually enough to make the diagnosis. In a significant number of cases, x-ray is more necessary for checking the results of reduction than it is for confirming the presence of fracture.

One exception is the fracture that does not reduce easily. Occasionally a bit of muscle may become caught between the ends of the fracture. When this happens prolonged traction is often required for proper reduction. X-ray may emphasize the fact that this has occurred.

Technique

An ordinary posteroanterior film of the shoulder is all that is needed.

Interpretation

The diagnosis of fracture is easy. Interpretation of a reduction may not be so easy.

The clavicle is a bone that heals well, and a 50 per cent apposition of the fracture ends is sufficient to give excellent functional results.

This is not a bad reduction of a severe clavicular fracture:

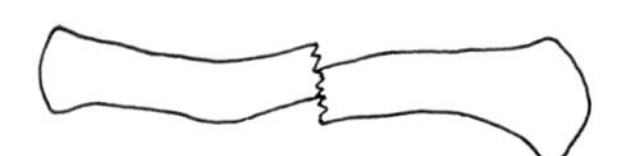

This is a bad result:

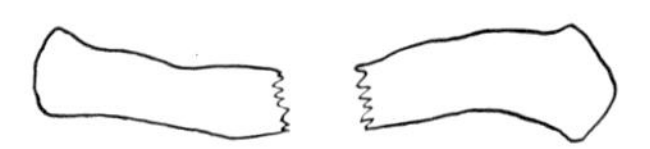

It shows that the fragments are separated, probably by a bit of muscle.

Errors

Errors are exceptionally rare.

ACROMIOCLAVICULAR DISLOCATION

The acromioclavicular joint is often subject to extreme trauma in the course of life. Its integrity depends upon the coracoacromial and coracoclavicular ligaments, as shown here:

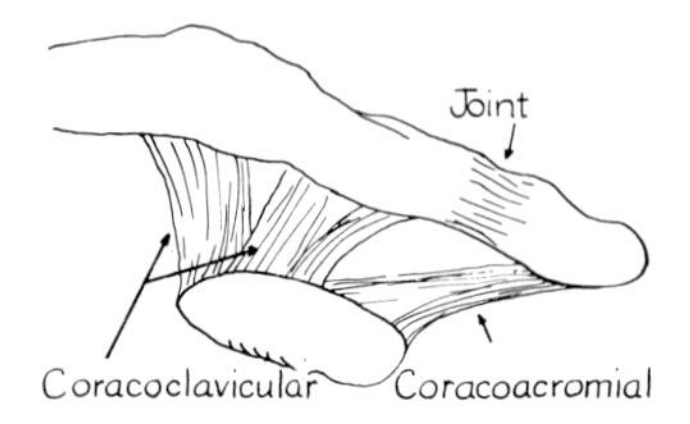

An injury involving only the joint capsule will usually heal without difficulty, but an injury in which the ligaments are also torn represents a potential crippling trauma and must be treated accurately and well. Differentiation between these two injuries is usually one of extent. The x-ray can be of great help in answering the question.

Technique

Have the patient hold a heavy object, such as a flat iron or a medical book, using the hand on the involved side. Then take an ordinary posteroanterior film of the shoulder.

Interpretation

Before you take the x-ray you will know that there has been some slippage in the joint. The question to be answered is "how much?"

Cases in which the ligaments still retain their integrity show slight displacement at the acromioclavicular joint, like this:

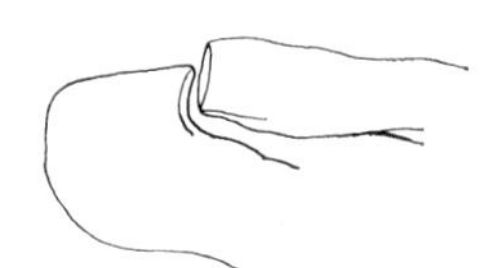

Cases in which the ligaments have been severed show a much greater displacement, like this:

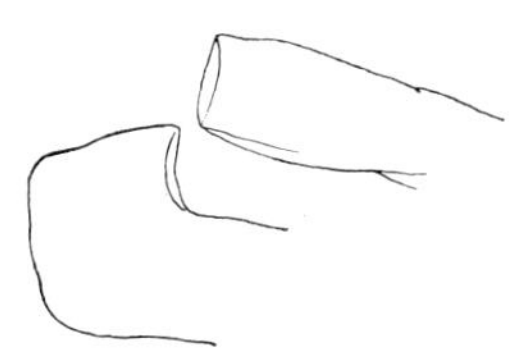

Occasionally the end of the clavicle will be torn off, like this:

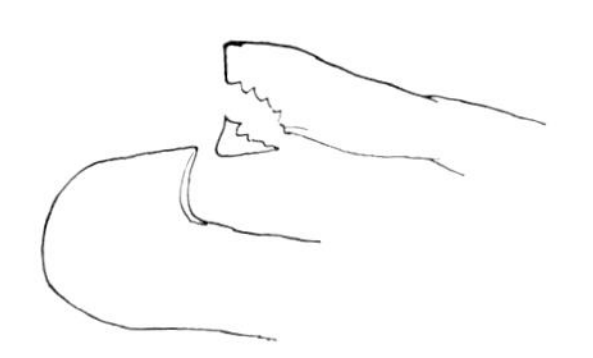

Errors

A common error is failure to follow such a case a sufficient length of time and to neglect making a repeat film after treatment is finished. Sometimes the lacerated ligaments do not heal properly and a chronic acromioclavicular dislocation results. This is an indication for surgery, but it will sometimes be overlooked if one does not do adequate follow-up x-ray studies, using the above technique.

DISLOCATED SHOULDER

Subcoracoid dislocation of the shoulder is the commonest dislocation seen. It has been estimated that at least 50 per cent of all dislocations occur here.

An x-ray is not necessary for diagnosis of the lesion but is usually taken to rule out a possible occurrence of a fracture along with the other pathology. This does happen in perhaps 2 or 3 per cent of the cases and it is wise for the physician to take it into account.

Recurrent dislocations can be diagnosed historically, but x-ray evidence of this condition usually exists to prove that the history is accurate.

Technique

The standard posteroanterior or anteroposterior film of the shoulder is entirely adequate to demonstrate the lesion.

Interpretation

The dislocation is obvious. One should, however, look for fractures here:

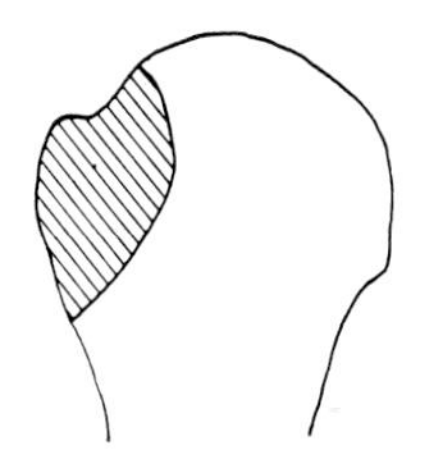

Approximately one in every five or six shoulder dislocations will show some fracture in the greater tuberosity area.

In recurrent dislocation there may be flattening of the humeral head due to a wide, shallow, V-shaped groove formed between the greater tuberosity and the head. The cartilaginous ring around the glenoid cavity, the labrum glenoidale, may be torn loose in a recurrent dislocation and parts of it may calcify, giving an appearance like this:

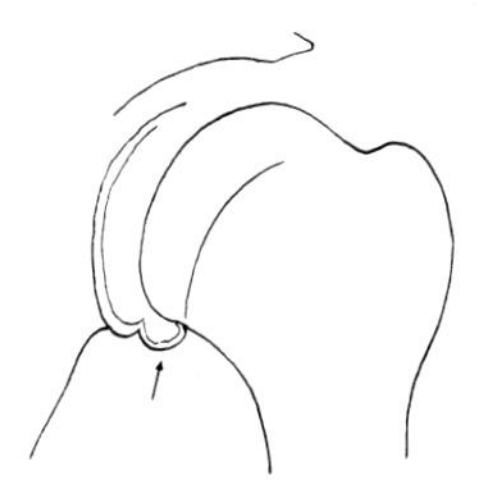

Errors

The most frequent error is overlooking an obvious fracture in the area of the greater tuberosity. If the tuberosity cannot be clearly visualized on the first films, repeat pictures should be taken ofter reduction in various positions so as to visualize the entire area.

FRACTURES OF THE HUMERUS

Fractures through the shaft or upper portion of the humerus are easily diagnosed on x-ray and require no comment here. There are two common humeral injuries, however, which are sometimes missed and, therefore, should be mentioned.

Epiphyseal separation or injury in youngsters from 6 to 16 is common. Certain points about these injuries should be remembered at all times.

First, there is a thick membranous layer of periosteum as shown here:

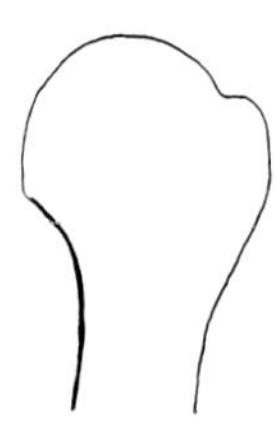

When the traumatic force applied is not of great intensity there may be only a loosening of the epiphysis and a stripping of the heavy periosteum. There is no way to diagnose this injury by physical examination. X-rays taken in such a patient are quite often negative. If there is pain in the proper location, along with negative x-rays, be very suspicious. Films taken of the same area a month after injury may show new bone formation where this heavy periosteum was stripped off. Always have the patient return in thirty days and look for a shadow here:

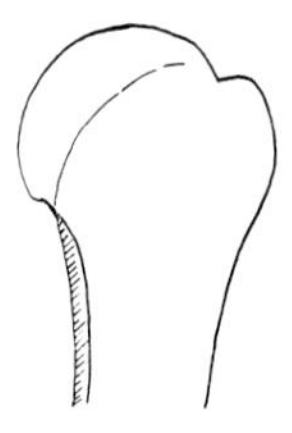

If the traumatic force is greater, the epiphysis may be completely unseated and a portion of the shaft may be torn off, like this:

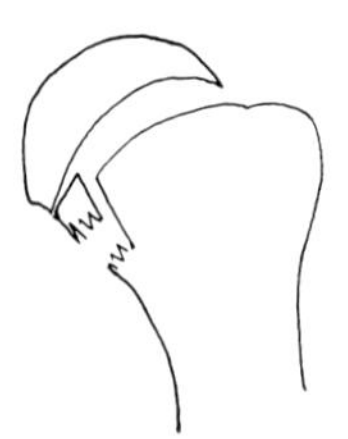

In adults, the greater tuberosity is frequently fractured or dented and may be torn completely free. When there is extreme pain on raising the arm, tenderness at the point of the shoulder, and a history of trauma, always examine the greater tuberosity carefully. In a surprising number of cases you will find evidence of bony pathology.

Errors

The commonest error is to confuse a bursitis of the shoulder with injury to the greater tuberosity. Usually the differentiation can be made easily enough clinically but occasionally an x-ray is required.

Unless one is fully aware that the greater tuberosity is often torn free, these fractures may be missed. This, too, is an error more common than you might suspect.

THE ELBOW

There are several facts which must be brought out in order to diagnose injuries about the elbow properly. In the lateral view, notice angulation of the humeral articular surface with regards to the humeral shaft, like this:

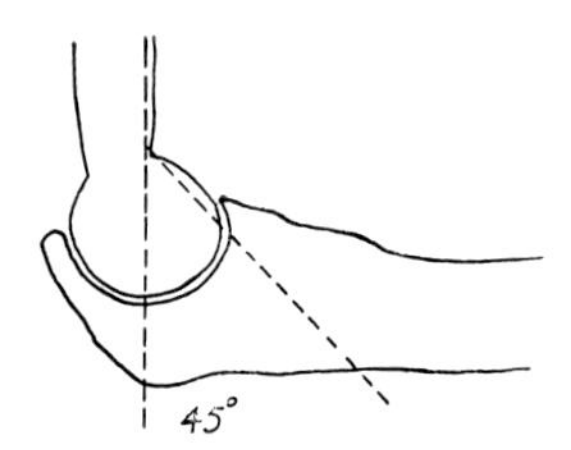

In the anteroposterior view the carrying angle is seen like this:

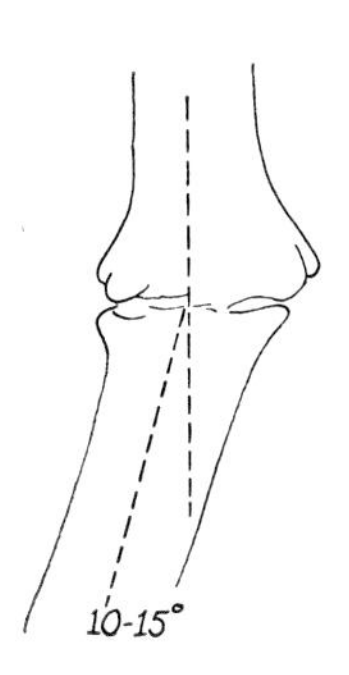

The integrity of these angles must be preserved in treatment if adequate function is to result. In children, ossification may be somewhat variable, and any picture of an injured elbow should be accompanied by a picture of the normal elbow for comparative purposes. If this is not done a fracture will sometimes be diagnosed when none exists.

Another extremely important point which must be kept in mind when considering fractures of the elbow is the possibility of soft tissue damage. A moment of consideration of the anatomy involved will reveal that there are many important structures lying in apposition to the elbow joint.

With the extreme displacement which often occurs in such fractures, sharp fragments of the bone may lacerate these structures and cause permanent impairment. Swelling must be combated, for it occasionally becomes gross enough to cause arterial compression and resultant ischemic changes in the hand or forearm.

Technique

Simple anteroposterior and lateral films of the elbow will supply all the required information. Occasionally when the patient cannot extend his elbow, pictures may be taken like this:

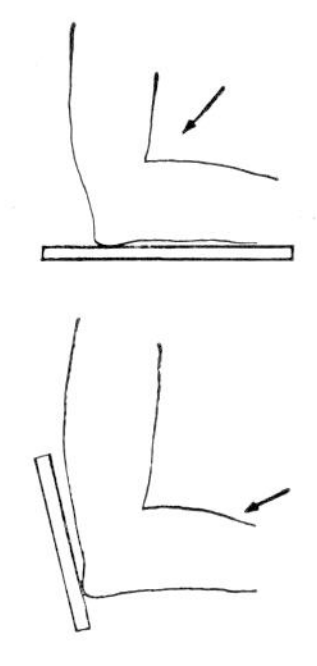

Most fractures about the elbow are easily detected upon roentgenologic examination. The commonest elbow fracture of children is the straight supracondylar fracture, like this:

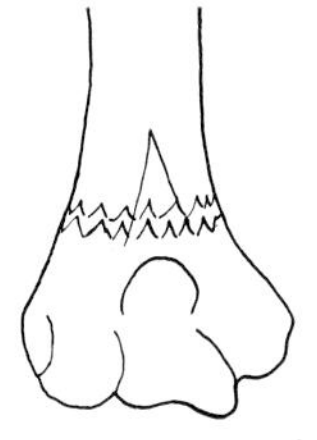

The next most frequent is separation of the lateral epicondyle, like this:

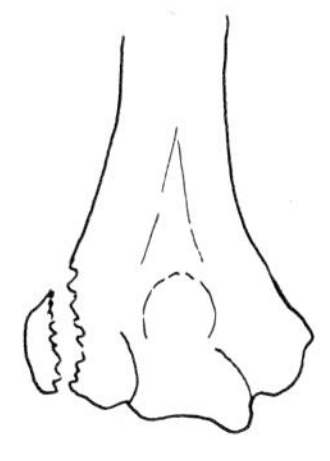

In adults, the one fracture that is likely to be missed is the fissure fracture of the head of the radius. It is simply a crack extending from the articular surface downward into the substance of the radius, like this:

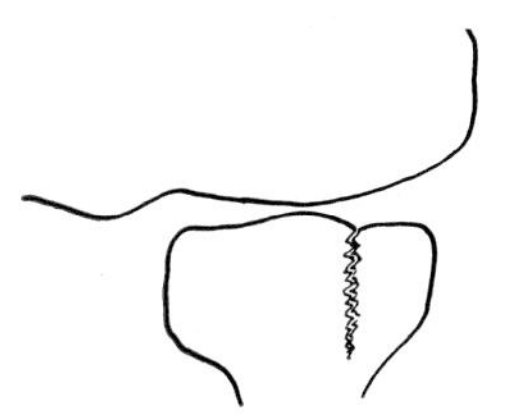

Epiphyseal changes are best detected by a careful comparative examination of the injured and normal sides.

Errors

The quality of the film probably causes more errors than anything else. Fractures about the elbow are not unduly difficult to detect, but one must have film sufficiently good to see bony structure in detail if detection is to be assured.

The second most frequent error is probably failure to compare the normal with the abnormal side in a young person. This, too, is imperative if one wishes to avoid embarrassing mistakes.

THE WRIST

Fractures about the wrist are so well known that extensive comment is certainly not necessary. There are, however, a few of these injuries that escape detection so regularly that they should be mentioned. Certain anatomic facts are also valuable in diagnosis. A normal anteroposterior view of the wrist shows this angulation:

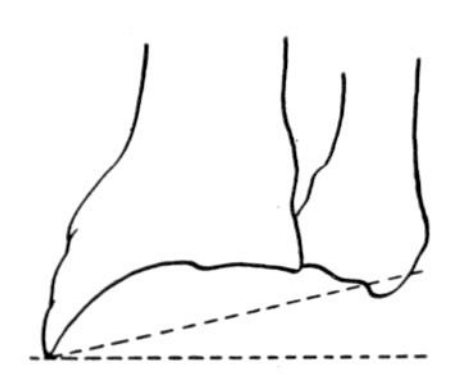

In the lateral view, the articular surface of the radius is inclined like this:

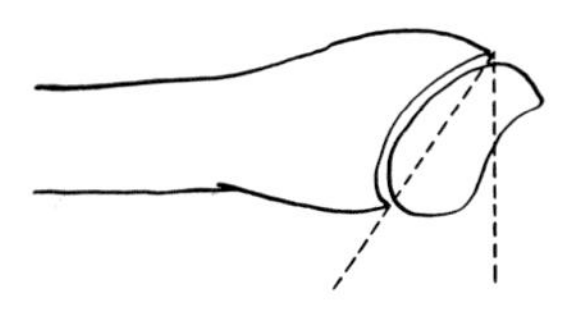

Any major change in this angulation results in an impairment of wrist function. It usually results from a recent or old fracture.

Technique

The straight anteroposterior and lateral films are usually all that are needed. When one is studying a navicular bone it is helpful to obtatin a partial oblique view by putting an ordinary two-inch child's block under the radius, like this:

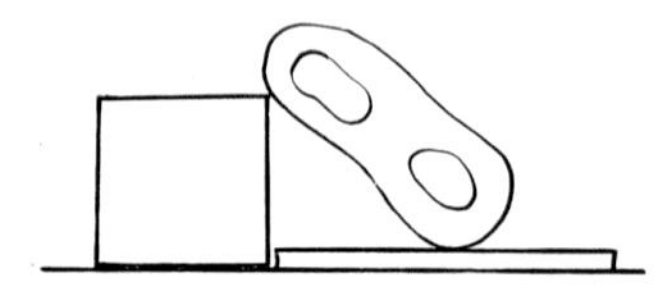

Interpretation

We see quite a few fractures that result from compression of the thin dorsal plate in the radius. This thin area is located here:

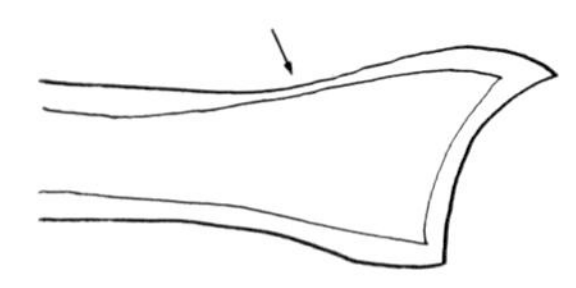

and a compressive blow will crush it. This changes the normal volar inclination of the radius and the lateral x-ray looks like this:

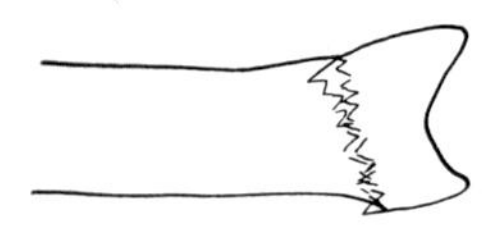

Fractures of the radial and ulnar styloid often seems to be missed. In the anteroposterior view one simply examines at these points:

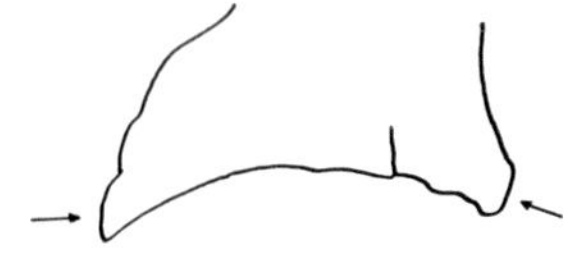

Fractures of the navicular are common but cannot be well seen in the straight anteroposterior roentgenogram. In the oblique film, as mentioned above, a thin fracture line may be made out. Sometimes one will not see the fracture line even after the most careful x-ray examination. In such cases and when clinical signs are present, we should splint the hand, treat the injury as a fracture for two weeks and take another x-ray. Usually there is an ovoid line of degeneration around the fracture line which in two weeks looks like this:

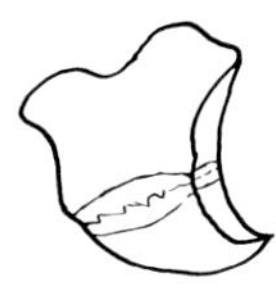

Another problem in an injury such as this is determining whether the injury is intra- or extra-articular. This can usually be told from the typical positioning of the fracture line, like this:

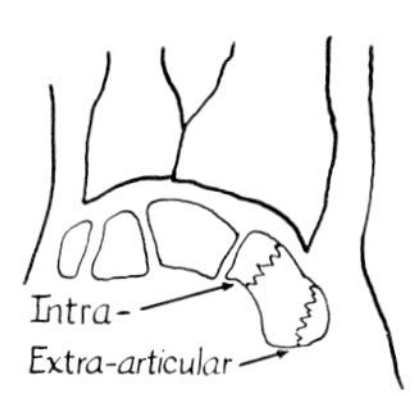

Errors

Errors occur most often from lack of careful inspection of the film. Occasionally even the best films will not show a fracture of the navicular. When such a fracture is suspected it is in error not to take films two or three weeks after the first pictures for further examination. In perhaps 50 per cent of these cases such fractures will be demonstrated on the second examination.

PELVIC FRACTURES

Most pelvic fractures involve the obturator foramen. They are usually so obvious that no discussion is needed here except for one point: If there is any extensive separation of the fragments almost always there will be a secondary fracture or a separation of the symphysis pubis. One must remember to look for this sometimes difficult-to-find second injury.

INJURIES ABOUT THE HIP

Traumatic dislocations of the hip are not infrequently seen by the practitioner. Most of these are posterior and can be diagnosed by physical examination alone. More rarely one will be seen in which the examination is not conclusive and the simple anteroposterior roentgenogram does not give all the information needed. A lateral picture taken as mentioned below will answer the question.

Hip fractures are common, particularly in older persons, and most of them may be diagnosed clinically. From the x-ray one can only obtain information as to the site of the fracture and, therefore, to its prognosis.

Technique

The standard anteroposterior film of the pelvis is sufficiently accurate for this particular view. A lateral film of the hip may be taken with the patient in this position:

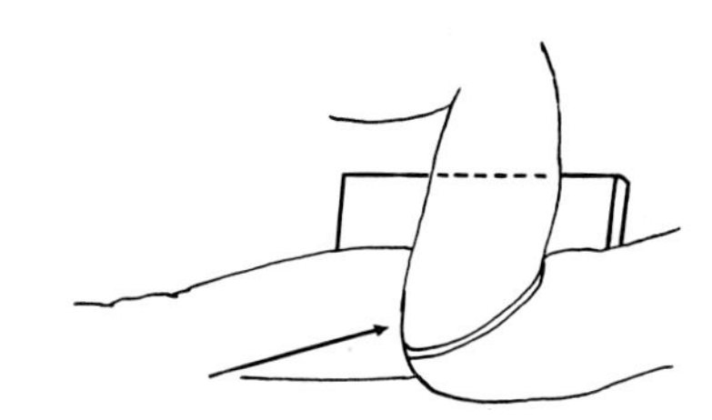

A properly aimed film gives this x-ray view:

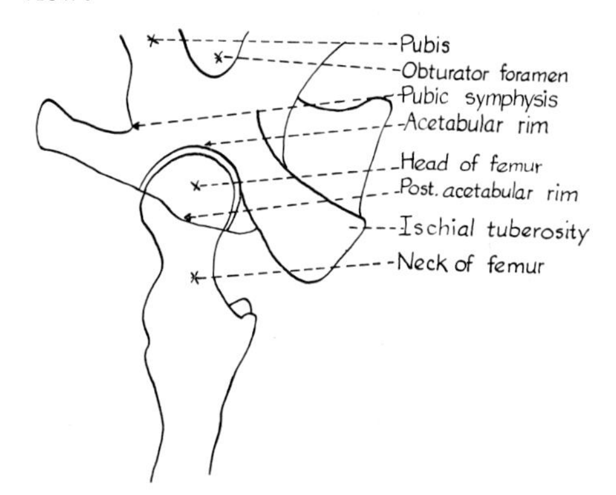

Interpretation

In addition to careful observation the application of Shenton's line test and the right angle test may be helpful.

This is Shenton's line:

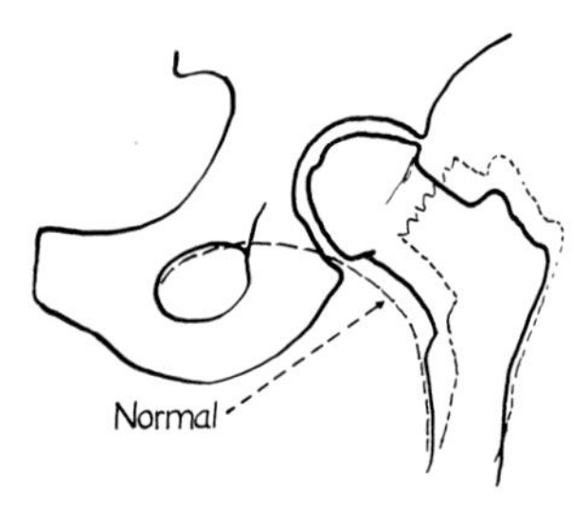

The right angle test is done as follows: Draw a straight line along the axis of the femoral shaft. At the level of the greater trochanter extend a right angle line inward to the acetabulum. In the absence of fracture, this line usually is below the fovea capitus. In the presence of some fractures (but not in all) the right angle will extend above the fovea capitus, like this:

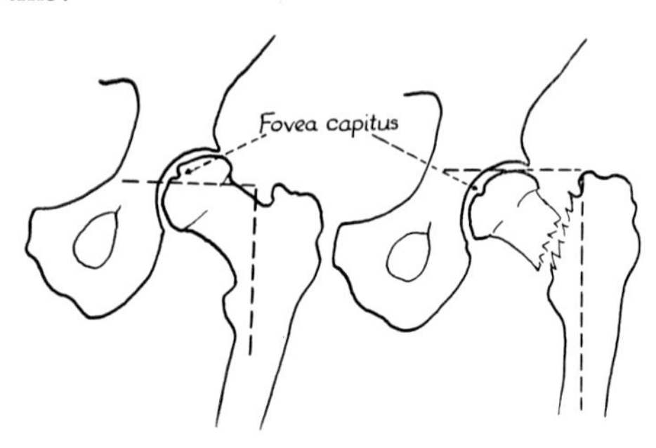

THE KNEE

Bony injuries about the knee are not difficult to diagnose, but ordinarily four views are required rather than the standard two. It is probably not necessary here to discuss the pathology seen in the x-ray plates so we will merely outline the technique for the two special views required. The tangential view of the patella, sometimes called the notch film, is taken like this:

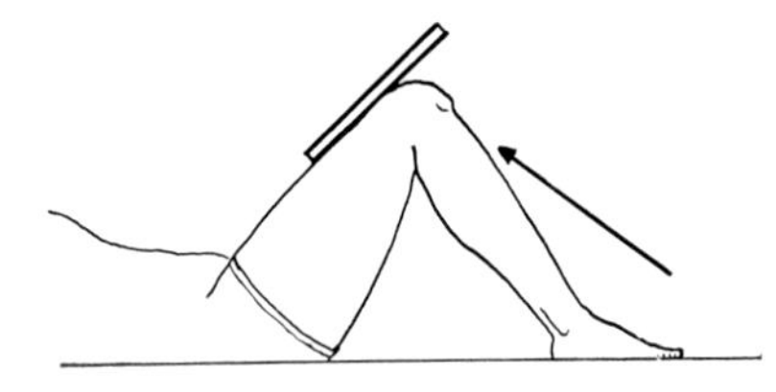

A view of the intercondyloid fossa of the femur—the tunnel film—is taken like this:

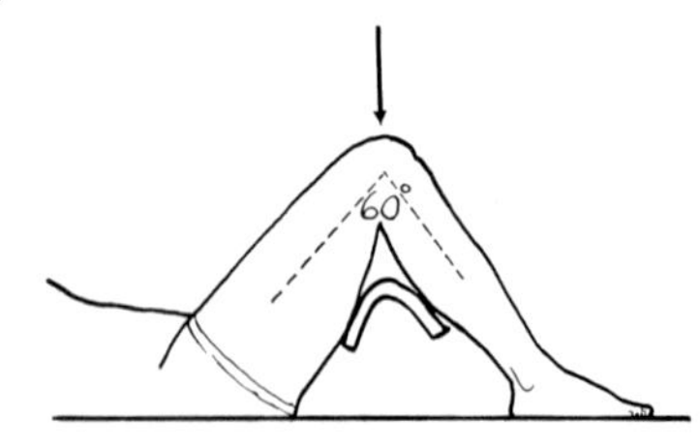

Do remember to look at the tibial spines in every case of knee injury. They are often torn away, the fracture line running through their base.

Fractures of the lower leg and ankle are so easily diagnosed from routine film that they need not be considered here.

CHAPTER THIRTY

Diseases of the Bones and Joints

In this chapter we will consider only the common diseases of bones which are seen often by the practitioner in his office and upon which he should be a diagnostic authority. Diagnosis of bone disease is not too easy and any film which does not fall clearly into one of the well-known patterns should be examined by an expert roentgenologist. Particularly is this true of unexplained densities or areas of rarification.

ABNORMAL CALCIFICATION

Calcium either may be deposited or true bone formed in any tissue of the human body. There have been reports of this on practically every area of the body, but only a few are commonly involved.

MYOSITIS OSSIFICANS

Myositis ossificans is a deposition of bone most frequently seen in the brachialis anticus or quadriceps muscles following severe trauma. Typical films look like this:

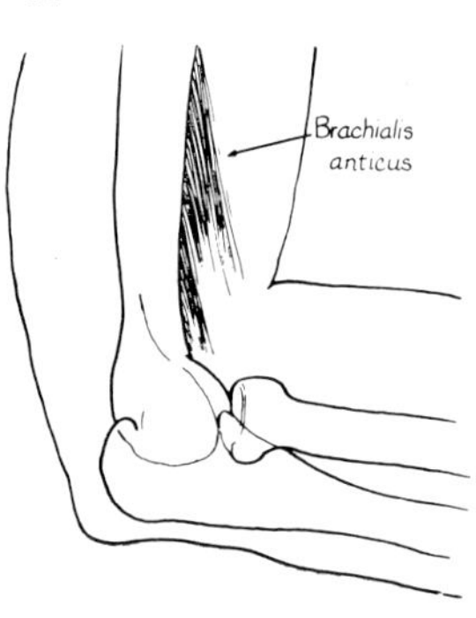

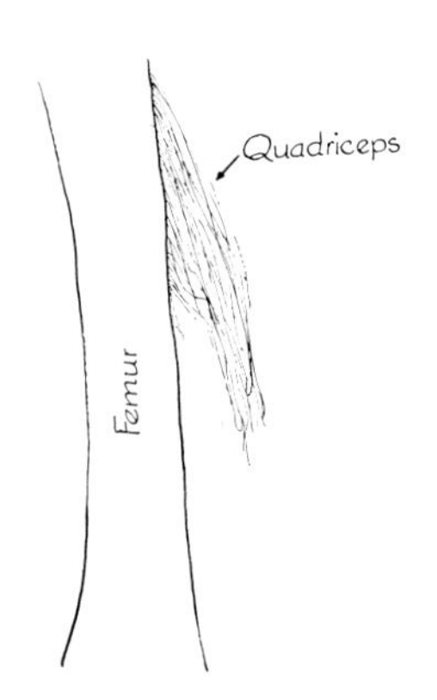

PELLEGRINI-STIEDA DISEASE

Pellegrini-Stieda disease is the calcification seen in the medial ligament of the knee joint, usually in its upper portion near the internal femoral condyle. Typically, it looks like this:

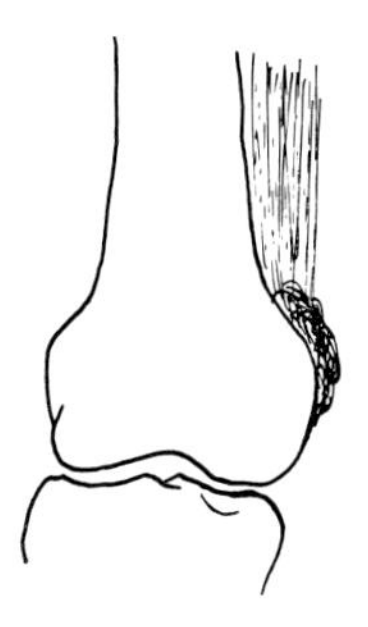

CALCAREOUS TENDONITIS

Calcareous tendonitis is a typical deposition of calcium in tendons often seen following trauma. Its most frequent location is in the tendon of the supraspinatus just above the humeral head. It looks like this:

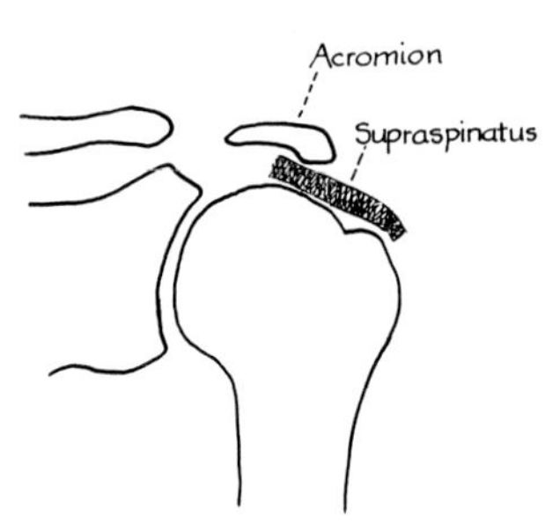

Similar depositions of calcium uncommonly occur in the tendons and the ligaments of the hands and feet following trauma. This is a typical ossification involving a flexor tendon of the finger:

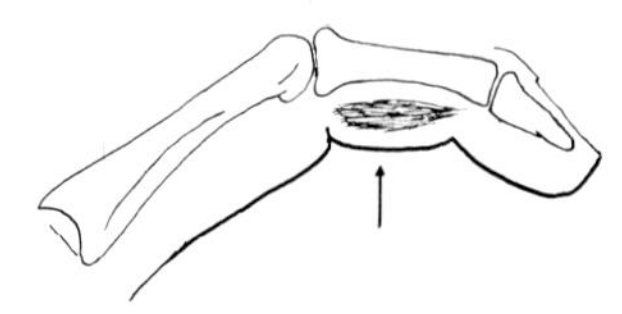

Bone is sometimes laid down in the attachment of tendons and ligaments to the normal bony surface with resultant formation of spurs. This is a typical calcaneal spur:

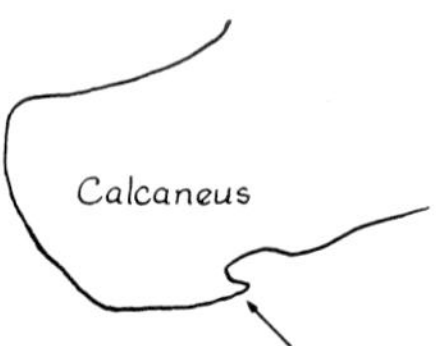

INFARCTS

There are many diseases which appear to be little more than typical infarcts of bone, known by a wide variety of names—Perthes' disease of the hip, Köhler's disease of the tarsal scaphoid, Osgood-Schlatter's disease of the tibial tubercle, and kyphosis dorsalis juvenilis, to name a few. I would advise the practitioner to become familiar with the typical appearance of infarcted bone and, at least until the problem is clarified, to forget the unusual names and let the process speak for itself.

The disease is most often seen in the epiphyses in growing children, but may actually occur in any part of the bone. It is apparently a result of trauma, although by no means do we know this to be the case.

To trace the process through a series of illustrations, some traumatic or other process stops up a vessel:

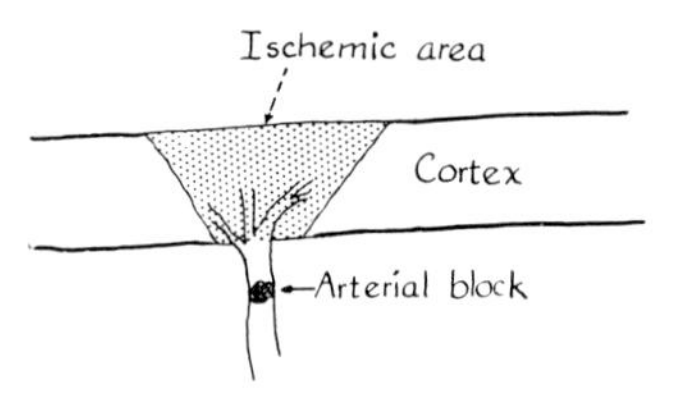

At first there are no clear-cut radiologic changes. There may or may not be clinical symptoms, depending upon the actual area involved. Sooner or later the dead bone collapses into a dense homogeneous mass in which normal markings are absent. It looks like this:

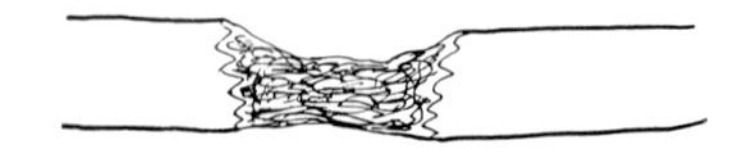

Osteoclasts migrate into the area and absorb the dead bone. The area is filled with fibrous tissue and becomes a defect in the x-ray film, like this:

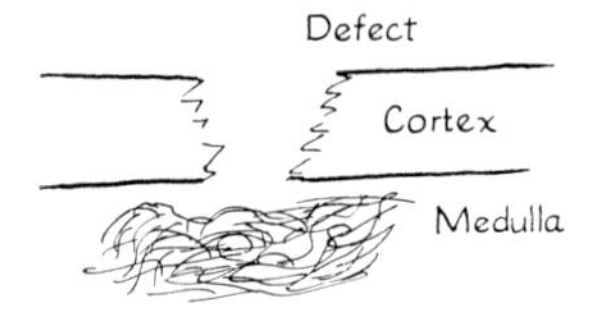

Next, osteoblasts move in from the surrounding normal bone and there is a gradual replacement of bone structure either with or without obvious changes from the previous normal pattern which existed in the area.

To summarize the point, there is (1) increased density with loss of normal structure, then (2) absorption with consequent rarification of the area, and, finally (3) regeneration.

Quite naturally, the exact character of this regeneration depends upon the mechanical pressures put upon the parts while it is taking place. A hip with Perthes' disease may regenerate a reasonably normal femoral head if kept immobilized and supported. If, on the other hand, the patient is allowed to walk and run about, distortion of the reconstructed bone may be extreme.

This, somewhat diagrammatically, is a typical early Perthes' disease:

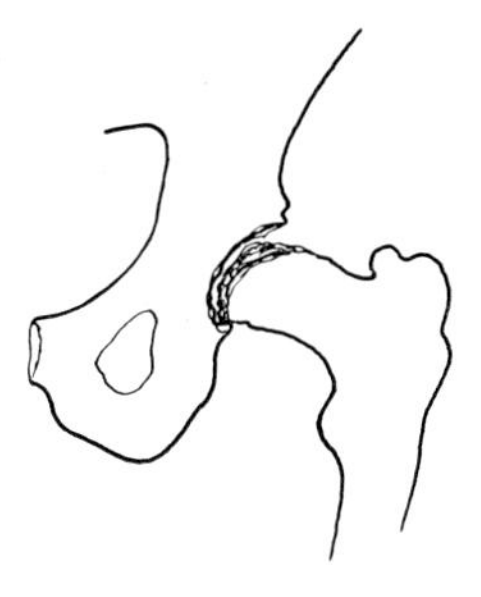

Notice the increase in density of the femoral head. Infarcts of bone are reasonably typical no matter where they occur. One should remember the usual sites: the tibial tubercle, the hip, the spine, and the tarsal scaphoid. This is a typical vertebral involvement:

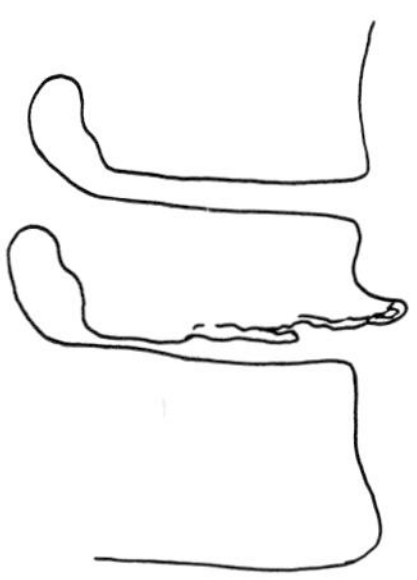

OSTEOMYELITIS

There are probably just as many cases of osteomyelitis as there ever were but those of us in clinical practice see progressively fewer. This, of course, is because the antibiotics are administered for any febrile disease and a significant number of patients are cured before they reach the point of clinical or roentgen diagnosis. Usually the sequence of events is about like this:

A transient bacteremia occurs from some trivial cause, but the majority of bacteria in the blood are promptly killed by the leukocytes. Perhaps a few enter the bones through the nutrient arteries and become established in the shaft of the bone near the epiphyseal end.

An inflammatory reaction is immediately set up, with local thrombosis of the vessels and the other concomitants of severe inflammation. At this stage, clinically, there is an acutely ill patient without many diagnostic signs.

The infection then burrows its way out through the cortex of the bone to become subperiosteal and inward toward the marrow cavity. A subperiosteal collection of pus is formed, which literally tears the periosteum upward off the bone, thus causing a diminution of blood supply in the cortex.

Meanwhile, the marrow infection has caused thrombosis in some of the marrow vessels, further slowing the blood supply to the already impaired cortex. Cancellous structure inside the marrow breaks down and portions of the cortex may be completely destroyed by the infection.

Within two weeks or so the elevated periosteum has made some progress with reparative bone formation although, since it is not in contact with the bone shaft, this results in a shell of periosteal bone from one to several millimeters away from the shaft itself. In the marrow cavity, reparative processes are also in progress, but bone laid down is irregular and does not conform to the typical pattern.

As repair becomes the dominant process, an increasing amount of new bone is laid down until the involved area is finally strengthened. This deposition of new bone, however, does not conform to the pattern of the previous normal bone.

The femur, tibia, and humerus are most often involved, although any area of the bony system is subject to the disease.

Technique

Ordinary roentgenograms will usually show all that one needs for diagnosis.

Interpretation

Primarily, the hyperemia of the infected area usually causes a haziness about the marrow cavity, making it look as though it were seen through a fine ground-glass screen. On x-rays this is simply not distinctive enough to allow diagnosis, although it may make one suspicious.

The first finding that offers a positive clue to diagnosis is a thin line of new bone formed by the elevated periosteum. It usually looks like this:

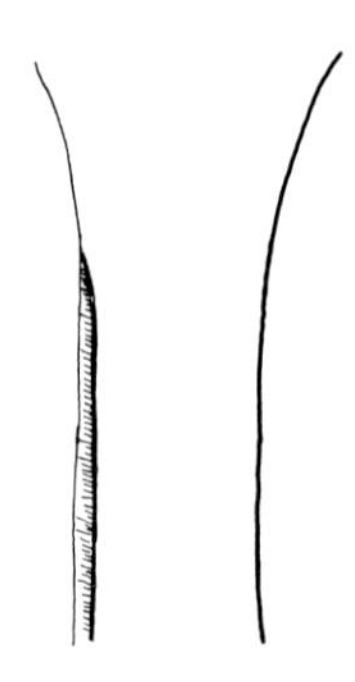

Next, areas of rarefaction appear in the shaft of bone, like this:

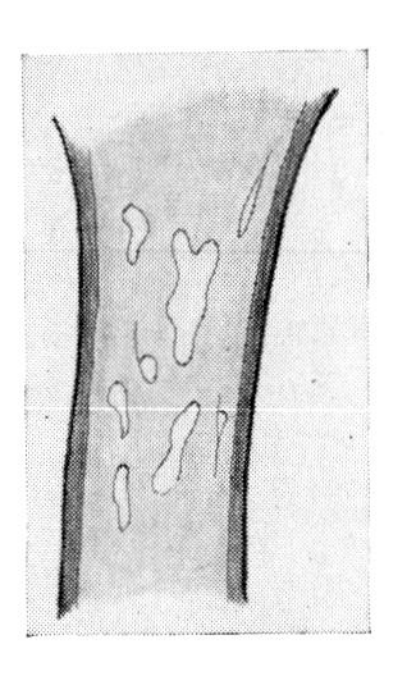

Finally, dense sequestra are formed, and soft tissue shadows of abscesses may be apparent.

During the healing stage there is, first, loss of the hazy opacity so characteristic of hyperemic bone. There is a gradual restitution of normal architecture, but this is seldom complete.

Errors

Osteomyelitis is one of the greatest sources of radiologic error regularly seen by the practitioner. The process itself is clear-cut and not difficult of radiologic diagnosis when well developed. There is one fact which, it seems, doctors just will not understand. *There are no radiologic signs observable* during the first ten to twenty days of the disease. To say that a patient does not have osteomyelitis because the x-ray is negative, unless twenty days have elapsed since the start of the disease, is to court error.

RHEUMATOID ARTHRITIS

X-ray is of little use in diagnosing late rheumatoid arthritis, for the disease is so characteristic clinically that x-ray films are simply a waste of the patient's money. In early cases, quite the opposite obtains. Often long before one can be entirely certain of the clinical diagnosis, x-ray evidence is conclusive, and the practitioner will find this technique useful.

There is no way to estimate the degree of activity from x-ray evidence alone. This is usually a clinical determination which is best made by an accurate history and sedimentation rate.

Technique

Rheumatoid arthritis most frequently begins in the joints of the hand and a simple anteroposterior x-ray of the hands will often give all the evidence that is needed for a positive diagnosis.

Interpretation

First notice the general appearance of the bones. Notice that they have an almost homogeneous density with loss of many of the characteristic variations seen in the normal hand. Notice, too, that there is great rarefication in the bone immediately adjacent to the involved joint. Here is a diagram of a typical normal joint compared with a joint affected with rheumatoid arthritis:

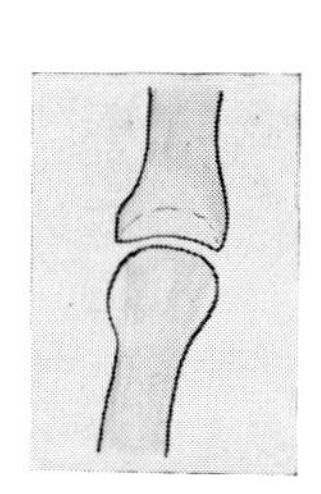

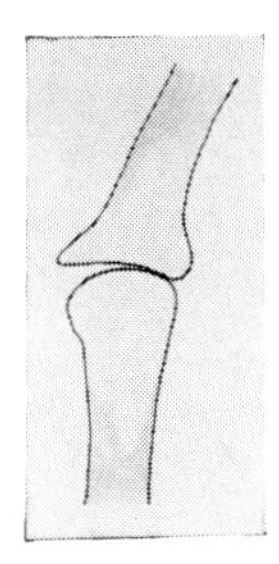

There is, first, an increase in joint space but seldom is this seen, for patients do not usually come to the doctor in this early stage of the disease. As the disease progresses and the cartilage is destroyed, the joint spaces progressively narrow. This is a normal joint alongside an arthritic one:

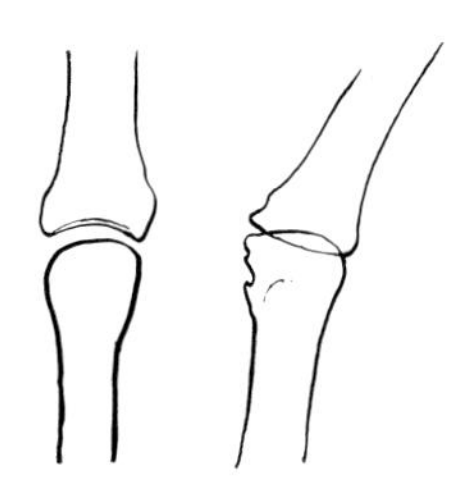

It is the rarefication previously mentioned which is the tip-off to rheumatoid arthritis in the early stages. Other signs occur as the disease progresses but are of little importance because roentgenologic evidence is no longer of great help in the advanced case.

Errors

This radiologic determination is practically not subject to errors if observation is careful and film technique adequate. One point does deserve comment.

The types of arthritis are clearly differentiated in textbooks but may not be so clearly differentiated in patients. Unquestionably both rheumatoid and degenerative changes can exist in the same joint and frequently do. It is sometimes a matter of deciding which process predominates rather than which is present.

OSTEOARTHRITIS

Osteoarthritis is a degenerative change, essentially a wearing out of the joints. Cartilage is destroyed and the bone reacts, as would be expected, to the trauma directly imposed upon it. The x-ray changes are entirely characteristic.

Technique

Ordinarily plain anteroposterior pictures alone or combined with lateral films are sufficient for diagnosis. Often the disease may be detected in films taken for another purpose.

Interpretation

Since we used the hand for interpretation on rheumatoid arthritis, let us use the same joint for osteoarthritis and emphasize the differential characteristics.

In the worn-out joint, the joint space is narrower and the angle at the articular margin is considerably sharpened. There is spur formation and lipping, like this:

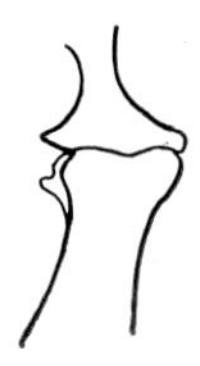

There is usually a dense area of sclerotic bone at the articular surface, like this:

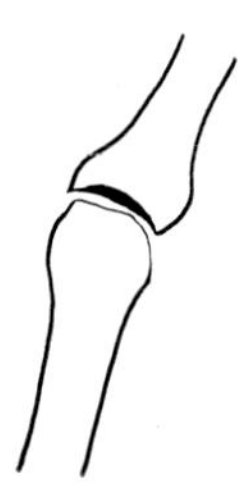

Odd, rounded, cystlike areas of rarefaction may occur near joints, but there is not the universal rarefaction seen in rheumatoid arthritis. Here are three illustrations for comparison: a rheumatoid arthritic joint, a normal joint, and an osteoarthritic joint:

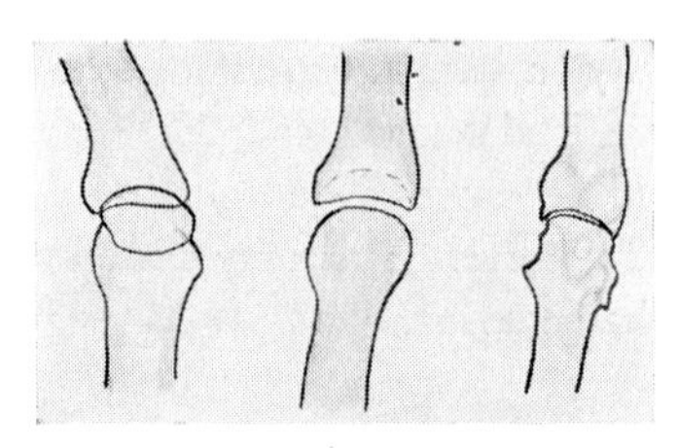

This is a knee joint, showing the typical changes of osteoarthritis:

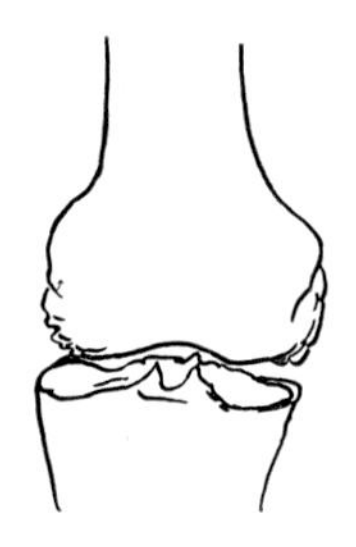

As you know, osteoarthritic changes may be found in any joint. They are, however, more frequent in the joints which suffer the greatest wear and strain. Seldom are asymptomatic lesions of much significance, although one often sees them in routine examinations.

Osteoarthritic changes in the spine are quite common. The edge of a typical vertebra might look like this:

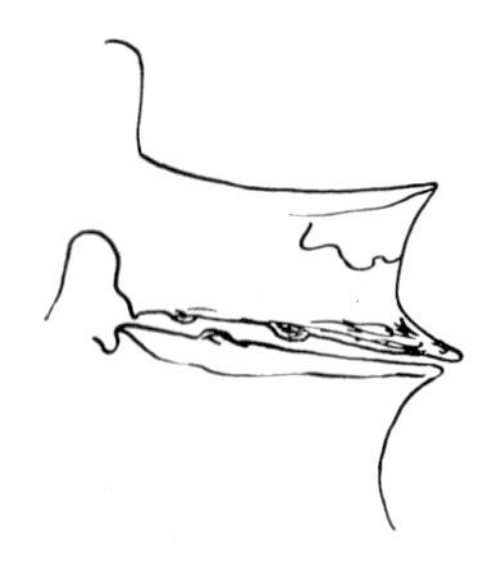

THE INTERVERTEBRAL DISCS

It is my belief that diagnosis of the intervertebral disc syndrome is a clinical matter insofar as the practitioner is concerned. X-ray changes are slight and interpretation difficult, and I have repeatedly seen experts make the wrong diagnosis from a well-taken film. To repeat, until we know more about the condition, the practitioner should leave its roentgenologic aspects alone.

This I believe applies to most radiology of the lumbosacral area. An obvious spondylolisthesis like this:

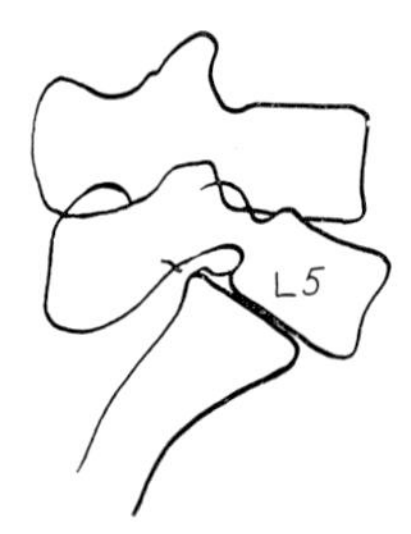

a fractured vertebra, and obvious gross changes in the area can be well interpreted by any physician. Roentgenograms of the area probably should be taken frequently by the practitioner, but he should base his preliminary treatment upon clinical findings and seek expert help in interpretation.

Epilogue

In medical practice there are many ingenious uses for the x-ray. The delineation of fistulas by injection of radiopaque dye, the localization of foreign bodies in tissues, and a hundred other minor but informative uses suggest themselves.

After the practitioner uses the x-ray for a year or two and becomes thoroughly familiar with it as a diagnostic tool, I would recommend that he purchase a modern and complete textbook on x-ray diagnosis and study it extensively. This book is only an introduction. There are several good textbooks on the subject.

In this book I have attempted to simplify, even to the extent of oversimplification at times, with the thought that one must make a beginning. It is written to be just that—a beginning—and nothing more.

If I have tended to scoff at some of our accepted x-ray and laboratory techniques (and I have), I must tell you why. The young physician finishes medical school with a touching faith in the miraculous omnipotence of the laboratory and x-ray. He has seen experts of the highest order use these tools to the gain of some patients and to the obvious detriment of others. In the hands of these experts the laboratory and x-ray provide facilities for doing wonderful things, but there is an obvious corollary. In the hands of the general practitioner they are good working tools that sometimes furnish information of value and sometimes do not. Perhaps the most important thing for the practitioner to learn is to recognize the occasions when the laboratory and x-ray would be useless and he must rely on his own judgment, not upon mechanical aid. If, in a decade or two, he can accomplish this without losing his respect for these wonderful mechanical devices, the value of his laboratory and x-ray to his patients will be doubled and he will practice a better kind of medicine.

Paul Williamson, M.D.

Index

8087788
3 1378 00808 7788